1986

Home Health Care

A COMPLETE GUIDE FOR
PATIENTS AND THEIR FAMILIES

Home Health Care

JO-ANN FRIEDMAN

W · W · NORTON & COMPANY · *NEW YORK* · *LONDON*

FIRST EDITION

The text of this book is composed in New Century Schoolbook, with display type set in Baker Danmark. Composition and manufacturing by the Maple-Vail Book Manufacturing Group.
Illustrations by Helen Algase and Sylvia Stone.

BOOK DESIGN BY MARJORIE J. FLOCK

The range-of-motion exercises that appear on pages 224–227 are adapted from the *Lippincott Manual of Nursing Practice, Third Edition,* Philadelphia: Lippincott, 1982. The tables for "Nonnarcotic Analgesics for Mild to Moderate Pain," "Narcotic Analgesics for Moderate to Severe Pain," "Antiparkinsonism Drugs," "Antianginal Drugs," "Antihypertensive Drugs," and "Arthritis Drugs Frequently Used," which appear on pages 268–270, 394–395, 448–449, 461–463, and 480–485, were adapted from *The Complete Guide to Prescription and Non-Prescription Drugs* by H. Winter Griffith, M.D., with the permission of HP Books. "Ostomy Care Techniques," which appears on pages 432–434, was reprinted with permission from *Nursing 83,* copyright by Springhouse Corp., 1983, all rights reserved. "The Five Stages of Dying," discussed on pages 289–295, is adapted from *On Death and Dying* by Elisabeth Kubler-Ross, copyright © 1969 by Elisabeth Kubler-Ross. The table for "Selecting a Nursing Home," which appears on pages 40–42, is from *Jane Brody's The New York Times Guide to Personal Health,* by Jane Brody. Copyright © 1982 by the New York Times Company. Reprinted by permission of Times Books, a division of Random House, Inc. The seven levels of cognitive decline listed on pages 364–369 are adapted from "Stages of Cognitive Decline," AJN, Feb. 1984, and are reprinted with the permission of the American Journal of Nursing Company. The guidelines for "Fighting Fatigue" on page 388 were reprinted from *Inside MS,* Fall 1983 issue, with the permission of the National Multiple Sclerosis Society. Material from the *Emotional Aspects of MS,* which appears on page 389, was reprinted with the permission of the National Multiple Sclerosis Society. The "Living Will," which appears on page 297, is reprinted with the permission of Concern for Dying, 250 West 57th Street, New York, NY, 10107.

Library of Congress Cataloging in Publication Data
Friedman, Jo-Ann.
    Home health care.

    Bibliography: p.
    Includes index.
    1. Home care services—United States.   2. Home nursing.   I. Title.   [DNLM: 1. Home Care Services. 2. Home Nursing.   WY 115 F911h]
    RA645.35.F75   1986   649'.8   85-5112

ISBN 0-393-01889-X

W. W. Norton & Company, Inc., 500 Fifth Avenue, New York, N.Y. 10110
W. W. Norton & Company Ltd., 37 Great Russell Street, London WC1B 3NU

1 2 3 4 5 6 7 8 9 0

To my late grandfather, Joseph H. Schwartz,
a wise and loving man

Contents

Tables   11

Foreword by Jane E. Brody   13

Introduction   17

Acknowledgments   21

I

HOME CARING

1   Why Home Care Is Better Care   25

What Is Home Health Care? • Can Home Care Really Help? • How It All Started • Home Care—No Wonder! • The Smorgasbord that Is Home Health Care • The Home Health Care Network Is Growing • Finding Home Health Care • Paying for Home Health Care • Are There Alternatives? • Institutions Can Be Hazardous to Your Health • The Future

2   Plugging Into the System   49

The Caregiver's Critical Role • The Home Health Care Team • Where to Begin • Home Health Care Agencies • The Three Pillars of Home Health Care • The Support Network: Therapists • The Doctor's Role • The Rest of the Home Care Team

3   Insurance! Insurance! Insurance!   85

Health Insurance Guidelines • Is Home Health Care Covered? • Medicare • Making up the Difference • Medicaid—When There Is No Money • Getting Your Money's Worth

4   Preparing for Home Care   103

The Patient • Current Home and Health Situation • The Fourth World • Dealing with Stress • Setting Up the Home • Setting Up the Bathroom • Setting Up the Bedroom • A New Look at the Kitchen • Living in the Living Room

II
DAILY LIVING

5   Living Each Day   139

Acute Onset—Expected Recovery • Managing Continuity of Care •
Tracking Progress • Tips to Consider • An Amended State of
Wellness • Goals Are Important • Conserve Energy and Plan
Ahead • A Perspective on Chronic Illness • Learning to Cope: Day
by Day

6   Nutrition, Plain and Special   192

What Is Good Nutrition? • When Eating Is Not Possible • Enteral
Nutrition • Parenteral Nutrition

7   Drugs and Medication   204

Drug–Drug Interactions • Food–Drug and Drug–Nutrient
Interactions • Self–Medication

8   Personal Health Care   220

Eye Care • Keeping Fit: Your Own Program • Special Considerations for Special Conditions • The Skin—a True Miracle Fabric •
Special Skin Care Problems • Incontinence • Oral Care • Oral Care
for Special Situations • Oral Care Aids • Sexuality • Sleep

III
SPECIAL CARE

9   Pain and Pain Control   263

What Is Pain? • The Preception of Pain • Pain Relief Through
Drugs • Pain Relief Without Drugs

10   Pressure Sores   274

Stages of Ulcer Development • Assessment of Risk • Treatment •
Prevention

11   High-Tech Home Care   280

Diabetes • Nutrition • Respiratory Disease • Renal Disease •
Chemotherapy • Guidelines

12 The Dying Patient   288
    The Stages of Dying • Relieving the Pain • Should the Patient Be
    Told? • Patient Stress • Caregiver Stress • Guidelines for the
    Caregiver • Preparing for Death • When Death Comes • Hospice
    Care at Home

IV

THE GAMUT OF HEALTH PROBLEMS

13 The Aging Person   309
    The Aging Couple • Hearing Loss • The Memory Lingers On • A
    Little More Light, Please • Watch Your Step! • Heat • Don't Stay
    Cool Too Long • Mental Calisthenics • Elder Abuse

14 Cancer   319
    Surgery • Radiation • Chemotherapy • Questions to Ask • Maxi-
    mizing Cancer Treatment Through Nutrition • Pain Management •
    Activity • Coping with the Cure

15 Eye and Ear Problems   331
    Eye Problems • Hearing Loss

16 Diabetes   344
    Treatment • Dangerous Reactions • Complications of Diabetes •
    Diabetic Testing at Home • The Elderly and Diabetes • Tips for the
    Diabetic

17 Neurological Problems   360
    Alzheimer's Disease • Amyotrophic Lateral Sclerosis (ALS) • Multi-
    ple Sclerosis • Parkinson's Disease • Spinal Cord Injuries • Stroke

18 Gastrointestinal Problems   426
    Inflammatory Bowel Disease
    Managing with an Ostomy

19 Circulatory and Cardiovascular Problems   437
    Heart Attack: Sudden Onset and Step-by-Step Recovery • Angina:
    The Pain that Warns • Hypertension

10   CONTENTS

20   Arthritis   468
     Rheumatoid Arthritis • Osteoarthritis • Joint Replacement
     Surgery • Gout • Managing with Arthritis • Good Eating and
     Arthritis • The Right Attitude

21   Renal Disease   487
     A New Life with Dialysis • Transplants • Living with Dialysis

22   Respiratory Disease   495
     COPD: A Major Disabler • Asthma • Engaging in Activity to
     Tolerance • Medications • Oxygen • Living Each Day

APPENDIX

A Resource Directory   509
Aging • Arthritis • Blindness • Cancer • Community Services
(Social and Legal) • Death/Dying • Dentistry • Diabetes • Diges-
tive Disorders • Equipment and Supplies • Hearing Disorders •
Heart Disease and Stroke • Home Care Services • Information
Services • Institutionalized Patient Services • Kidney Diseases •
Mental Health • Miscellaneous • Neurological/Neuromuscular
Diseases • Nutrition • Pain • Physical Disability • Recreation •
Respiratory Problems • Sexuality • Skin • Speech

Index   569

Tables

1	Types of Housing Facilities and Their Services	38
2	Evaluating and Selecting Alternative Residential Settings	40
3	The Home Health Care Team	51
4	Typical Cost of Home Health Care Services	60
5	Medicare Part A: Hospital Services	93
6	Medicare Part B: Medical Expenses	93
7	Medicare Part A: Payment Schedule	94
8	Medicare Part B: Payment Schedule	95
9	Tips for Daily Living: Grooming and Personal Care	166
10	Tips for Daily Living: Dressing	172
11	Tips for Daily Living: Food Preparation	174
12	Tips for Daily Living: Eating and Drinking	180
13	Tips for Daily Living: Household Chores	182
14	Tips for Daily Living: Sports and Recreation	186
15	Tips for Daily Living: General Activities	187
16	The Macronutrients	193
17	The Five Basic Food Groups	194
18	Nonnarcotic Analgesics for Mild to Moderate Pain	268
19	Narcotic Analgesics for Moderate to Severe Pain	270
20	High-Tech Home Care	281
21	Types of Cancer and Their Treatment	321
22	Antiparkinsonism Drugs	394
23	Antianginal Drugs	448
24	Antihypertensive Drugs	461
25	Arthritis Drugs Frequently Used	480

Foreword

WHEN ILLNESS and disability force people to leave the emotional and physical comforts of home for the sometimes cold, dehumanizing setting of a hospital or nursing care facility, the quality of their lives and their health often suffers. Institutions, with their tendencies to "take over" a person's life and treat all people with a frightening sameness, can quickly turn a once-vital, independent adult into a listless, vulnerable, and passively obedient child.

Particularly for an elderly person, the loss of familiar surroundings, the isolation, can be so disorienting and emotionally devastating that they strip away the will to recover and the strength to cope with illness and encroaching disability.

As Jo-Ann Friedman has so aptly shown in this extraordinarily insightful and practical book, for millions of people facing institutional care, there is a feasible alternative—health care at home. Although the home was once the setting for almost all medical care (until fairly recently, people went to hospitals only for surgery or acute, though not terminal, illness), the growing complexity of medical therapies and technology during recent decades has made the hospital the focal point of advanced care for most patients with life-threatening or disabling illness. Because American families no longer maintain three-generation homes, or even necessarily live in the same parts of the country as their parents and siblings, the role of caregiver for those no longer able to cope on their own with health problems has shifted from relatives to professionals in institutional settings.

It's time to go home again—and this book can show you how. It is a book for ordinary people who may lack prior experience with illness, who may never have dealt with health professionals, and who have not yet developed expertise in negotiating the bureaucratic maze of medical care. This invaluable guide takes you by the hand and leads you, step by logical step, toward establishing the home as the basis for recovery or continued care for someone you love.

If you are to be the primary "caregiver" for a sick or disabled person, this book will help you, first of all, to determine your willingness and ability to meet the demands of this consuming task. If you come to the realization that home health caregiving is *not* for you, this book will help you shed that inevitable feeling of guilt and take constructive steps toward finding an acceptable alternative. You, have to live too, after all, especially if there are other people central to your existence who demand and deserve your attention.

Next, Ms. Friedman's book will help you to define exactly what kind of care is needed and who should provide it. The primary caregiver is not expected to be doctor, nurse, physical and recreational therapist, chief cook and bottle washer, friend and relative rolled into one. Many—sometimes most—of these tasks can be fulfilled by specially trained experts who come to the home periodically. The caregiver's role may be primarily a matter of coordinating this outside help and providing an environmental constancy and emotional climate that promotes recovery or, for patients who will not recover, continued ability to enjoy what life still has to offer.

Home health care is clearly the wave of the future. The treatment of long-term and chronic illness and disability in institutional settings—combined with the growing numbers of people reaching ages where the need for this kind of care is commonplace—is breaking the back of governmental budgets and, in many cases, wiping out the personal savings of patients and their families as well.

Federal insurance programs are already being cut back. Medicare, for example, has established a new basis for reimbursing hospitals: diagnosis-related groups, or DRGs. This new system sets monetary allowances for various ailments or treatments, no matter how much time the patient actually spends in the hospital. Thus, for example, if a man who suffers a heart attack is hospitalized (without further complications) for six weeks, the hospital will get no more Medicare reimbursement than for a similar patient who goes home after three weeks. Needless to say, hospitals, to keep their own budgets balanced, will be encouraging patients to spend as little time there as possible so that the bed can be used for a new patient who will not be a financial drain. Families who may lack supplemental insurance to cover hospital costs beyond the DRG reimbursement, will be forced to take the patient elsewhere. But where? Nursing homes are crowded, the good ones have long waiting lists, and they are extraordinarily expensive—$30,000 to $50,000 a year in many cases. Moreover, by placing patients in an environment where sickness, not wellness, is the norm, nursing homes are too often a stepping stone to the grave for people who might otherwise have enjoyed years of good life despite illness or disability.

When circumstances permit, health care at home can be a financially and emotionally more desirable alternative. But it is not a task to be lightly assumed. Much preparation—emotional as well as physical—is needed. As Ms. Friedman repeatedly reminds us, patience and persistence are essential qualities in executing the role of caregiver. Once you have determined (using the book's guidelines) that this is a role you are willing and able to undertake, this book will serve as the essential aid to successful, even enjoyable, home health care. There isn't an important consideration left uncovered: forms and finances; physical arrangements and activities; feelings and frustrations; and the future. You name the problem, Ms. Friedman has provided a practical checklist and the resources to help you through it, including many simple things that you may never have otherwise thought of but that could greatly simplify the task at hand.

Most people, when they think of medical care, think only of doctors and nurses. You will learn in this book of the extraordinary medical benefits of various paramedical services: physical and occupational therapy, nutrition therapy, psychological and sexual counseling, rehabilitation and recreational aids, among many others. More importantly, Ms. Friedman tells you exactly how to enlist these services and what to expect in the way of results. You will be appropriately cautioned, too, on the costs of home care, which is, regrettably, inconsistently covered at present by medical insurance, both government and private.

In thinking about home health care, many people incorrectly associate it only with caring for the ailing elderly or dying patient. In fact, much of home health care can and should involve sick people of all ages who will eventually recover or who will live many years—even decades—with a disability that does not necessarily get worse. In effect, this book is for everyone with responsibility toward someone who faces a lengthy recuperation from a serious illness or who is afflicted with a permanent disability. Most people recover faster or learn to cope better if they can do so in a setting that most closely resembles "normal" life. Home is such a setting: the best place for most of us, well or ill.

JANE E. BRODY
Personal Health Columnist
The New York Times

Introduction

OME is growing in importance as a health care treatment setting. At one time we looked solely to doctors, hospitals, and extended care facilities to make us well before returning home. Today, there is increasing recognition that involving patients and their families and friends can contribute greatly to the patients' physical and emotional recovery. Medical professionals acknowledge that recovery quickens when patients take an active part in their own health care—certainly more possible at home.

The recent growth in the number of home health care professionals and agencies across the country is easing the way for people to shorten expensive hospital stays (or even avoid admission to a hospital) and recover in the comfort of their home, where they usually prefer to be.

Frequently, home health care can offer a less expensive alternative to costly extended hospitalization. With medical costs growing at the rate of over fifteen percent each year, the need for alternatives to long-term hospital or institutional care has become critical. Add to this the imposition by the federal government of fixed Medicare reimbursements to hospitals for specific illnesses or medical procedures. DRGs (Diagnosis Related Groups) have had a staggering effect on the health care scene. The average length of hospital stays is decreasing, not because patients are recovering faster but because they are getting discharged "quicker and sicker" to recover at home. Medicare and private insurers are forcing hospitals to discharge patients more quickly than they used to.

Still another factor contributing to the growth of home health care is the demographic change brought about because people are living longer. The fastest growing segment of the population is the over-75 age group. Many of these people have survived acute infections and illnesses, which were fatal to their ancestors, because of the aggressive and effective medications and treatments that have been developed during the last 40 years. Yet these people are coping with a variety of chronic health conditions in addition to the natural changes that accompany old age. For the elderly, the only alternative to long, costly stays in a hospital or nursing home is health care at home.

Whether it's for you, your spouse, or a mother, father, sister, brother, relative, or friend, the prospect of health care at home can be anxiety-provoking. For those immediately involved—the caregivers—the challenges which home care can present can be formidable.

Our health care and community support systems seem to have their own culture, their own vocabulary, and their own rules and regulations. Navigating through the system to develop a workable home-care plan can seem impossible.

I wrote this book to serve as your guide: to help you find the home health care help you need so that you manage the care, not martyr yourself to provide that care. I cover: what Medicare, Medicaid, and private insurance will pay for; how to find the right community resource support group or health organization to help you; how to organize your home to care for a sick person; how to set up a support network; what doctors can and cannot do; what to expect from the home health care professionals—the nurses, therapists, and aides; and how you, the caregiver, can ease your feelings of stress and guilt.

In the Appendix, "A Guide to Resources," I identify the variety of organizations and resources ready to help you; and I include descriptions of the kind of assistance and information they make available.

This book is intended to support, not replace the counsel and assistance offered by your family physician. The information and resources it offers may add options to the course of action for you, the doctor, and the patient to discuss.

A Personal Note

Although it was more than ten years and two career changes later, my training and experience in neurology and rehabilitation came in handy when I was hospitalized in 1982 with a sudden, paralyzing illness called Guillain Barre Syndrome, a viral attack on the nervous system. Muscle movement sparked by the affected nerves became progressively weakened. In some instances, the ability to actually move certain muscles disappeared.

I had seen patients with this illness before and I knew of its rapid onset. As my arms and legs became weaker and weaker and so-called simple activities such as eating and walking became almost impossible chores, I focused on my breathing. I knew if the virus impaired the muscles that control breathing in and breathing out, I would need to be connected to a respirator until that capability returned. Everyone, including me, would simply have to wait to see which abilities I would lose and which would remain. Fortunately, I knew that, with time and physical therapy, my weakened muscles would grow strong again.

As I checked into the hospital, I felt that I had a lot going for me. I had worked in a hospital and knew the language of doctors as well as the politics and protocol found in a hospital unit. Over the years I had often functioned as an ombudsman for friends and family who were hospitalized, helping them to request and receive the "little things" that can make all the difference when your total world becomes the four walls of a hospital room. I believed I knew how to make the system work for me. I was in for a big surprise. I discovered things are quite different when you're on the other side of the bed rail.

During that time in the hospital, I experienced the profound healing power of caring family and friends. And I discovered my own determination to use whatever abilities I had to regain what I had lost so suddenly.

Once the viral attack subsided, I knew that the road back to health and strength would take time. Without a doubt, the comfort and convenience of my own home seemed the ideal place to be. Clearly, I needed help just to get around: my eyes were paralyzed, my coordination and balance were reminiscent of a drunk's, and I was so weak that my then six-year old niece was able to push me over with the touch of her finger. And I knew I needed physical therapy to help me regain my lost strength and balance.

Years earlier when I worked at the Lubin Rehabilitation Center at the Albert Einstein College Hospital, I had become aware of the advantage of home health care. Although home health care services were not well organized then, on special request by the patient or his physician, some physical therapists did make home visits. Other members of the therapy team would also visit a patient's home and evaluate its safety and accessibility. Home health care made a dramatic difference. The patient's spirits would lift with the promise of returning home. And therapy in the home seemed logical. There a therapist would work with real-life situations rather than practicing in a therapy room. At that time patients and their families had to be quite assertive to arrange for their own home care. And they had to be able to pay privately, since insurance companies did not cover home therapy visits.

I had kept abreast of the changes that had taken place during the intervening years between my work experience and my own hospitalization. Arrangements for home care were now part of the hospital social worker's job description. Insurance coverage was now possible. Through various services and agencies, almost any treatment that was available in a hospital could be arranged for at home. Imagine my surprise when as a patient I learned that many health professionals lacked comprehensive information about home health care. They could not answer my questions about insurance coverage, housekeeper help, or arranging for physical therapy. Despite my expertise I was unsuccessful in my attempts to get the hospital to "offically" place me on home care. Eventually my wish to go home outweighed my wish to untangle the administrative web at the hospital. I arranged for my own housekeeper and was fortunate to have a dear friend, Tess Sholom, as my physical therapist.

In retrospect I can see that despite my expertise the turmoil of my sudden and unexpected illness and not having an extremely well informed advocate to act on my behalf contributed to my lack of success.

It's been three years, and the memory of the illness itself and the road to recovery has faded. While many people have suggested that my rapid recovery was almost miraculous, I knew that I had recovered faster because I recovered at home. Physical therapy treatments took place on my living room floor, and I could practice as often as I was able. Visits from family and friends were not dependent on hospital visiting hours. I was even able to give dinner parties by having the food delivered! Guests were only too happy to do the cleaning up.

I know that my familiarity with health care options was of great help. Had I not opted for taking charge of my own recovery, I may have spent too much time resting on a hospital bed rather than using to the fullest whatever abilities I had at the time.

My experience convinced me of the benefits of home care. It also alerted me to the frustrations and difficulties which patients and their families encounter in arranging and coordinating that care.

It is my hope that this book will provide you with practical information you can use to ease the road to recovery or the management of an ongoing illness in the best of all possible treatment settings: home.

Acknowledgments

WRITING A BOOK is an all-consuming activity, as my support network of devoted friends and relatives will agree. It could not have happened without their cheerleading and encouragement.

I owe special thanks to my aunt and uncle, Monte and Sidney Rogers, M.D. They always knew when a swim or a bit of indulgence was needed as a restorative. In addition, Dr. Rogers read through the entire manuscript, offering constructive suggestions and comments to ensure its medical accuracy.

I want to thank my staff at Health Marketing Systems, Inc., whose hard work allowed me the time and freedom to work on the manuscript. In particular, I wish to thank Pamela Lyons, R.N., who has given full measure to ensure the quality of the work. She read through the entire manuscript and provided the insight that comes from being a well-trained and experienced nurse. The painstaking research that was necessary to make the Appendix accurate complete and informative was done by my staff; thanks to Jacquelyn Goodrich, Muriel Morgenstern, and William Ortiz for pulling it all together. I'm grateful to Reima Sontup for her help in keeping the office together, and for numerous courier rides carrying my work to Danny Sontup for preliminary editing. A special thanks to Danny for a job well done.

I also want to thank my parents, Leonard and Frances Schwartz, and other relatives for offering encouragement in their unique way. I appreciate Frank Kramer's counsel as I tried to balance writing a book with running a company; I'm grateful to Michael Schwartz, D.D.S., for his informative help with respect to the chapter on oral care. Thanks to Michael, Marilyn, Sharon, Jill, and Judith for cheering me on.

I am grateful to the home health care professionals (nurses, physical therapists, occupational therapists, and social workers) who shared their knowledge and experiences with me. Thank you Mary Bartlett, Pat Bloomgarden, Ann Goldberg, Nadine Julius, Barbara Keyes, Iris Kimberg, Ilene Masser, Phyllis Shulman, Valerie Takai, and Jeanne Ussher. Ann Goldberg and Valerie Takai, two talented occupational therapists, who were particularly helpful in ensuring that the information contained in the book was practical from the patient's point of view.

The book benefited greatly from Margaret Maruschak's comments; her high spirits and those of Doris and Steve Colgate and Pamela Waters were the fuel that kept me going. Jane Brody pointed the way to many resources and offered me tips of the author's trade that were much appreciated. And to my other friends, especially Jane and Richard Engquist, Tess and Ronnie Sholom, and Cathi Hunt, thank you for your patience with me and for being there.

Most of all I want to acknowledge the assistance and encouragement of Mary Cunnane, W. W. Norton & Company's talented editor. Her clarity of thought and guidance helped to make molehills out of mountains. In addition, I appreciate her dedication and commitment to the success of this project. Her contagious enthusiasm had everyone at Norton, including Marjorie Flock, Andy Marasia, Fran Rosencranz, and Deirdre Dolan, involved in helping this book be the best it can be. Thank you.

I

Home Caring

1

Why Home Care
Is Better Care

A MANSION or a cottage . . . A spacious penthouse or a cramped apartment . . . A tract house or a rambling farmhouse . . . Take your pick. They all spell home—and there's no place quite like it. If you want to see this truth in action, spend some time in a hospital lobby. Look around you and listen. You are bound to come across someone like Frank Thomas.

There was nothing special about him—just another elderly man in a wheelchair, a common enough sight in any hospital lobby. He sat in the wheelchair, facing the outer doors, a young candy-striped aide standing beside him. Each time the outer doors swung open, he leaned forward and took a quick breath, as though testing and savoring the cool fall breeze that swept in.

The aide glanced at him. She knew he had just been through a major operation to remove an intestinal blockage. His recovery was going to be slow, and there would be much discomfort as well as some pain. He could have remained in the hospital longer, but he had been adamant. He had badgered his doctor to sign him out, and in the end he had prevailed. His doctor had discharged him, and now Frank Thomas sat bundled up in a wheelchair and waited for his daughter to bring the car around from the parking lot.

"Will you be staying with your daughter, Mr. Thomas?" the candy striper asked.

He shook his head. "Going back to my own apartment."

"Alone?"

He nodded. "Oh, we've made arrangements for people to come in and help me—a housekeeper a couple of times a week, some therapists, it's all been taken care of."

"Are you sure you'll be all right, Mr. Thomas? I mean, wouldn't you be better off going to stay with your daughter for a while?"

He shook his head and smiled. "I'll get better a lot faster this way," he said. "I'm going home."

Home.

There's no real substitute. It's where we turn to for warmth and security and the comfort of familiar surroundings. We know every nook and cranny, every sound and smell of where we live. It's an ingrained part of our lives.

It's not surprising, therefore, that people like Frank Thomas cherish the independence of living in their own home. Almost every family can find among its relatives a chronically ill or partially disabled aunt, uncle, parent, or grandparent who stubbornly insists on living alone in their own home, despite the conviction of other family members that this is a dangerous and unhealthy thing to do. The family and well-meaning friends, and sometimes even the family doctor, point with alarm to all the compelling reasons for not living alone—the disabled or ill person cannot shop unaided, meal preparation may be difficult, their diet is poor, the neighborhood is unsafe, and so on. As valid as some of these reasons may be, they cannot outweigh the undeniable sense of self-reliance that comes with having control of your own life.

Small wonder, then, that if we get sick or disabled, no matter what our age, we want to be in our own bed in our own home. We know where we are and we draw strength from being at home. We know, even in the darkness, where everything is—the door, the window, the dresser, the night table—even what the floor will feel like when we step down.

For some families there once was, in fact, a family home. It was the center of a full lifetime of activities. People were born there, grew up there, were sometimes married there, and went out and established their own homes not too far away. Generations shared their homes with each other when the need arose. Thus, there was always someone around to help care for a sick child or an elderly relative. Hospitals were for the poor and were few and far between. Rest or convalescent homes were for people with contagious or life-threatening illnesses.

Times have changed; families have changed; the way we live and when and why we die has changed. Today, sons and daughters often live far from the community in which they were raised. Fragmented families see each other only on "state occasions," and family members now live separate lives among different friends in different communities. The sense of family and the bonds of closely knit family life have changed.

At the same time, medicine has advanced to such a degree that many of the killer illnesses of the past—pneumonia, tuberculosis, and other infectious diseases—are now being treated and cured with a much higher rate of success. In 1900, the average life expectancy was forty-seven years, and the leading causes of death were influenza, pneumonia, diptheria, and tuberculosis. Between 1900 and 1980, advances in medical science and the availability of early detection and drug treatment dramatically reduced the death rate from infectious disease. Today, the major chronic illnesses, such as heart disease, cancer, and stroke, are the killers and cripplers. A recent study by the National Center for Health Statistics has shown that the average life expectancy in 1982 was 74.5 years, and the leading cause of death was heart disease. Only one person in twenty-five was over sixty-five in 1900; today, one in nine (11 percent of the population) is over sixty-five. By the year 2000, the figure is expected to grow to one in eight (13 percent of the population).

The combination of a more fragmented family structure and increasing life expectancy brought about the obvious result—an increase in ailing, elderly people living alone or far from their children. It was to be expected, therefore, that in the 1960s and 1970s institutions such as nursing homes and extended care facilities seemed to be the answer to the problem of how to care for the elderly. In such institutions, it was argued, necessary food, shelter, and medical care could be provided in the most efficient and humane manner. Moreover, the "old folks" could find the companionship of others with similar interests and outlooks on life.

It was almost too good to be true. Millions of dollars in government funds were allocated to subsidize the construction of nursing homes, and public assistance monies were made available through Medicare and Medicaid to pay for care of the ill or disabled elderly. But in all this rush to build nursing homes and extended care facilities and fill them with the ailing elderly, one question was not addressed: What would be the quality of life and the quality of care in these institutions? As a result, the way was left open for abuses, which not only occurred but became rampant.

Unscrupulous nursing home operators collected payments for their patients from government health programs (Medicare and Medicaid), from private health insurance carriers, from patients' personal funds, and from patients' families. Very little of this money was spent on the patients, who were badly housed, ill fed, medically neglected, often mistreated, and in some cases, died as a result of what had been done to them.

By the time the abuses were discovered and corrected, it was clear that, because of economic considerations and other factors, nursing homes would have only a limited impact on the situation. It also became clear that, in one aspect at least, the pendulum would swing back to the way things used to be—people would be cared for at home.

Home health care became the "new and preferred" alternative.

What Is Home Health Care?

Defining home health care is not as simple a task as it may seem. To begin with, the term *health* can cover so many categories—nutrition, physical fitness, general well-being. For our purposes in this book, therefore, "home health care" will mean the provision of care at home for a person who is sick or disabled to the extent that he or she is unable to function in the same manner as a "normally healthy" person in our society. This is broad enough to cover all aspects of what we want to consider in this book, but before we continue, let's also take a look at a couple of "professional" definitions of home health care.

The AMA Definition • The American Medical Association has defined home health care as follows:

The provision of nursing care, social work, therapies (such as diet, occupational, physical, psychological, and speech), vocational and social services, and homemaker-health aide services may be included as basic components of home health care. The provision of these needed services to the patient at home constitutes a logical extension of the physician's therapeutic responsibility. At the physician's request and under his medical direction, personnel who provide these home health care services operate as a team in assessing and developing the home health care plan.

This covers more ground and is a valid definition both from the physicians's point of view and from that of the individual. The emphasis, as you can see, is on giving the cared-for person the home equivalent of institutional medical care, with none of the often depressing or even hazardous effects an institution can have on a sick person. (More about this later on in this chapter.)

The AHA Definition • The American Hospital Association provides us with this listing of what constitutes home health care:

Medical care and supervision	Speech therapy
Nursing care and supervision	Inhalation therapy
Social work services	Medical technician services
Physical therapy	Appliance, equipment, and
Occupational therapy	sterile supply services

Availability of hospital in- patient services	Pharmaceutical services
Nutritional guidance	Transportation for patient and equipment
Laboratory and radiology services	Homemaker and health aide services

It's easy to see that this matter of defining home health care can become quite involved. Basically, all we are talking about in this book is taking care of someone's health at home rather than in a hospital or nursing home or other such institution. It's as simple—and as complex—as that.

Can Home Care Really Help?

Listen to the words of a home care professional: "A person who has initiative and an ability to communicate their needs will probably fare better at home than in an institution. They do not want to consider leaving their home. That's asking them to leave the house where their children grew up, the house where their husband died, the house where they cooked all their meals. I have seen patients do without many of the necessities of life to stay in that house. Their house is their whole identity."

According to experts in the fields of neurology, gerontology, rehabilitation, and psychiatry, the inner strengths and resources that many of have had to call upon in our daily lives will become essential when we get older and illness or disability strikes. With the wisdom of years of life experience and better knowledge of their own uniqueness, older people can guide others and help arrange the modifications that will assure them a high quality of home health care.

Setting goals, experiencing new things, and enjoying lifelong pleasures do not cease with an illness or chronic health problem, as some of the more zealous preventionists would have us believe. If fact, a health problem marks not the end but rather the beginning of a rededication to the principles that promote the good life. The gifts and treasures that life offers may well take on new meaning—and making the effort to maximize the skills, capabilities, and strengths that exist within each of us are vital steps to physical and mental health.

How It All Started

Home care is not a new concept. We have always taken care of ourselves at home. Organized home health care actually began in the 1800s with voluntary agencies in cities such as New York City, Buffalo,

Boston, and Philadelphia. These agencies later became the Visiting Nurse Association, which is still in existence.

Hospital-based home care services utilizing a multidisciplinary approach had its beginnings in the late 1940s. Montefiore Hospital in New York City started a program of using physicians, nurses, and other health professionals to provide personal health care to a number of community residents in their own homes. This program brought about a new realization of the importance of social factors and their influence on disease. By treating patients in their homes, home care professionals had to go beyond the treatment of the disease process itself. They found they had to consider such factors as how the patient's family reacted to his illness, where the patient lived, what kind of home environment was present, the type of food he ate at home, his employment status and how it was affected by his confinement to home, and a host of other conditions.

The basic concept of home health care remains essentially the same today.

Home Care—No Wonder!

Let's take a look for a moment at a medical "Shangri-La," the ideal model of medical care. To begin with, you and each individual would have a key primary care physician at every stage of your life. This doctor would function as your medical consultant and confidant. He would monitor, assess, diagnose, and treat all health-related problems. Should you become sick or disabled, your primary physician would, if necessary, call in specialists, who would help specify your health needs and care requirements. Medications would be provided, necessary therapy supplied, and any required convalescent support made available.

This primary care system, although attractive in concept, is not a reality for most of us, and even if it were, one person should not be made completely responsible for anyone's lifetime medical care. Except in cases of full dependency, such as a coma victim, all of us are, in essence, responsible for our own health care.

The longer life expectancy we now enjoy, coupled with advances in medical science, has resulted in growing numbers of older people who, while not subject to as many life-threatening infectious diseases as in the past, must now contend with health problems with a long-term disability, whose impact on an individual's life style can be devastating.

Many people now continue to live years—even decades—after suffering a disabling stroke, and an increasing number of older citizens are finding it necessary to adjust to the disabling effects of chronic pulmonary disease or neurological illnesses.

What is urgently needed now are cost-saving and quality-assuring alternatives to the institutional care of the past. Progressive organizations, both private and public, are beginning to test and develop new home health care delivery systems.

The one big stumbling block is money. At best, the government and other health care bureaucracies move slowly. Public and private facilities are presently geared to handle only patients requiring custodial or institutional care. Federal, state, and private insurance programs have limited provisions, if any, for the individual requiring additional assistance to remain at home. The ironic aspect of this, of course, is that it costs more to maintain a patient in a hospital, nursing home, or convalescent facility than at home. Yet the present laws governing Medicare assistance, for example, have limited provisions for home health care.

Every Congress in recent years has gone on record in favor of expanding home care alternatives to costly institutional care. Numerous proposals have been advanced for the purpose of expanding home health care benefits under Medicare and Medicaid. Some of these proposals have been enacted into law, but at present, home care benefits coverage is limited to only those patients who qualify for highly intensive medical or nursing services. In addition, still other restrictions require a prescription by a physician and a determination that the patient is truly "homebound."

As a result, the last twenty years have witnessed a rapidly growing consumer movement in which people are taking more responsibility as individuals, and as families, for their own health care. Doctors and health and science writers have produced a steady flow of books and articles on the subject of health and self-care. Most of this material has been written with the underlying assumption that people will be assessing their own health problems and will be actively participating in decisions that have an impact on their health and the care they receive. This proliferation of information has resulted in a more aware and health-responsible population.

In reaction to this new awareness on the part of the public, the present health care establishment is slowly becomimg more prevention oriented. The needs and rights of patients are being explored, and the health care system is gradually evolving to a point where it will have to meet these needs.

Currently available home health care resources are fragmented, but in the near future they will, of necessity, grow to meet the needs of informed consumers seeking assistance. Elected officials will rally around the cause once they realize the significance of the issues to their constituents. Thus, while home health care efforts right now are confined to pilot programs or otherwise limited efforts throughout the country, we will soon see some dramatic changes. Adding urgency to this movement is the fact that the over-seventy-five age group is the fastest growing group in this country. The National Institute on Aging estimates that by the year 2000 the number of Americans seventy-five and older will have increased by 53 percent since 1980—and this is the age group especially vulnerable to disabling illnesses such as arthritis, heart disease, and stroke.

The Smorgasbord that Is Home Health Care

At present, the term *Home Health Care* implies different things. In some cases, it involves something as simple as periodic visits by a housekeeper to do shopping, light housekeeping, and some cooking. At the other extreme, it can consist of the continuous operation of life support systems, such as intravenous feeding or kidney dialysis. Whatever the level of help required, though, the primary goal has to be to preserve and improve the quality of life at home for the individual patient.

Let's consider the various levels of home health care.

MINIMAL CARE

This is best typified by the example of a seventy-eight year-old woman struggling to live independently at home. Her disabling arthritis is sometimes so bad that she is unable to leave her home and shop for groceries or to prepare a meal for herself. Her spirit is strong, but her body at times is just too weak. The obvious solution is to have a part-time homemaker available to help out on a regular basis.

In still another case, a seventy-two-year-old man had a stroke ten years earlier but, with the help of his wife, he had been able to live an independent life at home. Although his activities were limited—meeting with friends in the park or just sitting on a bench and watching the world go by—he did function on his own. With the sudden death of his wife six months ago, he was left to fend for himself. Shopping and housekeeping were all but impossible for him, yet he was determined to make a go of it. He did not want to leave his home, his neighborhood, or his lifelong friends. Once again, a part-time homemaker was the answer.

INTERMEDIATE CARE

Consider the case of a sixty-five-year-old man slowly recovering from a stroke. He is in a hospital and needs assistance in bathing and dressing. He is presently getting physical therapy and speech therapy in the hospital, but he knows that he could recuperate effectively at home—and wants to. Because he lives alone, a range of "hands on" services has been recommended. A home health aide will help him with his personal care, and a physical therapist and a speech therapist will visit on a regular basis to give him therapy for his specific problems. An occupational therapist will be brought in to retrain him to dress and bathe himself. Supervision will come from a nurse and social worker responsible for coordinating the home health care for this individual. When necessary, transportation and escort services will enable him to venture out into the community where he lives and also help him keep his medical appointments. Finally, equipment and supplies prescribed by his physical or occupational therapist, such as special shoes, a cane, and equipment for his bathroom, will be supplied as needed. This is a perfect example of the efficiency and effectiveness of good home health care—and, moreover, obtainable at a much lower cost than keeping the patient in a hospital or other institution.

INTENSIVE CARE

This represents the highest level of home health care. In essence, it comes close to having hospital care full time in your home. For example, a young man in his early twenties was unable to eat regular food to obtain the nutrients he required. He had had sections of his intestine surgically removed and had to be fed intraveneously. His total parenteral nutrition (TPN, see Chapter 6) provided all the nutrition he needed—and all of this was done at home. Being at home in its pleasant surroundings and privacy meant a lot. With properly administered care, this person was able to live at home and receive the same level of care available to him at a hospital.

The Home Health Care Network Is Growing

Today, the major source of home health care is family and friends. This can be an enormous strain for them, however, and in many instances they cannot make a long-term commitment. However, with the growing awareness of the need for home health care on a reliable basis, a number of organizations and agencies and private companies are starting to provide the kind of care needed, or expanding the services they are already providing.

Nonprofit home care agencies, for example, are community-based, hospital-based, or freestanding agencies, that provide home health care services to people in their community. Funding for their services comes from Medicare and Medicaid, insurance carriers, and / or directly from the patient based on a sliding fee scale. Agencies such as the Visiting Nurse Association provide nursing, home health aides, physical therapy, occupational therapy, and other support services.

Proprietary home health care agencies often have a network of offices nationwide. They recruit, train, and supervise a full range of home health care workers, assign them to clients, and supervise their work. Companies such as Olsten Health Care, Upjohn Health Care, Quality Care, and Kimberly and Beverly are representative of this type of organization. The Yellow Pages lists those available in your community under "Nurses" or "Home Health Agencies."

Tax-supported home care services are a type of government-aided health care and can be found through your county or state health department or government offices on aging. Certain income and age requirements may have to be met to qualify for aid.

Employment agencies and nursing registries work for a fee, but unlike proprietary or nonprofit agencies do not act as the employer. The patient or his family assumes responsibility for obtaining, supervising, and paying for the type of health care services needed.

Finding Home Health Care

Patience and persistence are what's most needed here. The ease or difficulty of finding home health assistance depends upon a number of factors, and the channels of information and community resources vary considerably. The task can be frustrating.

If the patient needing home health care has been hospitalized or has been in a nursing home or other such institution, the medical social worker or discharge planner can be an excellent source of information and referral. Discharge planning usually begins right after a patient's admission to a hospital. The discharge planner's primary objective is to free the hospital bed as soon as possible. Acute care hospitals are under considerable pressure to justify long-term use of a hospital bed, and with the newly passed DRGs (diagnosis-related groups), which now dictate a flat fee for Medicare reimbursements, the pressure to expedite discharge may become even greater.

A typical patient in an acute care hospital occupies a bed for about a week. If the stay is much longer, the hospital may not be reimbursed for all of the additional costs under the DRG system. For example, in one special case where a stroke victim had to remain in a hospital for months because neither the family nor the social workers could find a nursing home to take the patient, the cost to the hospital and the insurance carrier was prohibitive. Under the DRG system, the long-term use of the hospital as an extended care facility will be reduced.

A hospital discharge planner has access to the appropriate forms and knows the local community agencies offering home care services, and thus can often resolve a situation so that both the patient and the hospital are well served. The rapid discharge of the patient (consistent with good medical progress, of course) frees the bed for the hospital, and the recuperating patient is delighted to return home.

The one significant problem in all of this is the great variance in home health care services that different private health insurance plans cover. The discharge planner cannot change this, but he can help interpret the patient's insurance coverage.

Obtaining home health care presents a more difficult challenge for the individual who has not been hospitalized. In this case, the individual usually has to seek out home health care community agencies on his own, or the family has to do it. Hospital discharge planners or social workers can sometimes offer help, but it will be limited assistance because they have to concentrate their efforts on the hospital patients in their care. At best, they can direct the individual or the family to certain agencies or organizations in the community.

In such a situation, the search for home health care usually begins with inquiries to various family services agencies or to a religious organization. If the individual is unable to cook at home, an organization such as Meals on Wheels can be contacted. In addition, consulting or "networking" with your physician, clergyman, neighbors, and friends often proves fruitful. If the individual's disability stems from a specific disease, such as cancer, arthritis, or diabetic blindness, the appropriate voluntary organization may be of assistance—the American Cancer Society, the Arthritis Foundation, the American Diabetes Association, for example. Also, assistance can be sought from the nonprofit agencies and the proprietary home health agencies directly. The National Home Caring Council (235 Park Avenue South, New York, N.Y. 10003) has lists of accredited home health care service agencies organized by state.

Mainly, you must have patience, be persistent—and keep asking.

Paying for Home Health Care

Most sources of financial aid for home health care services place limitations on the kind of services that can be used, the number of visits therapists and others can make to the patient, and the amount and frequency of other benefits available. In addition, there are varying and inconsistent sources of financial aid.

Medicare (available for people over sixty-five and for certain disabled individuals) pays for some health services in the home and not for others. For example, Medicare may pay for part-time skilled nursing care or physical or speech therapy but will not pay for home-delivered meals or homemaker services. Your local Social Security Administration office will have further details.

Medicaid is a state-administered program for those with low incomes. Each state sets its own eligibility requirements and its own schedule of assistance. Your local public assistance office or the Social Security office may have further information on the assistance provided in your state.

Some private health insurance policies may cover certain health-related home care services. Your insurance agent or the benefits manager at your place of employment should be able to help you sort through the services provided. You may not find the service you need specifically identified as home health care, so check carefully. In addition, special insurance, such as automobile insurance and workmen's compensation, may cover home care services if the need for home care falls under the specific coverage provided. In some areas, health maintenance organizations (HMOs) such as Kaiser Permanente Aid or the health insurance plan (HIP) of your area include some aspects of home care in their health plans.

Although home health care is significantly less costly than institutional care, it is important to check insurance coverage and other financial plans carefully in order to avoid unanticipated bills for home care services. Unexpected financial burdens will surely add stress to an already stressful situation.

Chapter 2 gives guidelines for keeping charts and records to sort out available resources and financial needs and requirements. The time and energy spent doing this may well make it possible to reap all possible benefits available for home health care.

Are There Alternatives?

There are some people who just cannot be helped by home health care. First there are the tragic cases, such as someone in a deep coma, who of necessity has to be cared for in an institution. Second there are those who live alone and whose disabilities, whether physical or emotional, are severe enough to prevent them from ever being able to manage on their own. They need twenty-four-hour care. Third would be those patients who, because of inner emotional difficulties, perhaps longstanding and deep-rooted, find the onset of illness or disability a ready excuse to give up completely. They literally abandon themselves and become completely dependent upon others, to such an extent that home health care, no matter how carefully planned, is not feasible.

In such cases, there are alternatives, financed either with private funds, through government subsidies (Medicare or Medicaid), or through private insurance policies. Table 1 lists various housing facilities available for those who need health care away from home. Table 2 presents guidelines for evaluating and selecting alternative housing.

If possible, the patient should participate in the choice of a home. Location is important if there are family or friends in the area who might want to visit.

Several resources can help you compile a list of appropriate facilities in the chosen area: the patient's physician, the local medical society, social services department, community welfare or aging council, Social Security office, and state chapters of the American Health Care Association (for proprietary homes) and the American Association of Homes for the Aging (for nonprofit homes). Ask for the names of licensed facilities that are eligible for the type of reimbursement you expect to rely on.

The next step is to visit the homes, both on an official tour and, if possible, as an ordinary visitor of a patient. The questions in Table 2 will help you evaluate what you find. Copy them and take the list with you; don't hesitate to ask questions about anything that is not immediately apparent.

It's important to understand that sometimes home health care doesn't work out, despite high hopes on the part of everyone involved. There is inevitable stress in a home care arrangement, and time may make it clear that the relationship between the care provider and the cared-for individual cannot stand up under the stress.

Sometimes an older person's illness and disability can become "contagious," in the sense that constant exposure to a chronically ill person can "infect" the care provider with a corresponding depression and other stress-related conditions. If this happens, especially in the case of close relatives (a son or daughter caring for a parent), it's essential that a calm and objective evaluation of all the options be made.

It may well turn out that alternative housing and health care facilities need to be found. In such cases, it's best to be realistic and admit

Table 1 ▪ TYPES OF HOUSING FACILITIES AND THEIR SERVICES

Services	Nursing home		Personal care and other homes	
	Total care. Presence of skilled medical personnel for continuous/intermittent care.		Nonmedical residential institution providing some or total assistance with personal care	
	SKILLED NURSING	INTERMEDIATE CARE	PERSONAL CARE	DOMICILIARY CARE
1. Shelter	X	X	X	X
2. Monitoring	X	X	X	X
3. Meal Preparation	X	X	X	X
4. Housekeeping and Chores	X	X	X	X
5. Shopping and Errands	X	X	X	X
6. Intermittent Personal Care	X	X	X	X
7. Continuous Personal Care	X	X	X	
8. Rehabilitation	X	X		
9. Skilled Nursing	X	X		
10. 24-hour Nursing	X			
% of Elderly	5	n.a.	.05	.5

that this may, after all, be the more desirable arrangement for all concerned.

Also, we must not overlook the fact that a sudden change in circumstances—for example, an unexpected transfer to a job in another city for the care provider—may necessitate a search for alternative housing for the chronically ill person. Unforeseen events have to be dealt with as they develop, and there's no real way to avoid or anticipate these situations.

	Caretaker environment		*Congregate housing*	*Independent housing*	
	Semi-independent living arrangement		Shared services and common areas, with independent living arrangement (i.e. retirement communities)	Homeowners and renters living on their own	
	FOSTER HOMES	WITH RELATIVE		SELF AND SPOUSE	SELF
1.	X	X	X	X	X
2.	X	X	X		
3.	X	X	X		
4.	X	X			
5.	X	X			
6.	X	X			
7.					
8.					
9.					
10.					
	n.a.	n.a.	n.a.	51	27

Source: William Scanlon, Elaine Difederico, and Margaret Stassen, *Long Term Care: Current Experience and a Framework for Analysis* (Washington, D.C.: Urban Institute, February 1979).

Table 2 ■ EVALUATING AND SELECTING ALTERNATIVE
RESIDENTIAL SETTINGS

INSTITUTIONAL FACTORS

Is the home licensed by the state or local agency? Ask to see the certificate. Is it accredited by the Joint Commission on Accreditation of Hospitals?

Is a medical examination required before or immediately after admission? This is *de rigueur* in good nursing homes.

Is there an arrangement with a nearby hospital for transfer and care of any patient who needs hospitalization?

Is the facility clean and relatively free of bad odors?

What are the visiting hours, and who can come?

Does each bedroom have a window and open onto a corridor?

Is there room to maneuver a wheelchair?

How many beds to a room? Four should be the maximum.

COSTS

Is the home eligible for Medicare and / or Medicaid reimbursement?

What is covered under the basic rate? What is extra? To guard against surprise charges, get a signed statement about coverage from the home you choose. Remember, however, that while the better homes tend to charge more, higher costs do not guarantee better care.

Are there refunds on advanced payments should the patient leave the home?

Does the patient's insurance policy cover any or all charges?

SAFETY

Is the building fireproof or fire-resistant, and are there a sprinkler system and clearly posted emergency exit routes?

Are there ramps for wheelchairs, and are the halls wide enough to permit two chairs to pass?

Are the floor coverings nonskid and the hallways well lit?

Are there grab bars in the halls, bathrooms, and elevators and call bells at bedside and in the bathroom? Do they work?

STAFF

Is there a doctor and a registered nurse on call twenty-four hours a day?

Is there provision made for regular dental care? What about an ophthalmologist, or any other specialist the patient may need? How often are they available?

Is the nursing staff trained in basic rehabilitation techniques? Is there a full-time physical therapy program directed by a qualified physical or occupational therapist?

Is there a social worker available to handle family and patient concerns and negotiations with other community resources?

Is the staff friendly and efficient in responding to patient calls? If possible, talk to a few current residents.

Does the staff encourage patients to be independent?

Are patients overtranquilized or restrained to minimize staff harassment? Often the patients who are the best candidates for rehabilitation are the most heavily sedated since they are more active and demanding than others.

FOOD

Are the meals varied, well balanced, well cooked, and appetizingly served? Are special likes and dislikes taken into account?

Is there a dietician who prepares meals for patients on special diets?

Are the menus prepared a week or more in advance, and does the food served match what's on the menu?

Are patients encouraged to eat in a group, or do they dine alone in their rooms?

Do those who need help in feeding get it, and get it promptly, before the food gets cold?

Is the dining room attractive and accessible to patients in wheelchairs?

ACTIVITIES

Is there a recreation program?

Are there rooms for socializing, physical therapy, and occupational therapy?

Are the grounds well kept, and are patients who are able to go outside encouraged to do so daily?

Do volunteers from the community work with and visit patients regularly?

Are patients kept busy and occupied? Are there activities like card games, knitting and sewing, conversation?

Are outings scheduled?

(Table 2 continued)

PERSONAL FACTORS

Are patients treated with dignity and respect, or are they talked down to as if they were small children?

Do patients have privacy—for dressing and undressing, phone calls, visits?

Are any personal possessions, such as a favorite rocking chair, allowed, and is there room for keeping personal belongings?

Are there arrangements for religious observances?

Are a barber and a beautician available?

Are patients allowed to wear their own clothing? Are they kept clean and well groomed?

Can patients leave for special outings or home visits?

Source: Jane E. Brody, *Jane Brody's The New York Times Guide to Personal Health* (New York: Times Books, 1982).

Institutions Can Be Hazardous to Your Health

Before her encounter with the small patch of ice on the sidewalk, Mrs. Barbara W. had led the kind of independent life many another widow in her sixties would envy. She had a small apartment in a good neighborhood, furniture that was worn but lived in and comfortable, and pictures of her children and grandchildren displayed on every available surface. Her financial needs were not great and were adequately met by the income from her husband's insurance, her own small pension, and Social Security benefits.

As with many older people, Barbara found security in the familiar daily routine of her life. She ate small meals several times a day, prepared by herself with food that she liked; she took catnaps whenever she felt like it; she read or watched television late at night if she couldn't sleep; she went for leisurely walks in good weather, stopping to chat with friends along the way; and she treasured each moment of the exhilarating visits of her children and grandchildren.

Then the nightmare began. She slipped and fell on a patch of ice. A broken hip put her in the hospital. Surgery followed, and then came painful recuperation in a nursing home. The pain she could bear—but not the way control of her own life had suddenly been wrested from her.

Life in the nursing home became a frightening and demeaning

continuation of the hospital life Barbara had deplored. While the physical therapy she was given did help relieve the boredom of the long days, the endless nights remained. She longed for the privacy of her own home and the ability to take her frequent catnaps. The regimentation of the nursing home seemed senseless, and the staff treated her as if she were a child. Her attempts to bend the rules even a little or to modify the regimen so it would closely resemble her own home life were met with criticism of her "stubbornness."

Barbara maintained her sanity and some semblance of dignity by telling herself that she was "getting out and going over the wall" as soon as she could. She channeled her tenacity toward her physical therapy treatment, attacking it with spirit and vigor. The effort paid off. She was able to walk independently with a cane much sooner than anyone at the nursing home had anticipated, and she wasted no time in getting back to her own home.

Any life change at any age, such as that undergone by Barbara W., results in a period of adjustment and stress. In some of our largest corporations, for example, management recognizes that there is a period of time required for readjustment whenever a young executive and his family are moved to a new position in a new home in a new town. Support is offered for the time needed to adjust to the new life and environment, even if it takes many weeks or months.

In the health field, however, there is no such universal recognition of the traumatic impact of change on a person who suddenly finds himself in a hospital or other such institution. Amazingly enough, some health professionals are often surprised when older patients become disoriented and unsettled almost immediately after admission. These misguided professionals feel that some degree of disorientation or inability to adjust can occur *after* surgery or other upsetting medical treatment but that there's no logical reason for this to happen so rapidly after admission. Consequently, adult patients who had been alert and functional prior to admission are soon described as senile and are treated accordingly.

Unfortunately for some patients, the behavioral change due to the sudden impact of institutionalization becomes a form of self-fulfilling prophecy. There still seems to be a limited awareness among institution-based health professionals that an environment so familiar to them can seem alien and terrifying to elderly patients newly arrived.

PROCEDURES, PROCEDURES, AND MORE PROCEDURES

Most health care facilties are beset with what seems like an endless procession of forms and procedures from the moment of admission to eventual discharge. Medicare forms, insurance forms, intake forms, release forms—a veritable blizzard of forms—are a major aspect of any health care institution. Unhappily, it's necessary.

The sheer number of people treated at hospitals and other institutions make all these forms absolutely essential. We have to live with that fact. The total effect, however, can be exhaustion on the part of the patient and unending paperwork on the part of the staff.

Practically every aspect of institutional life has been systematized into a procedure or a schedule. Patients are checked regularly; temperatures and blood pressures are recorded on a definite schedule; meals are delivered at set times. The goal is to have everything running like a smoothly oiled machine, despite the fact that the "raw material"— the patients—are human beings who are ill or injured or hurting and cannot function with machinelike regularity. In effect, to continue the analogy, a large hospital is little more than a factory that has divided up various aspects of its product—patient health care—into a series of bits and pieces and procedures that are handled in assembly-line fashion by the institution's staff.

The compartmentalized care given in most hospitals can and often does result in morale problems for the staff. It's difficult to feel good about the job you're doing if that job consists only of flitting in and out of patients' rooms in order to record blood pressures and temperatures or to change water in the pitchers. For the patient, the numerous people that wander in and out of the room become a blur after a while. There is often no sense of who is in charge or whom you can talk to should a problem arise. Even if the patient knows who is the charge nurse or doctor, that person may not be responsible for handling the patient's immediate problem or request.

The patient is expected to become the passive recipient of the fragmented, departmentalized, and impersonal care that is provided. Nursing home staffs perceive patients as socially dependent, childlike individuals who are somewhat "different" from the general population. The qualities considered least desirable in a patient are stubbornness and persistence—characteristics that generally would be considered admirable in the society outside the institution's walls.

It's no wonder, then, that Barbara W. felt imprisoned in the nursing home and that she was unable to effect any meaningful modification in her environment to create a more homelike atmosphere for herself. Small, frequent meals are close to impossible in a setting geared to deliver three meals a day at specific times—to say nothing of all the other aspects of Barbara's individuality and life style that she couldn't duplicate in the institution.

Hospital procedures may be necessary, but in certain circumstances some procedures can actually become dangerous to the patient. In many institutions, medications are dispensed by one nurse, who follows the orders on the patients' charts and doles out medication into little cups that she carries on a tray or a cart to the appropriate patient at the specified time. However, this nurse often doesn't know each patient personally, nor is she always aware of changes in the condition of each patient when she makes her medication rounds. Because of fragmentation of duties and responsibilities, there is always the potential for information not being available exactly when needed. Unfortunately, this has sometimes led to instances when wrong medications have been given to a patient because, through no one person's fault or negligence, the system lagged.

This is not a common occurrence, to be sure. However, it does point up the fact that systematized procedures in health care institutions are less than nurturing and often are in direct opposition to the care, support, recuperation, and rest the patient needs.

INSTITUTIONAL HIERARCHY

Whether you are in a hospital, nursing home, or other extended care facility, you are confronted with a pyramid of professionals providing your care. In a hospital, the captain of the team is the attending physician. He is responsible for approving and signing orders regarding all medical care for a patient.

At times, however, there is confusion about the coordination of this care. Although a family physician may have hospitalized a particular patient, he may not be the physician in charge throughout that hospitalization. If, during the course of a patient's stay in the hospital, another health problem or condition arises requiring the involvement of another physician or specialist, that doctor may become the physician in charge. The decision as to who is in charge often occurs without the involvement or knowledge of the patient or his family. The physician in charge is determined by a professional's perception of the patient's needs or condition. The new doctor, the one now in charge, may not have known the patient prior to his involvement in the case, which can lead to confusion and apprehension on the part of the patient.

To complicate matters further, the head nurse or supervising nurse often has little to do with direct patient care. This nurse is usually a seasoned professional, but she plays more of an administrative and management role. Her primary duties are frequently to supervise and schedule the assorted professionals—nurse aides, practical nurses, and registered nurses—on her staff. This is a formidable task under the best of circumstances and leaves the supervising nurse little time or opportunity to deal directly with any of the patients.

Established hospital procedures determine much of the routine for each of the health professionals involved. With beds to change and medications to dispense, blood pressures to take, and many other tasks to perform, it's no wonder that the nursing staff cannot always get to know their patients as people. Moreover, the nurses have virtually no time at all to accommodate the particular needs or requests of the individual patients.

HOSPITAL FOOD IS . . . ?

If you've ever been in a hospital, you can fill in the blank with whatever words you deem appropriate. Actually, hospital food is no laughing matter. In some cases, hospitalized or institutionalized patients have been found to be more malnourished when they left the institutions than when they were admitted.

If food is properly prepared and served, mealtime can become one of the more pleasant experiences in an otherwise depressing day in an institution. Yet it is difficult to become enthusiastic about a slice of mystery meat, instant mashed potatoes, overcooked and pale green beans, two slices of white bread, and a quivering square of red gelatin. Institutional food can be unbelievably unappetizing, causing hungry patients to pick listlessly at their plates and leave most of the meal uneaten. In addition, inferior ingredients and inadequate menu planning, which are much too prevalent in institutions, can result in poor nutrition even if the patient eats the food.

Recent attention to institutionally induced malnutrition has convinced some institutions to initiate changes. But at present most institutions serve few fresh foods and rely on processed high fat, high sodium alternatives. This is not the sort of diet that speeds recovery or builds strength in a patient.

Meal choices often must be made hours and sometimes more than a full day in advance from a boring and limited menu. And although many hospital patients are not bed-bound, meals frequently must be eaten in bed rather than at a side table or, better yet, in a dining room. It's difficult to measure just how much of the apathy and weakness frequently seen in patients living in institutions comes from poor nutrition, but it's a certainty that this is an underlying cause.

PRIVATE—COME ON IN

Privacy is nonexistent in most institutions, even in private rooms. The staff—doctors, nurses, aides, porters, maids—all seem to feel free to enter a patient's room at any time of day or night to perform their respective tasks. A patient may find himself rudely awakened at 5 AM to the sound of the nurse aide changing the water in his bedside pitcher.

Protests are usually silenced with the admonition that the patient is in the institution for his own health and that anyone healthy enough to care about his own creature comforts isn't really that sick.

Personal belongings are frowned upon, and patients are the passive recipients of decisions made for them by others. The feelings of passivity and resignation engendered by this sort of treatment rob the patient of the self-esteem and self-reliance needed for a speedy recovery. Many of these problems become topics of cocktail party conversation following a brief hospital stay, but they can become chronic and their impact can be considerable when the length of stay in an institution is indefinite because of the nature of the patient's illness or disability.

MAKING THE SYSTEM WORK FOR YOU

All is not hopeless. If you take the time to learn the functions of the professional staff and the constraints under which they must work, you can put this knowledge to good use. Once you understand why institutional care brings with it many annoying discomforts, you will be able to take a more assertive posture in assuring good quality health care for yourself or for someone close to you for whom you are providing care. By learning the hierarchy that exists in hospitals and other health care institutions, you can identify the individuals who have the power and authority to make changes. In addition, it is often helpful to enlist the aid of someone in a more junior position, a person lower down in the institutional pecking order. This person may be more accessible and can function as a channel to the one in charge.

In the depersonalized system of an institution, it's vital to become "known" to the health professionals around you. By interacting with you, on a more personal basis, they can't help but become aware of and acknowledge your individuality. The more they get to know you as a person, the more direct their involvement will be with you and the better you'll be able to make the system work for you.

Institutional life itself and society's attitude toward institutions encourage continued abuses, whether the institution is a hospital, a nursing home, or a rehabilitation center. The pervasive procedures and fragmented care dehumanize and depersonalize all who come in contact with the system.

During hospitalization or a stay in an institution, the individual must make every effort to retain a level of responsibility for his or her own care. The courage, tenacity, and positive emotions that are so important to us throughout life take on new importance in maintaining a sense of self in an institution.

It's up to each of us individually.

The Future

At some point in the not too distant future, home care will be a well-developed alternative health care delivery system—a comprehensive community-based program providing a range of services to those needing assistance at home. These services may include a multidisciplinary assessment of the patient's total needs, including individual and family counseling sessions, supervision of medication, rehabilitation therapy, home care services (meal preparation and light housekeeping), personal care services (grooming and dressing), the provision of medical equipment and supplies, and community and volunteer services.

There is no doubt that present health care systems will evolve and change. Increased demand for health care from the growing number of disabled elderly is already having an impact. Drug companies and equipment and supply manufacturers will give more attention to the chronically ill adults at home as important customers, and this will add to the health delivery revolution. In addition, reduced government expenditures for nursing home and hospital care will result in increasing numbers of chronically ill and disabled older people at home.

The pressures for change in the health care system cannot be ignored, but above and beyond these pressures we have, in this age of entitlement, a genuine awareness of the needs of the elderly and a growing desire to improve the physical, mental, and health status of our older citizens. There's also a growing realization of what has now become an obvious truth:

There's no place like home—for health care.

2

Plugging Into
the System

NONE OF US is truly alone. We touch each other's lives in countless ways each day, and our lives change as we interact with each other. This is nowhere more apparent than in home health care.

One person becomes disabled or chronically ill, and the effect spreads out in ever widening circles, encompassing and involving many others. Families, friends, associates, health workers—all of them become in some way touched or altered by what has happened to the person at the core, the one who must now be cared for at home.

And the one person most directly affected, the one with the heaviest responsibility, is the caregiver.

The Caregiver's Critical Role

The home care team can include registered nurses, home health aides, homemakers, physical therapists, social workers, occupational therapists, nutritionists, respiratory therapists and pharmacists. The key players on the team, however, are the patient and his family or close friends.

Very often a key issue in determining whether or not an individual will be able to remain in his own home is the availability and accessibility of family or close friends to be of assistance. Family or friends can be caregivers or coordinators of care given by others. Sometimes the family member lives nearby, in the same community or in the same home as the person being cared for. Often, family members live at considerable distances, and the job of orchestration and coordination of care and services then can become a formidable challenge.

In many ways, the caregiver's role in orchestrating and obtaining the needed home health care services, equipment, and supplies resembles a homeowner's role in redecorating a house. Once you decide to redecorate, you probably create a list of the tasks or projects involved. For each project, you decide whether to do it yourself or to hire someone to do the job for you. And in some situations you may decide to hire a decorator to plan, orchestrate, and coordinate the entire job. The degree of personal involvement varies, in each and every case, but the ultimate responsibility rests with the homeowner.

Orchestrating home health care services also demands that you identify the kind of help you feel may be required. You then need to decide which of the tasks you are prepared or able to do and which tasks will require the assistance of another member of the family, a close friend, or an outside resource. As you will see later on in this chapter, home health care services can be engaged on an as-needed basis, full-time or part-time. Some therapists, aides, and consultants work under the umbrella of a home health care department of a hospital or home health care agency; others are often available on contract basis for short-term or long-term assignments.

It should not surprise you to learn that the majority of home health care services are actually provided by family and friends. A recent government study reported that family and friends often provide the bulk of care either directly or as the important link to help connect with and coordinate the home care services for the person in need.

With each passing day—as needs grow for almost every conceivable type of home health care service—agencies, health care organizations, and companies are developing new ways to meet these needs. It's up to the caregivers to learn about available resources and keep abreast of new developments and programs as they become available.

As in the example of the homeowner, the ultimate responsibility for overseeing the home health care for someone close to you rests with you.

The Home Health Care Team

In many instances, home health care demands a team approach. The multiplicity of problems that are seen in patients—health, medical, emotional, environmental, financial—can be more than any one health professional can handle. No matter how well trained or experienced a health care professional may be, the expertise and coordination of the team is needed to provide effective and efficient home health care. While some members of the team can plan and implement medi-

Table 3 ■ THE HOME HEALTH CARE TEAM

Health care professional	Function
Physician	Writes or authorizes request for home health care services through a medical treatment plan • Supervises treatment
Nurse	Evaluates patient's condition and determines type of nursing or therapeutic care needed • Performs necessary nursing care (changing sterile dressing or catheter care, for example) and instructs patient and family in follow-up care
Social worker	Works with patient and family to cope with health problems, home situation, future planning • Recommends and obtains community services for the patient
Home health aide	Provides wide variety of assistance to patient—dressing, bathing, walking, meal preparation, light housekeeping • Administers oral medication and reports to nurse on patient's progress
Homemaker	Maintains the home; shops, cooks, light housekeeping, companionship
Physical therapist	Evaluates patient's strength, flexibility, endurance, ability to walk, and develops treatment plan and schedule for therapeutic exercises • Some exercises done during home visit by PT, others with help of family or homemaker-home health aide
Occupational therapist	Evaluates patient's ability to perform skills necessary to independent daily living—dressing, washing, bathing, and others • Develops treatment plan and schedule for teaching skills to reduce dependence • Counsels family and homemaker-health aide on follow-up program
Pharmacist	Fills prescriptions, rents or sells needed equipment, products, and supplies
Speech pathologist	Evaluates patient's ability to communicate—hear speak understand write • Develops treatment plan to help patient relearn language skills or communicate within limitations of disability

cal and rehabilitative care for the patient—changing dressings, for example, or teaching procedures for bathing and eating and for getting in and out of bed—the expertise of another team member regarding insurance reimbursement, community programs, and other resources is mandatory for making home health care work.

Coordinating all the medical, social and community health services is a formidable task. In many instances, hospital social service departments and community agencies and for-profit and voluntary home health agencies handle a great deal of the coordination of professionals engaged in home health care; at times, the coordinator's role falls to the caregiver.

Table 3 briefly describes the members of the home health care team. Each will be discussed in greater detail later in this chapter.

Where to Begin

What to do? Whom to call? Where to find help? What kind of help is available? What will it cost?

These are just some of the questions that bedevil the care provider as he or she sets out to arrange home health care for the person in need. The course of action taken will depend to a great extent on how the need for home health care first arose.

Basically, two avenues lead to the necessity for providing health care at home: prior hospitalization due to illness, accident, or injury; or a gradual decline in health that culminates in the need for more and more help to function. The realization that home health care will be needed can become apparent at different times and different points for different people.

STARTING POINT—THE HOSPITAL

The pleasant-faced woman in her early thirties who came into the hospital room wore a white lab coat and carried a clipboard, but there was no stethoscope draped around her neck. Ted, in his late sixties, looked at her, then glanced questioningly at his wife in the bed.

The woman smiled at them. "Hi, I'm Mrs. Olsen, the hospital discharge planner." "Discharge?" Ted Davis frowned. "My wife is only two days out of surgery. She can't go home yet."

"Of course not. A broken hip takes longer than that. If you can spare me a few minutes, though, I'd like to help you plan what to do when your wife is finally discharged. We want to make sure your care continues even after you leave the hospital, Mrs. Davis."

Mrs. Olsen pulled up a chair next to the bed, balanced her clipboard on her knee, and set to work. In a few moments she had cleared away the essential details, all of them carefully noted on her clipboard. Ted and Jane Davis were each sixty-eight years old, retired, and on Social Security and a small pension for Ted. They each had Medicare, and Ted had purchased additional health insurance to supplement the Medicare coverage.

Mrs. Olsen set down her clipboard and started to explain the kind of home health care services available to them. Ted and Jane soon realized that Mrs. Olsen's knowledge of hospital and community resources was of vital importance to Jane's successful recovery. They understood that Jane would not be completely recovered when she was ready to be discharged from the hospital but would, in fact, need to continue the physical therapy that had been started during her hospital stay. Also, she would require additional help during her first weeks at home.

Mrs. Olsen explained how the hospital's home care department would initiate the request for home care and follow up on it. She also told them what services Medicare would and would not cover, and she offered to help them review their additional insurance coverage. The policy might include home care, but under different wording.

Jane's recovery at the hospital was uneventful, and the transition to home once she was discharged presented no problems for her. After she had settled in at home, a nurse from the home care department visited her to check on her progress and evaluate her home environment. Jane's doctor had written an order for physical therapy, but the nurse requested that he approve an additional order for occupational therapy as well.

With the help of the occupational therapist, some minor changes in furniture location and bedroom and bath arrangements were made so that Jane would be able to get around the house, using her walker, easily and safely. The therapist advised Jane and Ted on how to manage some of the activities of daily living during Jane's recuperation. Additionally, she was able to make practical suggestions to the home health aide who would spend a few hours each day helping Jane with her personal care needs.

The physical therapist visited twice a week in the early period of Jane's home care in order to supervise the strengthening exercises Jane was performing as she learned how to walk again.

All of this care was coordinated by the home care department of the hospital under the supervision of the registered nurse in charge. Before long, Jane had made a successful recovery and the routine of her life with Ted returned to normal.

A fairy tale? Too good to be true? Real life doesn't flow this smoothly? Jane and Ted's story is not unusual. The road to home health care can be well paved when there has been a stopover at a hospital. When a patient is about to be discharged from the hospital, the discharge planner is in a position to identify the health care team members who can be called upon for either short-term or long-term assistance at home. She (discharge planners tend to be women) can consult with the doctor to learn when discharge from the hospital is planned. Then, depending upon the diagnosis, the medical problem, the condition of the patient, and the home situation for that patient, the discharge planner will make a recommendation and a referral to the home care department of the hospital or to a home health care agency.

The nurse in charge, either at the hospital's home care department or at the home health care agency, will evaluate the patient and the home situation. She will then recommend the health professionals who will be needed and will suggest and describe their assignments. In this way, there is continuity of care as the patient makes the transition from hospital to home.

STARTING POINT—ANYWHERE

Without the "benefit" of a prior hospitalization, the task of seeking effective home health care for an individual can become both complex and frustrating. Because of the fragmented, inconsistent, and often duplicated health care services available in a community, the care provider often doesn't even know where to start.

For most of us, our experience with health care begins with our doctor. The doctor examines us, prescribes medications, arranges hospital admissions, calls in specialists, and supervises our health care in the hospital. Physicians, however, are usually less knowledgeable about setting up systems of *home* health care. They are primarily concerned, as they should be, with preventing and controlling disease in their patients. The focus of the physician is primarily on the patient and the illness or injury involved.

Therefore it probably will be up to you to do the research and identify the home care resources that are available in your community.

DO YOU KNOW WHAT IS NEEDED?

As the caregiver, the awareness that some help is needed for a parent or relative living at home may sneak up on you. Her health problems probably have been longstanding, and while you were aware that her life had slowed down a bit and that she was not as active as she once had been, you actually gave little thought to her day to day life. You talked frequently by phone and visited periodically, but you may not have noticed or "wished not to know" just how difficult coping with day-to-day activities had become. Then one day you visit unexpectedly, you find her in her nightgown even though it's late in the afternoon, and her home is not just untidy . . . it's dirty and needs a good cleaning. Her refrigerator is almost empty and you wonder what she could have eaten that day because there's no evidence that any food had been prepared.

She now feels she has let you see that some problems are apparent. During that afternoon visit you learn of her increasing struggle and her methods and courage for coping with her daily existence. She didn't want to be a burden, and she absolutely does not want to consider leaving her home . . . but it is getting harder and harder. Her Parkinson's has progressed to the point where buttoning buttons, zipping zippers, shopping, or cleaning is just too difficult. She manages to muster up the energy to dress for a scheduled appointment, but otherwise it's just too much.

Cereal, tea, and toast have become her dietary mainstays. They're easy to carry and require no preparation. Her phone does not ring at all during that visit, and when you ask about her friends and neighbors, you learn that she sees them rarely because with her health problems she just cannot keep up with them.

As you realize the reality of her life, you may wonder why you ever stopped by unannounced. You may think that the only solution is for her to move in with you and your family. You know that this is not possible. There is no one home all day; you and your spouse both work; and your teenage children have active schedules of their own. With growing guilt you wonder what can possibly be done to help.

At first there seem to be only two choices: she can move in with you and your family; or she can move into a retirement home, something she would never do. Both of these choices are unacceptable. But she does need help.

Because it is Parkinson's disease with which she is coping, the local Parkinson's association or its self-help groups may be able to answer some of your questions. They seek to serve the thousands of people living with Parkinson's and probably are aware of the resources in your area. (Check the Appendix for the names and telephone numbers of Parkinson's organizations) They may be able to recommend home health care agencies their members have used successfully.

What kind of help can you expect in this type of situation? First, by describing her condition and home circumstances, you learn that she is an ideal candidate for home care. They review her health insurance coverage and outline what is and is not covered by Medicare and her supplemental policy.

She immediately needs a part-time home health aide to shop, prepare food, and help her dress and get out each day, and they are able to outline a group therapy program currently in place at your local hospital. There, under the supervision of occupational and physical therapists, individuals with Parkinson's disease meet once a week. The program includes an exercise program to improve flexibility, an occupational therapy program that covers techniques for dressing and food preparation, and a discussion group so that individuals living with Parkinson's can share information and provide emotional support for one another. They even have a special monthly group for the caregivers that is guided by the hospital social worker. There you meet other people who like yourself are struggling with conflicting feelings about doing what is best for the patient; you hear from other caregivers about the positive as well as the negative aspects of some of the community groups available.

This is but one example of a successful attempt to plug into the system of home care resources. The general scenario, however, is applicable to many situations.

Start with defining what you feel is needed. Housekeeping help? A nurse? Should a doctor be contacted to reexamine the person and check the medication? Know the patient's health insurance coverage. Is it Medicare? Is there a supplemental policy? What other financial resources exist to help pay for care that insurance may not cover?

Check health insurance policies carefully. You may find there is coverage listed under a heading such as "Home Care Benefits"—but the requirements may preclude the use of this benefit. For example, the policy may allow coverage for home care only if this care is begun within a set number of days (usually a week) after discharge from a hospital. If the person who needs home care has not been hospitalized, this benefit would not be available. Moreover, the home care benefits, even with prior hospitalization, may not be available unless a physician certifies that, because of the nature of the health problem, the only alternative to home care would be to confine the patient to a hospital or to a skilled nursing facility.

Some health care policies will provide limited disability coverage under the major medical provisions of the contract. When checking into this, or any other policy, make your initial contact by telephone (writing sometimes delays information) and try to speak directly to the benefits manager. If the health care policy is provided by an employer, you should be dealing with the person in charge of the company benefits program. Be persistent. It's the only way to get answers.

Remember, too, that coverage under an employer-provided health care policy doesn't always end on the day your employment terminates. Most such policies have a thirty-one-day grace period in which the coverage continues until you either sign up with a new group at your new place of employment or else take out coverage yourself under a direct payment policy.

If the person needing home care is sixty-five or older or seriously disabled, he or she may qualify for Medicare, the federal program of health care for the elderly and the disabled. A call to the local Social Security office may answer questions you have about coverage. If money is a real problem—if there are just no funds available—Medicaid may be of help. This is a state-administered program designed to provide health care for those who cannot afford to maintain themselves financially. (Medicare and Medicaid are discussed more fully in Chapter 3.)

Next, contact the agencies in your community that deal with the underlying health problem, if there is one. Consult the Appendix, which categorizes a wide variety of groups by health conditions, community agencies, and self-help networks. Each of the sources you contact, each of the people you speak to, can be of help—even though they may not be the ones to provide the home health care you are seeking. What they can do is provide you with leads, give you tips on who to contact next, what questions to ask, and what information to solicit.

There will be times during this search when you will undoubtedly feel that the telephone has become an integral part of your body, permanently attached to your hand and ear. You will be making many phone calls, continually copying down information and names and telephone numbers, and checking out one lead after another.

In an effort to keep the search for home care systematic, it might be a good idea to use a "Resource Record" such as the one on page 58. You can use this one or modify it to suit your individual requirements, perhaps putting the information on index cards for easier handling. Whatever method you use, get organized and be ready with your questions each time you make contact with an agency or an individual. Some of the questions you will want to ask are:

- What type of home health care is available for the person in question?
- What will it cost?
- Is the cost usually covered by most health care insurance policies?
- Are there government or community agencies that can be contacted for assistance and advice?
- If a special type of medical care or rehabilitation therapy is required, where would be the best place to find it?
- Who would be likely to have the most expertise in this field?
- Are there local institutions, such as teaching hospitals, where further help might be found?

There are no set questions to ask though. Much will depend on the individual who needs home care—his or her particular health problem, the extent of disability, the home situation (family members available for help, for example, or the amount of room available), financial considerations, and so on. One question is likely to lead to another; one answer may point to another line of inquiry.

HOME HEALTH CARE RESOURCE RECORD

Date _____

Organization and / or person contacted _____

Position or title _____

Address _____

_____ Phone no. _____

Questions asked   Answers

_____   _____

_____   _____

_____   _____

_____   _____

_____   _____

_____   _____

ADDITIONAL RESOURCES

Organization   Contact Person   Telephone

_____

_____

_____

_____

_____

_____

Next steps _____

_____

Persistence, patience, and a systematic approach will serve you well in this task.

Home Health Care Agencies

Although community agencies can provide valuable information about the resources and care available in your community, contacting a home health care agency can rapidly bring you the personnel help you may need. There are more than five thousand local offices of proprietary (investor-owned) and non-profit agencies throughout the United States. Some are affiliated with the out-patient department of a local hospital or medical center so calling the hospital and asking for the home care department or the social services department will connect you. Others are local offices of national networks of freestanding investor-owned or not-for-profit agencies. Some may be related to a nonhospital institution. Check your Yellow Pages for listings under "Home Health Agencies."

Home health care agencies employ registered nurses, licensed practical nurses, home health aides, homemakers, companions, sitters, and live-in personnel. Many offer physical therapy, occupational therapy, speech therapy, and other rehabilitation services. Speak with the nursing director or the intake coordinator. She should be able to answer your questions concerning the type of care they offer, whether or not they are Medicare- or Medicaid-certified agencies, and what types of health insurance will cover or reimburse you for their care. Be specific about the particular coverage you have. On request they should investigate the coverage provided for in your patient's policy and identify the extent and limitations of insurance reimbursement. If you decide to engage their services, they will usually assist you in completing and filing insurance claims.

Although their staff can provide home care twenty-four hours a day, seven days a week, in most instances that much help is not necessary. The nursing director will schedule an appointment to visit you, interview you and your patient, and develop a nursing / home health care plan. The plan may recommend periodic visits by a nurse supervising the care, while scheduling visits by a home health aide daily or two or three times a week. The aide may work a full day or just a few hours depending on the situation and the help that is required.

Fees for home health care vary depending on the type of care, the type of agency, and the town or city in which you live. Some rural areas have a half-day minimum for home health aides while others in more heavily populated areas may have a two-hour minimum. Table 4 lists

Table 4 ▪ TYPICAL COST OF HOME HEALTH CARE SERVICES

Fees and charges for home health care services are usually billed by the visit rather than by the hour. A home visit by a health professional varies, depending on the type of specialized care provided, the nature of the illness, and the requirements of the treatment plan. Listed below are fee ranges charged by home health care professionals.

Team member	Average length of visit (hours)	Range of fees*	
		Urban	Nonurban
Registered nurse	$1^1/_2$	$53.54–61.03	$62.15–69.70
Physical therapist	$1^1/_2$	$50.91–57.08	$61.26–68.81
Occupational therapist	$1^1/_2$	$54.76–61.21	$73.23–80.54
Speech pathologist	$1^1/_2$	$56.88–64.01	$71.47–78.70
Medical social services	$1^1/_2$	$85.01–94.09	$89.18–99.26
Home health care	2	$35.97–41.80	$39.87–45.20

*Based on Medicare reimbursement rates.

Housekeeper services are not covered by Medicare. This type of service may be covered through state-administered Medicaid programs. Private-pay agencies usually charge the same as Medicare, although their fees can be higher.

Source: Health Care Financing Administration.

the variety of home health care services offered by many agencies and the range of fees charged. Shop around. As home care grows and becomes more competitive, you may find quite a difference in fees charged in your area.

Substantial differences can exist among the variety of agencies providing home health care; there are state-by-state differences concerning licensure requirements for home health care agencies. Investor-owned home health care agencies, such as Beverly Home Health Services, Kelly Health Care, Kimberly Services, Olsten Corporation, and Quality Care, may or may not have a not-for-profit subsidiary that is certified to accept Medicare or Medicaid. According to the Home Health Services and Staffing Association, a trade organization representing investor-owned companies, the largest percentage of patients they treat are private pay, that is, the cost of their care is paid for by private insurance coverage or out-of-pocket payments by the patients or their families. They do report that an increasing number of their members do have Medicare- or Medicaid-certified subsidiaries whose patients are funded by Medicare, Medicaid, Social Services, and the Older Americans Act.

Other voluntary or not-for-profit agencies, such as the Visiting Nurse Association, or community-based home care agencies may have fee schedules based on a sliding scale according to the individual's ability to pay. In addition, they may be Medicare- or Medicaid-certified or be administering a specially funded program that subsidizes the home care costs—or expands the types of services offered at no additional cost to you.

Make a number of inquiries and stay with it. An investment of time at this point can identify a special program or organization that offers just what you need at the lowest cost for you. It's not unusual for a caregiver to waste a good deal of time and effort in trying to "plug into the system." The system itself is not too well organized, and as far as I know there is no one indisputable clearing house of information.

As you continue on the trail of available services and assistance, be a careful investigator. If a program and/or its coverage sounds too good to be true, that may well be the case. Ask to speak with the social worker or the intake coordinator and seek clarification (in writing, if need be) and speak with other patients or caregivers who utilize the service or participate in the program. You may want to ask whether or not the home health agency with whom you plan to do business is approved or accredited by the state or other accrediting organizations. Membership in the National Association for Home Care, a Washington, D.C.-based trade association will suggest a commitment and involvement in home care.

An organization that certifies home health aide training programs, the National Home Caring Council, Inc., has compiled a listing of approved or accredited agencies. They will respond to your written request for the names of accredited agencies in your area. Write to them at 67 Irving Place, New York, New York 10003.

You want to be sure that the agency you choose is a responsible agency that carefully screens and supervises its staff of home care workers. Do not hesitate to ask questions, such as the following:

- Is the home health aide carefully screened and trained?
- Has the aide received at least forty hours of training?
- Does the aide receive continuing in-service education?
- Has the aide been instructed as to the duties and any special tasks included in the plan for care?
- Does a professional assume responsibility for the care given? Is that person available in an emergency?
- Will a responsible person from the agency visit at regular intervals to make sure that everything is as it should be?
- If personal care is to be given as part of a medical plan, is nursing supervision provided to the aide?
- Are there professional staff members available at the agency who

have at least a current license to practice as a registered professional nurse and someone with at least a bachelor's degree in social work, home economics, or closely related profession, plus at least a year of related experience?

- Is there a written statement available from the agency that says who is eligible for service and under what conditions?
- If a person is not eligible for service from the agency, does the agency try to find service that is appropriate?
- Does the agency have legal authorization to operate?
- Has it been certified or licensed where that is required?
- Is the agency open about itself—its auspice, source of funds, cost of service? Does it issue an annual report and make it available to the community?
- Does the agency have a board of directors or advisory committee representative of the community? Is a list of those persons available?
- Has the agency been approved or accredited by an independent, voluntary national standard-setting body?
- Does the agency protect its workers with written personnel policies, basic benefits, and a wage scale for each position?

As of June 1983, twenty-nine states plus Puerto Rico had passed legislation with license requirements for home health care agencies operating in their state. In a number of states, licenses are limited to specific types of home health care agencies. Although a license is not a guarantee of superior care, it does indicate that certain basic criteria have been met for the home care agency to operate. In states without any licensure requirements, you will want to check references carefully. Speak with your local hospital discharge planner; she probably knows which agencies are more reliable. The states that do have licensure requirements are Arizona, California, Connecticut, Florida, Georgia, Hawaii, Idaho (for investor-owned home care agencies only), Illinois, Indiana, Kentucky, Louisiana, Maryland (for freestanding home care agencies only), Mississippi, Montana, Nevada, New Jersey, New Mexico, New York (for voluntary home care agencies only), North Carolina, North Dakota, Oregon, Pennsylvania, Rhode Island, South Carolina, Tennessee, Texas (for freestanding home care agencies only), Utah, Virginia, and Wisconsin, as well as Puerto Rico. If your state is not listed, check with your local state congressman to learn the current status of license requirements in your state.

Arranging for home care services can be an awesome task. You seek a caring, competent, compatible, honest, and dependable home helper for your patient. The process can take considerable time and can be frustrating. Seek out the assistance of what you know to be local reputable organizations and be persistent. You will find that before long you will know quite a bit about the available home care services in your community and be able to make an informed decision about arranging care for someone you love.

The Three Pillars of Home Health Care

There are three solid pillars on which the home health care system rests: nursing and home health aides; social services; and a support network of rehabilitation therapists. These are the mainstays of the system.

NURSING—PATIENT CARE AND EDUCATION

Whether a nurse working in a home health agency or home care department of a hospital is licensed as a registered nurse or as an independent community nurse practitioner, she is responsible for determining and supervising the nursing care the individual on home health care receives. Once the nurse completes her initial evaluation, she prepares a treatment plan that assigns all the nonspecialized nursing care to other members of the home health team. In addition, the nurse regularly reevaluates the progress of the patient and updates the clinical reports and progress notes. It is also the nurse's responsibility to keep the physician in charge informed of the patient's condition and progress and to request a home visit by the physician if she feels it's necessary.

An important part of the nurse's task is educating the patient and the family in how best to achieve effective home health care. The nurse guides them and is available for consultation on all medical and health-related matters. The nurse functions as a communications link between the patient, the family, the doctor, and the other members of the health care team. Additionally, the nurse performs such tasks as inserting feeding tubes and catheters and monitoring vital signs.

In most cases the nurse works under the supervision of the physician, who is in charge of the team. However, thre is a growing trend in many states to permit nurses to diagnose and treat illnesses and prescribe certain medications without a physician's supervision. These specialized nurses, called "independent nurse practitioners" or, in some cases, "adult nurse practitioners," are highly trained and experienced nurses with strong motivation who are capable of working with minimal direct physician involvement.

All nurses are not RNs, of course. Licensed practical nurses (LPNs), as well as nurse aides, work under the supervision of the registered nurse in providing home care services. LPNs are trained nurses and are graduates of practical nursing schools. They are expected to perform many nursing services, among them care of catheters, dispensing routine medications, and taking and recording blood pressure and other vital signs. In addition, in some instances LPNs supervise the aides and orderlies who provide care requiring less skilled nursing abilities. LPNs are licensed by the state and are an integral part of the home health care team.

It's important here to distinguish between nurses who specialize in home care and those more familiar to the public through hospital visits or perhaps through TV programs that glamourize the profession. The type of facility a nurse works in and the nature of the services she (or he) provides determine her expertise. RNs and LPNs on ward duty, operating room nurses (scrub nurses, circulating nurses, nurse anesthetists), and nurses in doctors' offices all have quite different backgrounds and experience from the nurse who specializes in home health care. Nurses with experience in home care programs must be particularly creative and inventive in order to utilize the home environment, which is noninstitutional, as a setting for providing health care.

Home care nurses are trained to guide the patient to undertake as much self-care as possible, and they also train and educate family members and others on the home health team in how to assist the patient and provide for his needs. The goal of a home health care nurse is to make the patient an active participant in his own health care, as contrasted with the hospital nurse, who often prefers a passive patient who will allow the hospital staff to take care of him and thus not disrupt "hospital routine."

HOME HEALTH AIDES: VITAL HEALTH HELPERS

When assistance with personal care is needed—bathing, dressing, and other activities of daily living—then the services of a home health aide are required.

Many voluntary and proprietary home health care agencies conduct training programs for home health aides, consisting of up to sixty hours of classroom work and supervised practice. Home health aides study such subjects as working with people, infection control in the home, basic body movements, rehabilitation, measuring and recording vital signs, personal care practices, basic nutrition, and a number of special procedures that may be a vital part of the daily health care of a client.

In home health care agencies, home health aides are usually

supervised by registered nurses. Once a patient is evaluated by the supervising nurse and a treatment/care plan is created, the home health aide becomes a vital part in implementing that plan. Whether giving personal care to the client, assisting the rehabilitation therapists with the various phases of physical and occupational therapy, or measuring and charting vital signs, the home health aide becomes the dependable "doer" of the home care team.

The home health aide usually reports to the nursing supervisor, but she often also assists the other members of the home health team and follows through on their instructions for the patient. The physical therapist, for example, may expect the aide to assist the patient in exercising each day. The occupational therapist may ask the aide to "sit on your hands this week" during meals because the therapist is trying to teach the client new self-feeding techniques and wants him to practice on his own.

The energy level and attitude of the home health aide working in your home or in the home of someone you care for can be an important aspect of the total care. Because of the day-to-day contact and "front-line" role of the home health aide, there is ample opportunity for a good rapport to develop between the aide and the person being cared for at home. If it does, the health care situation is immeasurably improved.

An example of this type of rapport is when a home health aide working four hours a day, five days a week for the initial weeks that a post-stroke patient is spending at home after discharge from the hospital finds her client in bed when she arrives in the morning. Although he is able to get out of bed and use the bedside commode, he prefers to wait for her watchful assistance, as he has been doing for the past two weeks, afraid that if he takes a step with his weakened right leg he will fall.

The aide doesn't chide him about this. She knows it will happen in due time if she's patient and does her job well. She has been trained to assist the patient to sit up in bed and slip on his socks and the long leg brace that he wears on his right leg. Using a walker to steady himself, he walks to the bathroom and steps inside and sits down on the chair facing the sink and mirror.

The aide sets out his toothbrush and razor and stays nearby to offer help as needed. After the patient has brushed his teeth and shaved, he's ready for a sit-down shower. The aide helps him remove the leg brace and get into the shower. She washes the body parts that seem unreachable to him (in a few days she plans to show him how to use the long-handled sponge for this purpose), and she watches as he shuts off the water and returns to the chair in front of the sink.

Once he is towel-dried, the long leg brace is slipped on again, and the two of them return to the bedroom to dress. Dressing will take the better part of the next hour, but the occupational therapist had been adamant about "sitting on your hands" during this time. The man has to learn to dress himself.

Sitting on a sturdy chair that faces his chest of drawers, he is able to open and close drawers as needed. He selects the underwear and socks he plans to wear and the front-buttoning sport shirt and Bermuda shorts. The aide watches, not helping, but offering encouragement as he dresses. He manages to do it in record time for him, and the aide feels a sense of satisfaction in his progress.

SOCIAL SERVICES—LISTENING AND TALKING

Although a nurse may, as part of the evaluation visit, explore the life circumstances of the patient, including the extent of his insurance coverage and his emotional needs, the knowledge and resources of the social worker are of vital importance in this respect.

Social workers perform an invaluable service in their ability to "tune in" to the needs of the patient and then, through their knowledge of available resources, identify the support systems needed and arrange for their use.

The social worker is required to have a master's degree and is especially trained to be knowledgeable about the available community resources. This allows the social worker to recruit the necessary services and provide the continuity of care needed for someone making the transition from hospital to home. In a hospital setting, the social worker is often the discharge planner, working closely with the physician during a patient's hospital stay. As part of the planning for discharge from the hospital, the discharge planner meets with the family and discusses their living situation, their needs and expectations, and their plans for the future.

The discharge planner often sets the wheels in motion with a referral to the hospital's home care department or to the appropriate home care agencies in the community in which the patient lives. The social worker is the chief "gatekeeper" who can pave the way for available community services such as the Meals-on-Wheels program or Friendly Visiting Services.

A social worker will focus not only on a patient's medical and functional problems and the patient's emotional state, but also on the home environment, the financial picture, and the existing network of family members, other relatives, and friends who can be called upon to help the patient. The outcome of the social worker's efforts will often result in a plan that will not only bring into play services provided by the social worker's own institutional facility but will also identify and recruit services from other outside agencies wherever needed.

A small but growing number of social workers are in private practice. They offer a positive program of emotional support for home care patients and their families. The readjustment to a severely disabling condition, or the slow adjustment to an illness in which the patient's functioning will continue to decline, is a difficult one at best. The dialogue and support that comes from sessions with a trained medical social worker can provide the insight and perspective needed to cope with the problem.

Special group therapy sessions can also be organized by the social worker in order to bring together a number of patients with similar problems to share insights and offer moral support. Major medical centers or home health care institutions conducting research among groups of people with special problems often have a social worker on the staff to meet with and counsel individual patients or groups of patients. Groups of people who have some disease or illness in common—Parkinson's disease, ALS, Alzheimer's disease, multiple sclerosis, emphysema—often provide each other with emotional support and information on coping with health problems. By helping to create a positive approach to a problem, social workers also create an environment for better health through their actions.

The strains and stresses of home health care act on both the patient and the caregiver. Depression is not an unusual development, especially in the patient, and this depression can be followed by anger, which is often directed at the person closest at hand—the caregiver. Add to all this the deleterious effects of being confined to home for long periods of time while recuperating, the frequent loss of libido in the patient, the daily frictions that can grow out of proportion between the patient and the person providing the health care, and you have a setting ripe for emotional turmoil.

Obviously, some form of counseling should be available for those involved in close association with each other in home health care, and this is where psychological therapy comes in. This counseling is not usually done by a psychiatrist, who does his work in an office or hospital setting. The health care professional who is most often called in to deal with these problems in the home is the social worker.

This social worker is specially trained in psychological counseling. He or she can step into a tense home situation and, by getting the patient and the caregiver to talk out their problems, start them on the way to a better understanding of each other and a more harmonious relationship.

None of this is easy. The social worker will often have to work long and hard to accomplish the goal of helping the patient and the caregiver deal effectively with the stresses of home health care. Some of the time the social worker simply needs to listen and, with skillful guidance, help the two distressed people come to their own realization of the nature of their problems and how they must deal with them. Other times the social worker may have to step in and take a more active role. The techniques used will depend on the circumstances and the people involved.

There will always be a need for counseling as long as the potential for emotional difficulties exists, and this potential is inherent in the very nature of home health care.

When everything is working properly—when nurses and social workers can blend their efforts and coordinate home health care—the system can be very effective. However, since nurses, social workers, patients, and caregivers are all human beings, the ideal situation cannot always be realized. People can be overworked and tired or have serious problems, and so not be effective or as pleasant to deal with as they might be. You'll have to understand this when things do not go altogether smoothly as you try to set up home health care for someone close to you.

You'll also have to understand that, as a new caregiver, you are going to do a certain amount of floundering around. Because of the nature of the health care system, there's no quick way for you to sort things out and get effective action right away every time you try.

The system doesn't always work as well as it should. Bear with it and work with it.

The Support Network: Therapists

The home care coordinator, whether the caregiver, home health nurse, or social worker, can call upon a wide network of supporting services in the community. Chief among these services are those provided by a group of highly trained rehabilitation therapists who use a hands-on approach and other special techniques to get the patient on home care functioning as normally as possible within the limitations of his illness or disability.

The rehabilitation therapist, working toward helping the patient regain function, is one of the most important members of the home health care team. One or more of the rehabilitation therapies (physical therapy, occupational therapy, and speech therapy are the most frequently employed) can make a significant difference in the quality of life and future well-being of a patient.

While the majority of therapists continue to be hospital based, a growing number of them are affiliating with home health care agencies, as well as working on their own in private practice, accepting referrals from a number of community home care agencies and private physicians. Because the effective use of rehabilitation is a relatively recent development, many physicians trained prior to the 1970s might not be completely familiar with the services and care the rehabilitation therapists offer.

Rehabilitation centers continue to be few and far between in the United States, and while it is more common for many acute care hospitals to offer rehabilitation services on both an in-patient and out-patient basis, the use of rehabilitation therapy is not yet universal.

The progressive physician, working closely with a home health care nurse, should be able to clarify the goals and potential benefits of involving the rehabilitation therapies in the treatment of his patients.

Which rehabilitation therapy, or combination of therapies, will be most effective will depend on the nature of the patient's disability or illness and just how severe he has been limited in his ability to function in his environment. The fervent wish of the patient is, of course, to get "better" and live a "normal" life. Unfortunately, except when home health care is undertaken as a temporary measure right from the start (broken bones or other injuries that will heal in time), the individual being cared for at home may have to face the fact that home health care will be a continuing process, lasting longer than expected.

The therapists, however, will usually be fully active only at the start of the home care and until the patient can function, even in a limited way, on his own. Once the therapy has been initiated and has accomplished the desired immediate results, the individual may need to maintain himself or be maintained at home with minimal follow-up. Therapists can then be available for help when needed or on a reduced schedule.

There's a certain degree of overlap in the various therapies. Home health care is a team effort, and this is especially true where therapists are concerned. The functions of the physical therapist and occupational therapist often complement each other, and the two therapists will often consult with each other to work out a program that will best serve the needs of the patient. In the attempt to restore function and mobility to a patient, the physical therapist may note, for example, that certain devices would be helpful in the kitchen or bathroom and will discuss this with the occupational therapist. The goal of all therapists is the same: the patient's well-being and restoring function in the activities of daily living.

Let's take a closer look at how the various therapies are set up so that therapists can reach this goal.

PHYSICAL THERAPY

It was the first meeting for the two of them.

The physical therapist smiled at the woman in a robe and slippers in the wheelchair, extended her hand, and said, "Hello, Mrs. Enrico. I'm Jean Harvey, and I'm—"

"I know, I know," Martha Enrico interrupted. "The doctor told me you'd be here today." She looked down at the floor, still ignoring Jean's outstretched hand. "You really expect me to believe you'll get me out of this chair and walking again?"

"If it's possible for you to walk again, Mrs. Enrico, we'll certainly do our best to get you there."

"What do you mean *if* it's possible for me to walk again?"

Jean pulled over a straight-back chair and sat down. The two women were alone in the kitchen. Martha's husband Frank had deliberately gone out for a long walk after he had let Jean in. He had briefed Jean earlier about his wife's emotional state in a hushed and hurried phone call, and they had agreed that it would be best if the two women were alone for the first meeting.

"You've had a stroke," Jean said quietly. "Your left leg is very weak."

Martha looked away.

"I'm sure the doctor has told you the weakness in your left leg may not be permanent," Jean went on. "This sometimes happens, but the doctors can't really tell anything yet."

"So what can you do for me?"

"I can help you exercise your legs so your muscles will stay strong and in tone. We can fit your left leg with a brace, which will keep it steady, and you'll be able to walk with a cane. In time and by following through with your exercises, your leg may get strong again, and you'll be able to walk without the brace."

Jean knelt by the wheelchair and took off Martha's slipper and held her left foot, her fingers gently exploring and touching, "Can you feel me doing this?"

Martha nodded. "Just a little."

"Try moving your foot against my hand."

Martha's upper body tensed and she gripped the arms of the chair. Her face showed the strain of her effort.

"Yes, there's some movement there," Jean said. "We'll work on getting even more. It'll be slow, but I'll show you how to strengthen your muscles and we'll take measurements of just how much movement you have so you'll be able to see your progress."

Physical therapists like Jean are specially trained and licensed health practitioners who are concerned mainly with restoring function or preventing loss of function following acute illness or injury or development of a chronic disease. And as with Martha, the therapy often includes comforting and offering encouragement.

The goal in physical therapy is to help a patient achieve maximum mobility within the limitations imposed by illness or disability. Dealing with and minimizing pain is also involved. A physical therapist may use therapeutic exercise, hot or cold applications, massage, or traction as part of the treatment. Each particular injury or disability requires its own form of treatment, and the therapist is trained to deal with all of them. If, as often happens, a stroke victim has difficulty walking, the therapist will work actively with the patient to increase leg strength and, where necessary, prescribe a brace to steady a particularly wobbly leg. With an amputee, the physical therapist will concentrate on helping the patient learn to use an artificial leg, as well as on strengthening exercises designed to accommodate the new type of walking motion involved.

Much of the work of the physical therapist centers around the "ambulating capabilities" of a patient. The ability to walk and move about is vital to all of us, and, unfortunately, illness and disability frequently attack this important function. Not only is such a disabling occurrence severely limiting, it also brings on heavy emotional stress. With the possible exception of blindness or deafness, few disabilities can be more disheartening than finding yourself unable to move about. If not treated properly and promptly by the therapist, this can lead to a loss of will in the patient to fight the disability.

It's for this reason that the physical therapist very quickly assesses the patient's ability to get around in his own home. If there are stairs in the house, the therapist will evaluate the patient's safety in attempting to maneuver up or down the stairs. If managing the stairs is not possible on the therapist's initial visit but can be considered a reasonable goal, the therapist will work with the patient during subsequent visits in order to accomplish it.

Strength and flexibility are another concern of the physical therapist. If a patient becomes discouraged and lapses into depression, making little effort to walk about although clearly able to do so, the unused body muscles will start to weaken. The physical therapist now has the additional task of emphasizing the critical importance of maintaining flexibility so as to prevent loss of range of motion in someone who is already weakened and disabled.

The therapist does not work alone. There are physical therapy assistants, mostly in hospital settings, and additional help can come from the family of the patient and the home health aide, if available. The therapist instructs the family in how to help the patient exercise and follow the program set up by the therapist. In Martha Enrico's case, Jean, the therapist, enlisted the help of Martha's husband, Frank. He was not only the natural choice for the hands-on work needed in helping Martha with her exercises, but his involvement helped bring the couple closer and alleviated Martha's fears that her husband wouldn't want to touch her because she was disabled.

Restoration of muscle function is only part of the benefit physical therapists bring to their patients. When someone has been badly burned, for instance, a physical therapist will supervise the whirlpool treatments designed to help the burn victim regain good motion in the injured parts.

Physical therapists are licensed by the state in which they operate. They must have a detailed working knowledge of human anatomy and physiology and be able to apply this knowledge for the benefit of the patient. In accomplishing their goals, physical therapists often use as a basic working guide the example of normal development in an infant. A newborn child slowly develops strength and muscle coordination and flexibility by constant repetition of various movements until these movements become automatic. A baby reaching for a toy in a crib will learn through repetitive efforts how to extend his arm, grasp the object with his fingers, hold it, bring the object closer, and of course try to put it in his mouth and chew it. After a period of time, the child's reaching and grasping movements are automatic and skillfully executed. The program the physical therapist sets up for the patient has this same goal of automatic, skillful, and positive movements.

OCCUPATIONAL THERAPY

Many people still believe that an occupational therapist is concerned solely with providing vocational training for the patient—basket weaving or ceramics being the most popular activities. Perhaps this may have been true at some time in the past—and there's nothing wrong with basket weaving or ceramics as forms of therapy—but occupational therapists today focus on improving and maintaining the quality of life of the individuals in their care. Occupational therapists are wizards at finding the most efficient way for a disabled patient to accomplish the activities of daily living.

When an occupational therapist enters a patient's home for the first time, she performs a thorough evaluation of the setting in which the patient will have to function. Home may be a comfortable place for most of us, but it can be a difficult environment for the newly disabled.

The therapist will first take note of any barriers or other obstacles that might in any way inhibit the patient's functioning. The therapist will notice the number of steps the patient has to mount or descend when entering or leaving the house. If the patient is in a wheelchair, it will be important to note whether the outside door is accessible and can be opened and closed by the patient from the wheelchair. If access through the front is not possible, an attached garage or a ramp constructed at the back door can sometimes be used to allow the wheelchair patient to come and go independently.

If necessary, the occupational therapist will consult with the physical therapist in order to evaluate the patient's ability to use the outside stairs when a wheelchair is not a factor but the patient does have limited mobility. Inside the house, the occupational therapist will observe the placement and arrangement of the furniture and suggest any rearrangement that might make it easier and safer for the patient to move about the rooms and function as normally as possible.

Where the patient sleeps is of particular interest to the therapist. Is it in the patient's own room, or is it in the living or dining room, which has now been furnished with a hospital bed delivered before the patient was discharged from the hospital? Unless there is no other alternative, the family's living quarters should not be converted into a substitute hospital room for the returning patient. The patient on home health care should sleep in his own room and use the same bathroom as before—as long as this is feasible and within his functional ability.

Since the occupational therapist is mainly concerned with the patient's quality of life, the therapist will seek to help the patient become as independent as possible. The therapist can judge whether the individual is capable of taking care of all his personal needs, such as dressing, washing, shaving, using the bathroom, preparing food, and eating independently. If so, the occupational therapist will urge the patient to continue these tasks on his own and not ask for, or come to depend on, the assistance of other members of the family. If some or all of these tasks seem too difficult to accomplish at the moment, the occupational therapist will work with the patient to devise methods and techniques to overcome any difficulties. Ingenuity often comes into play here.

One therapist had an elderly man as a patient on home health care. Crippling arthritis had taken away much of the man's ability to move around. Nevertheless, he still managed to care for himself in his small apartment, using special devices to feed, dress, and bathe himself. He had no family but did have many old friends, some of whom were neighbors. He didn't lack for help, and the occasional visits of the therapists were sufficient to help him keep going on his own.

His one pride and joy had always been his full head of white, wavy hair. Despite the pain, he would shampoo his hair daily, blow-dry it, and comb it out in the bathroom. Since he couldn't stand on his feet for long periods of time, he had a folding chair in the bathroom and a small mirror suspended above the sink from the bottom of the medicine cabinet. After each shampoo, he sat in the chair and blow-dried his hair. Since the hair dryer was too heavy and awkward for him to hold, the occupational therapist devised a simple rack and clamping device that held the dryer at the proper height and angle, and the old man would turn on the dryer and move his head about in the stream of warm air. It was painful, but the pleasure he derived from his hair was worth it to him. After the hair was dry, he would face the mirror under the sink and carefully comb his hair until it waved and set exactly as he wanted it. He had always been conscious of his appearance, and he had no intention of slacking off at this stage of his life, arthritic or not. He thrived on the compliments friends and strangers alike paid him at the sight of his gleaming white hair, full and wavy and the envy of many a younger man, to say nothing of some of the women.

The occupational therapist had worked with her client to fulfill the main goal of the therapy: allowing the man to function as normally as possible in the activities of daily living. To this man, caring for his hair was one of the important activities of his daily life. Despite his disability, he was able to continue with it.

Once the activities of daily living are evaluated and the therapist has identified goals for the patient, she will work to keep the patient active and interested enough to make optimum use of the therapist's plan. Occupational therapy does not end with getting the patient to perform his own personal care. There have to be other goals and activities beyond this to involve the interest of the patient. Otherwise, the quality of life will surely suffer and diminish.

Through counseling sessions and discussions with the patient and family members or friends, the occupational therapist is often able to identify a hobby that had been put aside or a new activity that might be attempted. Watching television is, of course, one of the favorite pastimes of the disabled, but it should by no means be the only activity available. Often, the therapist's gentle encouragement can bring about renewed interest in outside events and activities.

An important role of the occupational therapist is to instruct the caregiver in how to be an observer instead of a doer in aiding the disabled person to attain independence. Tasks are not necessarily learned rapidly but usually by constant repetition. The therapist understands that sometimes the caregiver will find it easier to step in and help the disabled person accomplish a task. It's more important for the patient's well-being if he performs the task by himself, though no matter how many times he has to try it. The occupational therapist can show the caregiver when it's best just to "sit on your hands" and let the disabled person work things out for himself.

The caregiver has to ask himself what he would be willing to do in the future. If, at the moment, he wants to help the disabled person to, say, put on a shirt, is the caregiver willing to do this all the time? The individual has to learn how to help himself, and the less the caregiver interferes, the better.

If some activity is important to the self-image of the disabled person (such as the man who wanted to be able to shampoo and comb his own hair), then no matter how trivial it may seem, the person should be encouraged in that activity.

The creed of the occupational therapist can best be summed up by this statement from an experienced professional: "The occupational therapist works on the assumption of *ability* rather than disability."

SPEECH THERAPY

The speech pathologist held up the sheet of clear plexiglass and showed it to the patient seated in front of him. "This is an eye-link board, Mr. Castle," the pathologist said. "It will allow us to communicate."

Mr. Castle stared at the board, then at the pathologist. Only his eyes moved. He had been striken with ALS (amyotrophic lateral sclerosis, a disease that causes loss of motor control) and had now lost the ability to move or speak. His spirit was still strong, though, and the pathologist knew this.

"You'll notice, Mr. Castle," the pathologist said, "that there are letters of the alphabet and the numbers one through ten, arranged in a circle on the plexiglass. "I'm going to hold this board up in front of me so it's between the two of us. We can look through it and see each other as well as the letters and numbers. What I want you to do, Mr. Castle, is to select a word or phrase you want to communicate to me and look steadily at the first letter of the word. I'll move the board around as I look at each of the letters in turn and at you at the same time. You keep your eyes on the particular letter you want to communicate to me. When the letter is directly between us and both of us are looking at it at the same time, our eyes will link and I will know this is the letter you selected. If you're ready now, let's get started."

After a few moments of maneuvering and sighting through the plexiglass board, the pathologist announced, "Got it. The first letter is H." He knew from the way Mr. Castle blinked that it was correct. "Now for the next letter, Mr. Castle."

It went slowly, but finally the pathologist smiled as he repeated the message: Hi there.

"Hi, yourself, Mr. Castle," the pathologist said.

Mr. Castle gave him a satisfied wink.

Speech involves basic communication. People who have problems with speech because of accidental injury or neurological disease often must resort to what is called "augmentative communication," which involved devices and techniques that can be used to replace normal speech. The speech therapist, more commonly known as a speech pathologist or speech-language pathologist, teaches the patient how to use augmentative communication.

Speech therapists work closely with people who have lost the ability to communicate, usually because of neurological disease or accident. Stroke victims often lose the ability to articulate their thoughts. They just can't get the words out. They are cut off from their families and others, and the effect can be devastating. The isolation experienced by stroke victims in this respect is terrifying to them.

Following a stroke, there is often a period of "return" in which the patient does regain some of the expressive and receptive language functions. A well-trained speech pathologist can, at this point, identify the areas in which the patient still retains some communicative ability—reading, speaking, writing, or understanding the spoken word—and the therapist then works with the patient to maximize the use of this remaining ability.

Patients with Parkinson's disease can lose the ability to produce enough volume in their voice to allow effective speech. The speech therapist may suggest an amplifier that can be carried or even attached to the patient, and this simple device can make a world of difference.

Another difficulty Parkinson's patients encounter is pacing their speech. The words tumble out too rapidly. In this situation, the speech therapist can provide a "pacer board," a simple device with spots (hills, valley, and bumps) on the board that the patient can touch as he speaks. In this way, the patient monitors the pace of his speech, using the board-touching technique to help ingrain a slower rhythm of speech.

New techniques and devices are constantly being explored, and the professional speech pathologist has many resources at his command to aid the patient. Because the focus of activity of the speech is communication, he may find himself at times functioning as a translator for the patient. His ability to do this for a stroke patient can be significant in helping the patient interact with his family and acknowledge his frustrations and express his needs. The speech pathologist, because of his expertise and his objective perspective, often helps the family and friends of a stroke victim to adjust to the changed method of communication the patient must now employ.

RESPIRATORY THERAPY

Respiratory therapists, sometimes know as inhalation therapy specialists, are called upon to treat patients with various respiratory problems. These can range from emphysema or chronic asthma to severe respiratory emergencies that arise because of heart failure or stroke. The therapist is knowledgeable about the equipment and the techniques used to help his patients and works under the supervision of a physician.

In a hospital setting, the respiratory therapist may be ordered by the pulmonary specialist or the attending physician to do "postural drainage" treatments on patients who are recovering from open heart surgery. The therapist will position the patient and guide him through "breathing and coughing" exercises in order to keep the airways clear and prevent the development of pneumonia. In some instances, the respiratory therapist is called upon to assist patients with chronic obstructive pulmonary disease to take their medications, often administered with the help of a device called an inhaler. In this way the medication can be delivered deep into the airways as a fine spray, increasing its effectiveness in opening the airways.

In addition, respiratory therapists are usually familiar with the wide variety of breathing aids so important to patients with asthma or emphysema. Oxygen, oxygen concentrators, humidifiers, and air purifiers are complex pieces of equipment that must be used correctly and cleaned and maintained regularly.

One of the peculiarities of the insurance reimbursement system of Medicare is that it does not cover home visits by respiratory therapists. Although coverage for the other therapists can often be provided when there is a referral order signed by a physician, respiratory therapy requires the presence of a physician on the home visit to qualify for coverage.

Coverage does exist for the respiratory equipment and for the oxygen. Most reputable respiratory supply companies have a credentialed therapist on their staff who will provide the initial training as the equipment is delivered. In addition, a number of respiratory supply companies have therapists on staff who conduct regular follow-up visits. When home respiratory assistance is needed, the respiratory therapy service under the supervision of a pulmonary specialist will write up the evaluation of the initial and subsequent visits. The evaluation will include complete information on the respiratory vital signs, the medications administered, and the equipment that is to be used. If this evaluation is made during a hospital visit, the patient or his family will usually be given a referral card with complete information and instructions. The proper equipment can then be leased, rented, or in some instances purchased at a respiratory supply dealer. The therapist in the hospital or your physician will usually be able to give you the names of a number of reputable suppliers in your area who operate the mandatory twenty-four-hour, seven-day-a-week service for respiratory care. Be sure to ask about insurance coverage when you arrange for home respiratory therapy. Once the patient is at home, the referral card can be given to the respiratory therapist accompanying the delivery of the equipment and supplies. The therapist can record the information on the card, sign it, and return it to the hospital or to the patient's physician, thereby assuring the proper continuity of care confirming that the requested equipment is being used.

NUTRITIONAL THERAPY

People unable to tolerate regular food can be well fed at home. Special formulas and solutions can now be prepared for home delivery to patients who, in the past, would have had to remain in the hospital in order to obtain the needed nutrients. These people are not eating in the normal manner but being fed liquid solutions and formulas through tubes. Depending on the method of administration, these tubes may connect to some part of the gastrointestinal tract, allowing for a mode of feeding called enteral nutrition. The other form of feeding—parenteral nutrition—sends the nutrient solutions directly into the bloodstream through the main vein of the body.

Nutritionists provide counseling to patients with illnesses requiring special nutritional therapy and education. Diabetes educators, for example, spend much time counseling patients. They may do a nutritional profile, requiring the patient to list every morsel of food eaten over a specified period of time. Glucose levels and activity levels, as well as insulin use, will also be monitored and the data correlated and compared with the nutritional profile. Special meal plans and diets can then be customized to meet the personal tastes and nutritional needs of the patient.

Because nutritionists seem to come from a variety of different backgrounds, it is best to consult your doctor, the hospital home care department, or a certified home health care agency if you wish to locate a trained professional nutritionist in your area. The letters "R.D." do indicate that the person is a registered dietician, but you will need to explore that person's experience further to make sure her experience and background apply to your particular needs.

The Doctor's Role

You've been prepared for the possibility, but now it's finally happened. Home health care has now become a present necessity. How do you and the doctor work together?

First, you and the doctor sit down and talk it over. Assuming that someone close to you needs home health care and that his doctor has been the one taking care of him, you, as the caregiver, will have to work with the doctor and the patient to determine what type of care will be needed. The doctor will be in charge of the health care team. Nurses, therapists, home health aides, or other health professionals will ultimately be responsible to the doctor for the care provided. As is true in most cases, a nurse will be the one to supervise the health care team. She will be the liaison with the doctor, keeping him informed of the progress of the patient and suggesting when it might be necessary for the doctor to see the patient, either at home or in the doctor's office.

Although the doctor will be in charge and will periodically review all that has been done, you as the caregiver will have your work cut out for you. You will have to set up the house or apartment as required for the patient. You will have to see to it that the bedroom, the bathroom, and the kitchen are all accessible, safe, and convenient. You will have to coordinate with the social worker, the therapists, the aides— anyone and everyone who becomes part of your home care team.

At the core of all this home health care, however, will be the doctor. He may not be seen as often as he would be in acute illness or emergency, since long-term home health care often involves an individual who has more or less stabilized or whose health care does not require the frequent presence of a physician. But on those occasions where the doctor has to be seen or consulted, the dividends of a solidly based health care partnership will start to pay off. Let's put the home health care scene in proper perspective:

Without a caring caregiver, it won't work.

Without good health professionals, it won't work.

Without the physician-partner, it won't work.

The Rest of the Home Care Team

Home care doesn't end with the services of physicians, nurses, therapists, and the other professionals previously described. There's a range of other services available in the health care system, and they should not be overlooked in obtaining home health care.

THE HOMEMAKER / HOUSEKEEPER

Consider these three examples:

Sylvia and Sam had lived as husband and wife for forty-eight years. Until Sam retired a few years ago, the care and maintenance of their home had been Sylvia's domain. She would have it no other way. After his retirement, Sylvia would call on Sam to drive her to the supermarket to wait as she shopped. Or she would often ask him to help with the cleaning chores in their house. He was happy to do it. Sadly, over time, Sylvia became more and more forgetful. Now, instead of just driving her to the supermarket, Sam had to come inside with his wife to help her remember to check the grocery list she had made. Also, instead of offering a helping hand around the house, Sam noticed that the management and cleaning of the house now rested on his shoulders. Sylvia's memory was unreliable, and she needed his continuous attention. Sam needed help to care for his wife and their home.

Ella lived alone in a one-room flat in South Miami Beach. Her daughter lived thirty miles away. Once a week, the daughter shopped and filled Ella's refrigerator with food. As the years passed, the food shopping visits were extended so the daughter could attend to minor housekeeping chores. Ella's arthritis was getting worse, and her hearing loss was a complicating factor. As she became more and more hard of hearing, it became almost impossible for the daughter to talk to her and check up on her by telephone. The weekly visits now became twice weekly, then almost daily, in order for the daughter to be sure Ella was eating the food that had been left for her. Before long, Ella's daughter found her life and plans revolving around the needs of her mother.

Fred's parkinsonism seemed well controlled by the medication he was taking. Although he lived alone, his apartment was in an area in which he had many friends, among them Mary and her husband Dave. Mary often invited Fred to join them for dinner or for an evening out to hear their favorite symphony orchestra. At first, Mary found that Fred needed help knotting his tie. She was only too happy to do it for him. Even Dave sometimes needed help, and he didn't have Parkinson's disease. In time, however, Mary and Dave found that they had to arrive at Fred's fifteen to twenty minutes early to help him with the buttons on his shirt and with tying his shoes. It was only when Fred, with great embarrassment, asked Dave to help him zip the fly on his pants that they realized Fred's illness was having a profoundly disabling effect on him—and help was needed.

In none of these situations was there an acute or raging illness. In each case, the day-by-day or month-by-month changes in health and independence had an increasingly involving effect on family and friends. Then, one day, the dramatic difference in health and independence was noticed. The people involved realized that unless some kind of help or assistance could be found, they would become increasingly locked in to caring for their friend, relative, or spouse. All at once, the burden became overwhelming, too demanding on their own time and independence. Yet each of them knew that without their help (or someone's help) the one being cared for would end up in a "home."

The kind of help that would make a significant difference in the lives of all the people involved would be to find someone to help out in the home. Homemakers and housekeepers can shop, cook, straighten the house, and be that extra pair of eyes and ears that are so necessary when someone is being cared for and needs assistance.

Although homemakers perform a vital service, insurance carriers often exclude this type of maintenance care. Many insurance companies, as well as Medicare, will not provide coverage for home health care unless part-time intermittent skilled nursing care is required—and certified by a doctor. In the examples just given, none of the three—Sylvia, Ella, or Fred—needed nursing care. But they did need assistance.

In most cases, the homemaker/housekeeper's primary responsibility is maintaining the home environment. Dusting, cleaning floors and rugs, washing dishes, cleaning bathrooms, and doing the laundry all can be part of a homemaker's job. Shopping and food preparation also may be needed. Sometimes, when a taxi or car service or public transportation is scarce, the homemaker may drive her employer or "client" to the doctor's office or even to attend recreational events.

Even when there are other home health care people involved in providing the care, it is the homemaker (or the home health aide, see p. 64) who will spend the most time in the home. She is often the first to notice changes in the health or emotional status of the person being cared for at home.

When you hire a homemaker to assist in maintaining the living environment of someone you love, be sure to define and describe the duties and tasks to be performed. Also, set up a reporting system to keep you informed of any changes in condition or behavior.

Part-time homemakers can be found through the services of a proprietary home health agency in your community. Check the Yellow Pages under "Home Care" or check the Appendix under "Home Care Agencies."

Agencies screen, supervise, and bond their employees. They will review your insurance coverage to determine whether or not you have coverage for a homemaker. If you don't, they can send in a homemaker for a few hours each day for as many days during the week as needed. Rates for homemakers can be six to seven dollars an hour, and some agencies have a four-hour minimum.

You may try hiring your own homemaker through a regular employment agency or by advertising in a newspaper. If you do, be sure to check references and previous work experience.

If you live near a college and have room in your home, you might try putting a notice on some of the bulletin boards at the college, offering room and board in exchange for a certain number of hours of household help per week. Once again, be sure to check references and previous work experience or any background in health work.

DAY CARE CENTERS

Fortunately, home care services are not necessarily restricted to one's own home. Each of us needs to get out, to interact with other people, and simply to socialize. For the patient who is able to travel the day care center will be a welcome change from the home environment. Many hospitals, social service organizations, churches, and Ys have organized day care programs. Some operate on a full-day basis, providing a respite for the caregiver and an alternative means for the patient to receive care during the daytime hours.

Full-day day care centers may provide a comprehensive range of services Monday through Friday thereby eliminating the need for a full-time companion if other members of the household are at work or are unavailable. Many of the hospital-based or institutional-based day care programs can offer meals, transportation, counseling, rehabilitation therapies, recreation, and socialization programs. Other programs may offer more limited services on a two or three times a week basis.

When checking into the availability of day care centers in your area, be sure to contact your local office on aging, as well as the organizations concerned with your patient's particular disease or health condition. Special programs may be available for patients with Alzheimer's disease, Parkinson's disease, or other neurological problems. Check the listing of state adult day care associations in the Appendix and contact your states day care association.

In some instances you will need to provide transportation or pay privately for car service or an ambulette. The social worker at the institution in which day care services are offered can be of great help in sorting out costs for these services. Many of these programs are part of a comprehensive home care program that provides for the cost of day care. More frequently, however, the fees for day care will need to be paid privately. For the families of patients with Alzheimer's disease, the respite from caring for a possibly very demanding and debilitating patient even for brief periods each day can be well worth the cost.

MEALS-ON-WHEELS

Meals-on-wheels delivers food to the person over sixty in need. Many organizations operate meals-on-wheels programs and deliver a hot meal each day, which can be crucial to an individual without the full-time assistance of a housekeeper. Funds for meals-on-wheels programs are provided by various sections of the Older Americans Act passed in 1965 and by other local fund-raising sources as well. A wide variety of voluntary and civic organizations (family service agencies, neighborhood associations, and women's clubs) sponsor meals-on-wheels programs. Some hospital auxiliaries, church groups, and even nonprofit agencies such as Visiting Nurse Association also sponsor programs. The meals are usually simple but nutritious, and the charge to the patient for the service is usually nominal. Your referral network can be used to identify the meals-on-wheels program in your area. In some areas the program operates seven days a week. In others, five meals a week are delivered. Consult the White Pages under "Meals-on-Wheels" or check with your local office on aging.

GROUP MEALS

In some communities where there are a large number of elderly people, group meal programs have been organized. These programs can assure that at least one hot nutritious meal is offered each day, in a group setting. Group meal programs may be a part of a community day care program or they may operate independently. The social benefits (as well as the nutritional benefits) are significant for the participants in group meal programs. The group meal gives the individual the incentive to leave the house and interact with others. Often the group meal will be far more nutritious than food bought and prepared to be eaten alone at home. Like meals-on-wheels programs, group meals programs may be federally funded and/or paid for by local fund-raising resources. Once again the charge to patients participating in established group meal programs is usually nominal.

TRANSPORTATION

Few patients on home health care are actually homebound or confined to their home. They may not be able to get around as easily as they used to, but they usually would be able to enjoy the emotional lift that comes with "going out"—if the services needed to transport them from point A to point B are recruited. Unfortunately for most people, the costs for transportation services usually are not covered by Medicare or other insurance. (Medicaid does reimburse for transportation costs to and from the doctor.) Local volunteer groups may provide transportation services. Of course, taxi services, car services, and ambulette services can be hired. It may prove to be cost effective for a few neighbors to plan appointments and excursions together. In some communities, volunteer van services are offered by local church groups, women's auxiliaries, and other community agencies. Finding local resources that provide transportation will take a good deal of networking. Ask the local office on aging, the discharge planner at your community hospital, and the social workers connected with any of the health care programs in which your patient participates. One notable exception to the rule in New York City, Cancer Care reimburses for the cost of transportation to and from chemotherapy treatments. Individual programs for cancer or other health conditions may well exist. Persistence here may provide great dividends in mobility.

3

Insurance! Insurance! Insurance!

SUPPOSE a good friend came to you and asked for advice on how to go about buying a new car—which make and model to choose, what options to add, how much to pay, how to negotiate with the dealer, and so on. In all probability, you'd tell your friend to proceed with care. After all, a car represents a major purchase and the more informed you are about what's available and what kind of quality you can obtain, the more certain you'll be of getting your money's worth. As for car insurance, you'd certainly tell your friend to begin by determining the kind of coverage most suited to his needs. Then, after that, he would have to begin the search for a reliable insurance company offering the desired coverage at the most affordable rates.

How about a house? This is an even larger purchase than a car. For most people, a house represents the most expensive item they will ever buy, and it may well be a one-time purchase to last a lifetime. Your advice to your friend would be to move even more carefully this time. Check the prevailing market thoroughly. Know in advance just what kind of a house you want and what kind of compromises you're prepared to make. Plan for the future. Will there be enough rooms for a growing family? Will extensive renovation be required? Hire an expert to inspect the house. Get a termite check. Hire a good real estate lawyer. Make sure a title check is performed. The list of things you'd advise your friend to investigate would be long and detailed. Insurance for the new home would require just as much diligence. Your friend would have to be certain there was sufficient coverage in his homeowner's insurance to take care of any foreseeable problems.

This is all common-sense advice, and in view of this it seems rather ironic that far too many of us don't give as much consideration to our health insurance coverage. There's an old saying that the only things we can be sure of are death and taxes. Add to this list one more item— health care. The longer we live, the more likely we are to need some kind of health care as we get older. The financial impact of a long-term illness coupled with inadequate insurance coverage can be disastrous and can involve many times the cost of even the most well-researched major purchase.

The time to research health care coverage is *before* it's needed. Unfortunately, too many people find out what is and isn't covered by their health insurance policy in a moment of crisis, and by then it's usually too late to do much about it. It's far too easy for many of us to accept the hospital and medical insurance provided by our employers or labor unions and assume that this is all we need, especially if the company or the union is paying all or most of the premium. We neglect to ask questions about the specifics of the policies or to find out whether we have options that could add to the coverage being offered to us.

There can be no excuse for not being as knowledgeable as possible about so vital a matter as health care insurance. All of us need it, and you can't just go out and purchase it and then sit back and forget about it. Health care insurance is a growing and changing aspect of our society and has its greatest effect on our lives when illness or accident or other health crises suddenly strike.

Health care insurance has changed considerably over the years and is still changing. If the coverage was purchased five, ten, or fifteen years ago and if it hasn't been reviewed and updated periodically, it will undoubtedly contain many outdated exclusions and lack important types of coverage current policies now offer. According to the Health Insurance Association of America, commercial health insurance policies written prior to 1970 did not provide coverage for home health care, whereas today approximately 40 percent of such policies include some form of home health care benefits. Prior to 1979, less than half of the Blue Cross plans covered home health services. Today, virtually all basic Blue Cross plans offer some home health care benefits.

The key word here is "some." There are still so many exclusions, limitations, requirements, and exceptions that it's almost impossible to sort things out on a first reading of the contract or policy. To help you become more knowledgeable about insurance coverage, as well as the availability of other forms of financial assistance for home health care, we'll start with a review of some basics about health care insurance and then go on to examine the major home health care insurance carriers and the coverage they offer—or do not offer. Most of all, you need to know what questions to ask, whom to ask, and how best to go about making sure you get the answers you need.

Health Insurance Guidelines

Fred S., a thirty-five-year-old executive, was suddenly stricken at his desk with severe pains in his lower abdomen. He called his doctor from the office and described the pain and was told by the doctor to go immediately to the emergency room of the local hospital. Fred wasted no time in following his doctor's instructions.

At the emergency room Fred filled out the appropriate forms, showed his health insurance identification card, and was then examined by the resident doctor on duty. Fred's doctor had called ahead to alert the resident about the possibility of acute appendicitis. Once the diagnosis had been confirmed, Fred was admitted to the hospital for emergency surgery.

In a few days, Fred was ready to go home. As he went with his wife to the cashier's office, he already had in his hand the bill from the anesthesiologist. Fred had been somewhat surprised to find it in an envelope on his bedside table the day after his operation. Fred was even more surprised when the cashier informed him the anesthesiologist's bill had to be paid in full before leaving the hospital, along with charges for telephone service and the rental of a television set in Fred's room. Fred started to explain that the services of an anesthesiologist were covered by his health insurance policy, but the cashier smiled and explained that since the anesthesiologist was on the hospital staff, it was hospital policy that his bill be paid at the time of discharge. On receipt of Fred's check, the cashier would give him a receipt and a completed insurance form, which Fred could send to his insurance carrier for reimbursement directly to himself. Since the cashier's tone seemed to imply that it was preferable that Fred wait for reimbursement rather than the anesthesiologist, Fred decided not to argue the point and made out the check and went home.

While the hospitalization itself had been uneventful, the period afer his hospital stay provided quite an education for Fred on the subject of health care insurance. That education had really started with the anesthesiologist's bill at the hospital and now continued at home.

A flurry of bills arrived. First came the bills for the use of the emergency room and the lab tests that had been performed in the outpatient department. Next, his personal physician's bill arrived. A few days later, the hospital bill came in the mail with a detailed itemization of the charges for the medication Fred had received and the lab tests and other services that had been provided to him during his short hospital stay. The hospital bill had been efficiently divided into two sections, one titled "Covered by Insurance" and the other designated "You Pay." It was comforting to Fred to find out that he owed the hospital only a nominal sum since his health care insurance policy covered just about all the charges for the hospital room and the meals he had eaten and most of the drugs and other medication he had received. However, the other bills represented a tidy sum of money, and Fred quickly discovered that, as with the anesthesiologist's bill, he was expected to pay in full.

Fred paid the bills and sent along with each a copy of his insurance company's claims form to be filled out by the physician or the lab that had supplied the service, requesting in a covering letter that the claims form be filled out and mailed to the insurance company. Only Fred's personal physician honored this request. The others returned the claims forms without having filled them out. Instead, a multiple-form receipt for Fred's payment was enclosed, one copy of which Fred was to keep and the other sent to the insurance company.

On the back of each multiple-form receipt, in almost indentical language (although the receipts and the forms were set up for different types of medical services) was the notation that the fee for medical services rendered was considered as being charged to Fred, the patient, and not to the insurance company. Fred was to fill out his portion of the insurance claims form and attach one copy of the multiple form, which would be sufficient to validate the claim. The doctor's signature would not be required on the claim form itself. Moreover, if Fred required additional paperwork, the doctor's office would have to charge extra.

All this was a real eye-opener to Fred, who had never been hospitalized before. He had always thought that checking in and out of a hospital with his insurance identification card would be almost like using his American Express card when staying at a hotel. It would be merely a matter of showing his card and signing the bill.

While the additional costs and the inconvenience did not have too great an impact on Fred or his life style, it did cause him to think about health care insurance. He carefully examined not only his own policy but also that of his parents, who were active people living on a fixed income and for whom an unexpected hospitalization could be a catastrophic experience.

As Fred delved deeper into his research on health care insurance, he soon discovered that most basic health insurance was divided into two main categories of coverage—hospitalization and surgical-medical. The hospitalization portion of a policy basically covers the cost of a hospital stay for varying periods of time and for varying levels of service. The cost of the hospital room, meals, laboratory tests, X-rays, staff nursing care, medications, and other charges associated with the hospital stay are generally included in the coverage. A fixed number of days are usually paid for in full, although some policies will pay a percentage of the bill (usually 80 percent), while others will pay a specified amount for each day of hospitalization. In most cases, private duty nurses, private rooms, television rental, and telephone charges are not covered and must be paid by the patient.

The surgical-medical portion of the policy generally covers physician's fees, therapist's fees, and charges for other services by medical professionals. Although hospital-based care is the focus of the surgical-medical coverage, some policies include a certain amount for out-patient visits to the doctor and even some home health care. Individual policies vary, and the only way to be sure of coverage is by carefully reading the policy and questioning the insurance carrier on any unclear points.

While some doctors will file for and accept direct payment from the insurance company, many more request that patients pay their fees directly to them and then file a claim for reimbursement from the insurance carrier. The actual amount paid toward doctors' fees and medical procedures varies with each company. Some insurance carriers pay an established fee for a particular medical specialty or service in a given geographical area. This is known as the "prevailing charge." Other carriers will pay charges only up to a predetermined maximum for a given service.

Most health insurance policies include a number of exclusions, offering no coverage at all for certain medical procedures or denying coverage until a specified waiting period has elapsed. Although this may seem unfair in some cases, from a purely business point of view the exclusions are necessary to protect the insurance carrier from losing excessive amounts of money or even going bankrupt. For example, except for health maintenance organizations (HMOs) where a yearly fee provides for most medical needs, routine medical checkups are excluded from coverage in most policies. Insurance carriers fear that if they provide coverage for routine medical checkups, far too many clients will avail themselves of this "free" service. No insurance carrier could afford to pay the fees for such examinations for all of its clients. Also, basic home health care in general and certain specific home care services or supplies in particular are excluded from coverage in many policies for the same reason. The insurance carriers, in general, have to concentrate on providing coverage for unexpected illnesses or accidents or injuries that usually require serious medical attention and possible hospitalization.

Many health care insurance policies exclude coverage of any preexisting health conditions entirely, or for a specified waiting period. The waiting periods vary and can be as long as a year. This means, in the language used by many insurance carriers, that a person will not be covered for any medical condition for which advice or treatment from a physician was received during the specified period of time prior to taking out the policy.

Major medical policies, another form of health insurance, are designed to cover serious medical problems or catastrophic illnesses, which can pile up expenses in the five- or six-figure range. Most such policies have a deductible—up to $1,000 or more—and a waiting period before the policy can go into effect. The amount of the deductible must first be paid by the client, and then the major medical policy takes over. The type of coverage, the length of coverage, and the lifetime maximum limits on payments can vary considerably. Many major medical policies reimburse 80 percent of the costs for hosptial charges, medical fees, prescribed drugs, medical devices, and rehabilitation services.

Clearly, all health insurance policies are not created equal. Therefore, when reviewing coverage, or when considering a new policy, it is imperative that you itemize the coverage the policy includes and, equally as important, what it does not include.

It would be very helpful in this respect to set up a hypothetical situation, an illness or disease that requires treatment or hospitalization, and evaluate the policy under consideration by identifying what medical services would or would not be covered in such a situation. This could be very revealing. If any questions should arise, you could then discuss them with the company benefits manager or the insurance agent, or with any qualified professional. Anticipating what might happen is the best way to prepare for it.

One of the most important guidelines to keep in mind when investigating home health insurance is: "Don't assume." Do not ever assume the policy provides a certain type of coverage. Check it out and make sure. First, read the policy—not the brochure describing the policy or any other such literature put out by the insurance carrier. Read the policy itself. Brochures, advertisements, and descriptive literature are not what will determine coverage. Only the actual policy can do this.

When you've made as much sense as you can out of reading the policy, get on the phone and call the insurance company itself. Even if it's a long-distance call, it pays to make the initial contact by phone. Insurance carriers are understandably reluctant to be fully responsive to questions posed in a letter. You might have better luck with a direct one-to-one phone contact.

Have your questions ready in advance. Get the name of the person you're talking to (ask for it to be spelled if necessary), and write down the answers you receive to your questions. If the answers are not complete or are not fully responsive to your questions, call again and try someone else. Be persistent. Don't assume anything. Don't even assume that you've been given the correct answers. Write a confirming letter to the person you spoke to. State your understanding of the conversation and request that, if your understanding of the answer is in error, you receive a reply by return mail clearing up the matter. You may not get full satisfaction in the reply (it's possible you may not even get a reply), but you will at least have on record the name of the person you spoke to and your letter requesting confirmation or clarification of the telephone conversation. Make sure you keep a clear copy of your letter (a photocopy would be best) so it can be reproduced and sent out again, if necessary.

If all this sounds somewhat paranoid to you, don't be misled. It's not a matter of the patient and the insurance carrier being natural adversaries or of the insurance carrier deliberately trying to keep the patient from getting what he is entitled to. Rather it's a matter of leaving nothing to chance, of making sure there is a clear understanding of the purchased coverage. Your complaint or your query will receive much more respectful consideration if you can show that you are knowledgeable in this area and that you've done your homework.

Is Home Health Care Covered?

Unfortunately, the wording of health insurance policies often isn't very clear on this. Even if you request clarification, you may find that any answer you receive is hedged with so many qualifications and restrictions that it is extremely difficult to determine what kind of home health care, if any, is covered. Since the life situation and the health and medical needs of each individual are unique, the determination of type and length of any home helath care benefits provided in the policy will often depend on an item-by-item review of the policy with the insurance carrier. It's a complex matter, and you have to proceed with care.

Coverage for home health care services frequently hinges on whether the care ordered by the physician includes specific tasks that must be performed by various health professionals and is often specified in terms of "visits." A visit usually consists of one session or treatment by a home health care professional. If two professional services are required on the same day (the services of a nurse and a physical therapist, for example), this would be counted as two visits by the insurance carrier. It would also be considered two visits if the nurse had to return on the same day to change a dressing or perform any other nursing function.

The careful recording of visits is important because home health care benefits often have a limitation placed on the number of visits that can be covered under the policy or contract. Blue Cross indicates that it will provide reimbursement for up to 200 home health visits per year for a subscriber. However, this benefit applies only if the home health agency supplying the services has an agreement with the Blue Cross plan and if the subscriber (patient) has been hospitalized within a specified period of time prior to the start of home health care.

Blue Cross of Greater New York indicates that when home health care is provided by an agency that does not have an agreement with the Blue Cross plan, or if the subscriber has not been recently hospitalized, reimbursement will be made only for a maximum of forty home health care visits per year at 75 percent of the "reasonable charges"— after the subscriber has paid a fifty-dollar deductible. In addition, a nursing evaluation of the patient is required, and part-time skilled nursing care or physical therapy must have been ordered by a physician before the plan will provide reimbursement for the additional services of a part-time home health aide.

As has been stressed before, your responsibility as the subscriber or as the caregiver of a subscriber on home health care is to examine each policy in depth and ask pertinent questions until you know exactly what will be covered under certain circumstances and what will not be covered. Unless you are thorough in this policy examination and evaluation, you may inadvertently lose out on coverage that should be available, or you may find it necessary to pay charges for services that you mistakenly thought were covered by the policy.

Remember: *Don't assume!*

Medicare

Statistics show that most of the people requiring home health care are elderly, and since almost all of them are entitled to Social Security benefits after age sixty-five, the health coverage provided by Medicare is of major concern to individuals involved in home health care. It has been estimated that about 40 percent of all hospital bills are paid for through Medicare, which gives some idea of the extent to which Medicare has pervaded the health insurance scene in this country.

Medicare is a federal health *insurance* program (not a *welfare* program) that has been in existence since 1965. Part A of Medicare covers hospital insurance; part B covers medical insurance. Tables 5–8 give the essential details of Medicare coverage. You can use these tables for background information to supplement our discussion of how you can obtain home health care coverage under Medicare.

Table 7 indicates that benefits under part A of Medicare are available for a total of 150 days; however, you should be aware that the last 60 days in this total represent what is known as a "lifetime reserve." There is no limit to the number of 90-day benefit periods you can use. Once you are out of the hospital or skilled nursing facility for 60 days, a new benefit period will start all over again. However, if you are unfortunate enough to be hospitalized beyond 90 consecutive days, you then draw on the reserve of 60 additional days, which is available as a one-

Table 5 ■ MEDICARE COVERAGE PART A[a]: HOSPITAL AND SKILLED NURSING FACILITY SERVICES AND HOME HEALTH CARE

Covered in full	Not covered
Semiprivate room and board	Doctors' fees[e]
General nursing care	Private duty nurses
Operating and recovery room[b]	Private room (unless medically
Intensive care unit[b]	necessary)
Lab tests	Television, radio, telephone
X-rays	First three pints of blood
Drugs and medication	
Anesthesia	
Medical supplies	
Rehabilitation services[c]	
Home health care[d]	

[a] Part A coverage applies only to Medicare-approved hospitalization or confinement to an approved skilled nursing facility.

[b] Operating room, recovery room, and intensive care units are not covered in a skilled nursing facility.

[c] Rehabilitation services include physical therapy, occupational therapy, and speech pathology.

[d] See page 97 for qualifying conditions.

[e] Doctors' fees are covered under Part B of Medicare.

Table 6 ■ MEDICARE COVERAGE PART B:[a] MEDICAL EXPENSES

Covered expenses[b]	Not covered
Doctors' and surgeons' fees	Routine physical examinations
Medical services	Dental care or dentures
Medical supplies	Hearing aids
Diagnostic tests	Examinations for eyeglasses
Physical therapy	Eyeglasses
Occupational therapy	Cosmetic surgery
Speech therapy	Routine foot care
Ambulance service[b]	Routine immunizations
Home health care[d]	

[a] Part B pays 80 percent of the approved charges for specified procedures and services (see Table 7). All services must be Medicare-approved.

Part B of Medicare is optional. At the time you are eligible for Medicare Part A, you are given the option of selecting Part B, for which a quarterly fee is charged.

[b] Both in-patient and out-patient services are covered.

[c] Ambulance service must be medically necessary.

[d] See page 97 for qualifying conditions

Table 7 ▪ PAYMENT SCHEDULE FOR MEDICARE PART A[a]

Benefit period[b]	Medicare pays	You pay
HOSPITAL[c]		
Days 1–60	All costs above first $356	$356
Days 61–90	All costs above $89 a day	$89 a day
Days 91–150	All costs above $178 a day	$178 a day
Beyond 150 days	Nothing	All costs
SKILLED NURSING FACILITY[c]		
Days 1–20	All costs up to approved amount	Nothing
Days 21–100	All costs above $44.50 a day	$44.50 a day
Beyond 100 days	Nothing	All costs
HOME HEALTH CARE		
Unlimited as medically necessary	Full cost	Nothing

[a] All services must be provided in Medicare-approved facilities.

[b] A benefit period begins on your first day in the hospital and ends after you have been out of the hospital or skilled nursing facility for sixty consecutive days. A new benefit period starts after the sixtieth day.

[c] Hospital and skilled nursing facility costs are for 1984. These costs are subject to change every year.

To obtain skilled nursing care benefits, you must have been hospitalized for at least three days and have entered the skilled nursing facility within thirty days after discharge from the hospital.

time benefit and is not renewable.

The deductible amount mentioned in Table 8 is renewable each year and is subject to change. At the beginning of each calendar year, a new deductible has to be paid before benefit payments can start. Remember, this is for part B of Medicare, which covers medical expenses not incurred as part of the charges for your stay in a hospital or skilled nursing care facility, as outlined in Tables 5 and 7.

After the deductible is paid, Part B of Medicare will pay 80 percent of the approved amount of the covered medical expenses. The phrase "approved amount" means that Medicare regulations determine what are reasonable charges for all covered medical expenses, including physicians' and surgeons' fees, medical services and supplies, as well

Table 8 ▪ PAYMENT SCHEDULE FOR MEDICARE PART B

Medical expense[a]	Benefit	Medicare pays	You pay
Doctors' and surgeons' fees, medical services, medical supplies, diagnostic tests, physical therapy, occupational therapy, speech therapy, ambulance service	Medicare pays for medical services in or out of the hospital	80% of the approved amount	A one-time $75 deductible,[b] then 20% of the balance of the approved amount
Home health care	Unlimited as medically necessary	Full cost	Nothing

[a] If the doctor or the supplier of medical services "accepts assignment," this means the Medicare-approved amount will be accepted as the full amount of the fee. In that case, you pay only the 20 percent balance.

  If assignment is not accepted, you will have to pay the difference between the total charges and the amount Medicare pays.

[b] The $75 deductible is for 1984.

as the other items listed in Table 8. The reasonable charge is calculated by taking into consideration the usual charges for these particular medical services by the doctors and suppliers in the patient's geographical area. The patient is responsible for 20 percent of these charges; Medicare pays the other 80 percent.

If, for example, a surgeon charges $1,500 for an operation and Medicare considers the reasonable charge for this operation to be $1,000, Medicare will indicate that the approved amount is $1,000 and will pay 80 percent of that amount, or $800. If the surgeon has accepted assignment from Medicare, then the patient will owe the surgeon $200, the difference between the approved and accepted fee of $1,000 and the $800 that Medicare has paid. On the other hand, if the surgeon has not accepted assignment, the balance of $700 (the difference between the surgeon's original fee of $1,500 and the $800 that Medicare will pay) will have to be paid by the patient to the surgeon.

In some cases, the surgeon (or any other physician) will agree to accept assignment and will tell the patient that he will also accept Medicare's 80 percent payment as payment in full. In that case, using the example given above, the surgeon would accept the $800 Medicare payment and the patient would owe nothing.

All of this applies equally to all the medical services in Table 8, whether the charges are surgeon's fees, therapists' fees, laboratory charges, or consultants' fees. It's important, therefore, that you determine in advance whether your doctor, medical supplier, or health care professional will accept assignment and what payment arrangement he wishes to make with you.

The reimbursement from Medicare will go either to the patient or to the doctor or supplier, depending on the arrangements made with these individuals. If they have been paid in full at the time of the service, then they so indicate on the Medicare form and the reimbursement check comes directly to the patient. If they haven't been paid, this is also indicated on the form. Medicare pays them the 80 percent reimbursement and notifies the patient of the amount paid, and the patient then knows the balance owed to the doctor or supplier. In either event, Medicare sends the patient a separate form indicating the amount of the original charge, the amount approved by Medicare, the amount of the reimbursement check, and to whom it has been paid. Thus, the patient will always have a complete record of medical expenses and proof of payment.

Part of the medical expenses, after hospitalization or care in a skilled nursing facility, may involve charges for care in a nursing home. It's important to distinguish between the medical services and health care provided by a skilled nursing facility and a nursing home. In a brochure published by the Department of Health and Human Services, "Guide to Health Insurance for People with Medicare," the distinction is made as follows:

A skilled nursing facility is a special kind of facility which primarily furnishes skilled nursing and rehabilitation services. It may be a separate facility or a part of a hospital. Medicare benefits are payable only if the skilled nursing facility is certified by Medicare. Most nursing homes in the United States are not skilled nursing facilities and many skilled nursing facilities are not certified by Medicare.

Medicare Part A will not cover your stay in a skilled nursing facility if the services you receive are mainly personal care or custodial services, such as help in walking, getting in and out of bed, eating, dressing, bathing and taking medicine.

As you can see, this pretty accurately describes the kind of care received in a nursing home—and Medicare will not pay for this. As stated in another part of the same brochure: "Medicare and private insurance will pay for most nursing home care. You pay for custodial care and most care in a nursing home."

Hospitalization or care in a skilled nursing facility or nursing home obviously is not home health care. However, treatment and care in these institutions is quite frequently the necessary prelude to home health care, and it's for this reason that I've gone into some detail about the Medicare coverage of the services offered by these facilities. The more you know of the expenses and procedures involved in health care, the better able you'll be to set up a good home health care program.

Medicare does cover home health care. However, as with private insurance companies, the Medicare literature is a bit evasive when describing its home health care coverage. In the same brochure, "Guide to Health Insurance for People with Medicare," a chart indicates that Medicare will pay the full cost of home health care and that the extent of this benefit is "unlimited as medically necessary." It's really not explained, though, that this benefit is a qualified one.

Certain requirements have to be met before the benefit can be obtained. In "Your Medicare Handbook," published by the same government department, the reader is told:

Medicare can pay for home health visits only if *all* of the following four conditions are met: (1) the care you need includes part-time skilled nursing care, physical therapy, or speech therapy, (2) you are confined to your home, (3) a doctor determines you need home health care and sets up a home health plan for you, (4) the home health agency providing services is participating in Medicare.

By way of explanation, the booklet states: "Medicare can pay for covered home health visits furnished by a participating home health agency." A home health agency is defined as "a public or private agency that specializes in giving skilled nursing services and other therapeutic services, such as physical therapy, in your home."

It's only when you combine the information from these two sources that you get a clearer picture of the requirements for home health care coverage by Medicare.

Once the four conditions cited above have been met, either Medicare hospital insurance (Part A) or medical insurance (Part B—if this optional service has been selected) will pay for an unlimited number of home health visits. When there is no longer a need for part-time skilled nursing care, physical therapy, or speech therapy, Medicare will continue to pay for home health care visits by an occupational therapist, if needed.

We now come to another catch. One of the four requirements for eligibility for home health care under Medicare is that the patient is homebound—confined to his home. What constitutes being homebound, however, is not at all clear in the Medicare regulations. According to a recent government report, the patient must have a "normal inability" to leave home and that if he did attempt to leave it would involve a "considerable and taxing effort." On the other hand, if the patient is confined to home because of "feebleness and insecurity brought on by advanced age," he is not considered sufficiently homebound to meet the elegibility requirements for home health care.

The regulations do permit the patient to leave his home if the occasions are "infrequent" and of "relatively short duration," especially if he is going out "for the purpose of receiving medical treatment." There are many more distinctions and qualifications in the regulations, but this should suffice to give you a good idea of what you have to contend with.

Medicare does not cover general household services, meal preparation, shopping, assistance in bathing or dressing, or other home care services furnished mainly to assist people in meeting personal, family, or domestic needs. Also, Medicare will not cover full-time nursing care given to the patient at home. Such nursing care, according to Medicare, must be provided in the "proper" institutional setting—a hospital or a skilled nursing facility.

While most of us would consider all of these items an integral part of home health care, necessary to maintaining the quality of life at home, Medicare regulations dictate otherwise.

Making up the Difference

Since Medicare does not pay in full for medical services received, many people decide to supplement their Medicare coverage with private health insurance. One thing to bear in mind right from the start is that word "private." Health insurance that supplements the coverage provided by Medicare is not sold, sponsored, or serviced by the government. Deceptive advertisements or insurance agents' sales pitches to the contrary, the government provides only Medicare coverage, not any supplemental insurance to close the gaps.

It's in the effort to close these gaps that people turn to private insurance carriers. All of the precautions mentioned earlier about checking policies and not assuming anything apply equally when investigating health insurance designed to supplement Medicare coverage.

A good way to keep track of the various policies and what they offer is to use the tables giving the essential details of Medicare coverage (Tables 5 through 8). Next to each item in these tables, place a check mark if the supplemental policy you're investigating supplies coverage for the item and, if so, what the cost is. Be especially thorough in finding out if the policy in question provides coverage for those services not covered by Medicare. In this way, a complete checklist can be constructed for each supplemental insurance policy being considered.

The following is a brief guide to the different types of private health care insurance coverage available. Some of them will fill the Medicare gaps, and some won't.

Medicare Supplement Insurance • Generally, this type of insurance policy will cover only the Medicare deductibles and the additional 20 percent costs the patient has to pay. Some of these policies may provide coverage for services not covered by Medicare. Check each one out carefully.

Major Medical Insurance • This type of insurance is designed to assist in paying for medical services and supplies when catastrophic illness strikes. After a large deductible requirement has been met, the policy pays a certain portion (usually 80 percent) of the expenses up to a specified amount. Since the coverage is for "major" medical expenses, the upper limits of the coverage can be quite high, sometimes in six figures.

Group Insurance • This is insurance coverage provided by an employer or by an organization (professional or fraternal associations, for example) who, because of the large numbers of subscribers involved, can obtain lower group rates for various forms of insurance coverage. This insurance can include benefits for hospitalization, surgical-medical, major medical, and dental coverage, as well as the services of optometrists and chiropractors.

Group contracts vary both in benefits provided and availability. The main thing to determine here—after checking out the coverage— is the matter of convertibility. After employment is terminated (hopefully for well-earned retirement) or after the person leaves the association, will he be able to convert his health care policies to an individual direct payment policy of equivalent coverage? Check this point carefully and thoroughly. Some employers have union contracts that require the company to pay the premiums for the health care insurance for retired employees and their spouses for the rest of their lives. Recently, however, such contracts have been terminated under special circumstances, which once again points up the warning: *Don't assume!*

Health Maintenance Organizations (HMOs) • This is a special type of coverage in which a person joins a HMO for a set fee, in return for which the organization provides the subscriber with specific health and medical services from physicians and suppliers affiliated with the HMO. Since the services are prepaid, there is no need to file a claim for reimbursement each time a covered medical service is used. The subscriber cannot select his own personal physicians or suppliers under this type of arrangement, but many people are pleased to have the convenience of prepaid health and medical services. As of February, 1985, qualified HMO's can accept Medicare and will be reimbursed by the government.

Medicaid—When There Is No Money

As has been mentioned in our discussions of how to obtain financial assistance in paying medical bills and other expenses associated with home health care, the patient or the caregiver almost always has to pay some money. Modern medical technology and the multitude of medical services and facilities available today take their toll financially. Of course, a good private health insurance policy, or the government-sponsored Medicare program, absorbs the major portion of the tremendous expenses that can arise from even a short hospital stay. Nevertheless, these insurance contracts do not pay everything in full, and the subscriber usually has to bear a part of the cost.

But what about those people who cannot afford even a small portion of the cost? What do they do?

That's where Medicaid comes in.

Medicaid is a joint federal–state welfare program that pays for health care for what has been estimated at over 22 million people who are too poor to pay even part of their own health care expenses, many of whom are elderly and disabled. Government figures for 1981 show that of the total Medicaid expenditures, 37 percent were for the aged, 30 percent for blind and disabled people, 28 percent for aid to families with dependent children, and the remaining 5 percent for other types of need.

As is to be expected, there are stringent financial requirements for Medicaid eligibility. The person applying for Medicaid was to be able to prove need and cannot have income or assets of sufficient worth to put him above the predetermined level. Medicaid does not work in conjunction with Medicare and does not have separate coverages for hospital and medical expenses. Medicaid coverage includes all necessary services.

The requirements vary among the states, and regulations change frequently. It's very important that you check all regulations carefully with a social worker or case worker with the local Social Security office, or with any source of professional help and guidance you can find, for example, a home health agency or a hospital discharge planner.

THE LAW—RULES AND REGULATIONS AND WAIVERS

As you must have realized by now, there are so many laws and rules and regulations, both federal and state, that it's almost impossible to keep up with them. One thing to keep in mind when Medicaid is concerned is that various states can request waivers—specific exceptions—to the Medicaid regulations. These waivers will allow the states to offer more services than are provided for by Medicaid. The more waivers a state requests, and the more of them that are approved, the more health care services, supplies, and resources that state can provide for its people on Medicaid.

As of December, 1984, 213 requests for waivers had been received from forty-six states (Arizona, Arkansas, Alaska, and Wyoming had not submitted any requests). Of the requests submitted, 130 had been approved, 41 were pending, 19 had been withdrawn, and 23 had been disapproved. These figures are constantly changing, of course, but this will give you an indication of the efforts the various states are making to provide health care services where they are most needed.

Getting Your Money's Worth

Making sure that all the home health care benefits and services provided by government and private sources are taken advantage of require virtually a continuing effort on the part of patient and caregiver. The following items are guidelines to use when encountering problems or attempting to evaluate health care insurance policies:

1) Do not accept at face value the benefits as described in a brochure about home health care policy coverage. Only the policy itself can provide a reliable description of the coverage provided.

2) Home health care coverage should be provided for as long as is necessary to achieve the goal outlined in the physician's health care plan.

3) Maintenance care, custodial care, and long-term care for the chronically ill usually are not covered.

4) The level of coverage will depend on the home health agency providing the care and its relationship with the insurance carrier. Medicare and Medicaid coverage is available only at certified agencies. Be sure to check with the home health agency to determine its status with the funding source.

5) Even though an illness or medical condition may be initially covered by an insurance carrier, the coverage may be terminated if, in the opinion of the carrier, it is no longer justified. For example, if the patient has reached a plateau and it's clear that continuing home care will be mostly maintenance or custodial, the carrier may decide to end the home health care benefit.

6) Be sure to submit bills for reimbursement promptly and often. If reimbursement checks suddenly stop arriving, get on the telephone

and contact the carrier to determine the reason.

7) Keep in mind that premiums for health care insurance are tax deductible above a certain percentage (now 5 percent). Also, if the caregiver provides over half the support of the one receiving the care (and this includes room and board), then the cared-for person can be claimed as a dependent by the caregiver. The separate income, if any, of the one being cared for has to be taken into consideration before the caregiver can claim dependency. Check the current tax regulations carefully on these points.

8) The subscriber has the right to appeal a refusal of claim from either the insurance carrier or Medicare. With Medicare, a review of the claim can be requested. The local Social Security office can help with filing the request. If the Medicare claim is for $100 or more, a formal hearing can be requested. For Medicare cases that involve claims of $1,000 or more, the matter can eventually be appealed to a federal court.

9) There are many excellent booklets and other materials on Medicare and Medicaid (many of them put out by the government) that are available at the library, bookstore, or the local Social Security office. Since the regulations are constantly changing, it's a good idea to consult these sources and keep up to date on what kind of coverage is available for home health care.

4

Preparing for Home Care

THE SOCIAL WORKER left the old woman's bedside and stepped out into the hospital corridor. The doctor was leaning against the wall, filling out the patient's chart.

"About three more days," he said in answer to the social worker's unspoken question. "Mrs. Eagleton should be ready for transfer to the nursing home." He closed the cover of the chart holder. "She can't stay by herself anymore. We can't send her home. This last stroke did it for her."

"How long will she need constant care?" the social worker asked.

"Indefinitely. You sure she has no family?"

"None. She's lived alone for many years, and she's always been an emotionally frail and fearful person. She's lucky we were able to place her."

The doctor nodded. The social worker made some notes in her folder. They walked together down the corridor while in the room Mrs. Eagleton stared at the ceiling and, despite her sedated condition, wondered what her life would be like in a nursing home.

It would have been nice if Mrs. Eagleton could have gone home after her hospital stay, despite her stroke, but she clearly was not someone for whom home health care would have been feasible. Generally, only a patient who doesn't require constant medical and nursing supervision—and who has a home to go back to—can benefit from being cared for at home.

Other factors have to be considered, of course, and medical and social work professionals have to evaluate all pertinent conditions when deciding whether or not to recommend home health care for a patient about to be discharged. Many questions have to be answered.

The Patient

The first consideration when evaluating the feasibility of home health care has to be the patient herself. Who is this person? What was she like before the onset of illness? What kind of life did she lead? Was she an independent person? What kind of family life did she have? These questions, and similar ones, help the health professionals determine the parameters of the patient, the essential characteristics that give an insight into the person herself.

The next step is to consider the disease or the illness or injury that brought on the necessity for home health care. In Mrs. Eagleton's case, her stroke made it impossible for a woman with her life and family characteristics to manage home health care, even with some assistance.

On the other hand, a woman like Janet R.—forty-three years old, divorced, with one child, a son now grown up and living on his own half a continent away from his mother and able to visit her only infrequently—presents a different picture.

Janet had always been independent, resourceful, and an active person who enjoyed life and had many friends. She had recovered well from her operation for stomach cancer, but the doctors could give her no guarantee about the future. Moreover, she would continue to need health care for a long period of time, perhaps always, and it was evident that she couldn't possibly return to her physically taxing job as an international fashion consultant. Constant air travel was definitely out of the question. Nevertheless, Janet was full of plans for setting up some kind of business for herself at home while she was cared for by a nurse and a part-time housekeeper. She had some savings and disability insurance she could fall back on, and she hoped her home-based business would provide for the rest of her needs. She had her moments of apprehension about the future, but she was determined to make it on her own at home.

Janet did not present a difficult case for the doctors and the hospital discharge planning team evaluating her potential for home health care. She was an ideal candidate.

Willard H. represents the other side of the coin. A diabetic in his mid-forties, Willard had cataracts in both eyes and had ignored his doctor's advice to have them removed until he could barely see. Then, frightened at the thought of going blind, Willard had finally consented to a cataract removal on his right eye.

The removal of the cataract disclosed extensive diabetic retinopathy—hemorrhaging of small blood vessels in the retina of the eye—caused by the diabetes. The ophthalmologist had warned Willard of this possibility, explaining that just as Willard could not see out of the eye because of the cloudy cataract, the doctor could not see into the eye for a thorough examination of the retina until the cataract had been removed.

The ophthalmologist wasted no time. Willard found himself back at the hospital, this time as an out-patient, undergoing laser surgery on his right eye to stop the hemorrhaging. The doctor was blunt. It would be some time before they would know if the laser treatment had been successful in sealing off the leaking blood vessels in Willard's eye, and there was no way to determine at the moment just how much vision Willard would retain in the eye. Moreover, another cataract operation on the left eye was imperative, since the retinopathy might be progressing unseen there.

Willard, unfortunately, was not the kind of person who could deal with such a situation. Discouragement and depression had been part of his life style for many years, and now, when he needed inner strength and resources to help see him through the crisis, he had nothing to fall back on. He became even more depressed and apathetic, certain that he would soon be completely blind—and then die from the ravages of diabetes.

In evaluating Willard's adaptability to home health care, the staff professionals took into consideration the fact that Willard was married and that his wife worked part-time and could arrange her work schedule to be home with him when she would be most needed. They had no children, and Willard was on short-term disability from his company, drawing two-thirds of his pay, which was not too great a financial hardship on them.

It would seem, on the surface, that Willard had a good chance of benefiting from home health care. But then, when his attitude and his mental state were evaluated, it became clear there was much work to be done. Willard's depressed emotional state would seriously hamper any efforts to provide effective home health care.

A program was set up with the main emphasis on psychological therapy. Intensive counseling, along with a medical regimen to control his diabetes and an occupational therapist to help him cope with his limited vision, eventually brought Willard out of his depressed state sufficiently to enable him to participate more actively in his own home health care.

Current Home and Health Situation

In evaluating the patient's current health status and his home situation, many questions have to be answered. Does this person live alone or with others? Are any of these people willing and able to be of assistance following discharge from the hospital? Are the wishes of the patient realistic?

A review of the home life situation will reveal whether or not assistance is available. Shopping, cooking, cleaning, and other daily activities may require some assistance. Ideally, this kind of help should come from an able person living in the same household.

Prime consideration has to be given to the health problem itself, its duration and prognosis, and the patient's current and projected ability to function on his own. Often, older people have more than one health problem. For example, a person who, unlike Willard, had been successfully managing his diabetes—taking insulin and watching his diet for years—might suffer an unexpected stroke. A new factor will have entered the picture, and the patient's continuance in a home health care program would have to be reevaluated.

Discussing the answers to numerous questions about the health problems with all concerned—and especially with the patient—will help determine the level of self-care attainable and the frequency and type of assistance that may be required. Methods for determining answers to the necessary questions will vary with the individuals and the health professionals involved. Personal contact and one-to-one interviews are generally very effective.

Questionnaires A and B and the functional profile pages 108 and 109 give you some idea of the type of information required when considering the feasibility of home health care. You can use these as a guide in reaching your own decision on how to proceed if you are facing the need to provide health care at home for another individual.

Questionnarie A covers items concerning the person requiring the care, and Questionnaire B covers the health problem itself. As you'll note, the questions are not exhaustive. They are intended here only as guides and as a representation of evaluation techniques employed by health professionals.

The same is true of the functional profile. (See p. 108.) Use of such a profile (some refer to it as a functional inventory) can serve as an objective tool to assist both the patient and the caregiver in identifying patient capabilities and in specifying needs that may arise during continued living at home. It will help you in examining the total picture in order to identify what's needed and to arrange for the required assistance.

In using these tools (the questionnaires and functional profile), do not expect to be able to intepret all the answers yourself. As mentioned, these are merely guides to prepare you for the type of questions health care professionals seek to answer. Obviously, a professional evaluation will be required, for example, before the need for any of the

QUESTIONNAIRE A: THE PERSON

Is the patient aware of the nature and extent of her health problem?

Has she indicated what her goals are in relation to her health problem?

Are these realistic goals?

Does she see herself as a dependent or independent person?

Does she wish to live in her own home?

Is she alert?

Does she have friends and neighbors with whom she had had frequent contact and with whom she has socialized?

Is she able to manage her own affairs?

Does she have a realistic concept of what her needs will be?

Will she be able to direct others in obtaining the assistance she requires?

Is her memory good?

Will she be able to follow written instructions?

QUESTIONNAIRE B: THE HEALTH PROBLEM

What is the health problem?

Is there more than one illness or disease involved?

What is the physician's evaluation and prognosis?

What improvement can be expected in coming weeks?

Will the patient's condition remain essentially the same once it has stabilized?

How can any further loss of function be prevented?

What rehabilitation therapies or training are appropriate?

> Physical therapy?
> Occupational therapy?
> Speech therapy?
> Psychological support?
> Respiratory therapy?
> Nutritional therapy?
> Recreational therapy?
> Other?

What are the possible benefits of each course of treatment?

What medications have been prescribed?

What is the purpose of each medication?

What are the possible side effects?

What is the schedule for taking the medication?

rehabilitation therapies (Questionnaire B) can be determined. But if you are aware that this question is being considered, and if you have attempted some evaluation of it yourself, you will be better prepared to understand the determination made by the health professional.

As you'll note, the functional profile concerns itself mainly with the mobility, flexibility, and capabilities of the patient. Use this profile in conjunction with the "Tips for the Tasks of Daily Living" (see Chapter 5) to point the way for overcoming many of the difficulties that might afflict the patient.

A positive attitude will be helpful in analyzing the results of the questionnaires and the functional profile. Focus on what the patient *can* rather than cannot do. Whatever problems may be indicated by the answers you put down can be dealt with by taking things one step at a time. Break the problem down into smaller parts and deal with each part separately. By analyzing and, where possible, resolving the individual parts of the problem, you will be able to deal effectively with the problem as a whole.

Functional Profile: Determining How Much Care Is Needed

	Functional ability		
Type of activity	Normal	Minimal impairment	Needs help
Vision (with or without glasses) Hearing (with or without hearing aid) Able to speak and communicate Breathing ability Heart function			
Use of dominant hand (right or left) Use of dominant arm (right or left) Use of other hand Use of other arm			
Use of right foot Use of right leg Use of left foot Use of left leg Walking Moving about safely (with or without special equipment)			

Functional ability

Type of activity	Normal	Minimal impairment	Needs help
General coordination Getting around the house Going up and down stairs Going outside Using house keys Getting out of bed			
Getting up from a chair Getting to the bathroom Using the bedside commode Using the toilet Bowel control Shopping			
Carrying things Preparing meals Eating and feeding self Washing Shaving Brushing teeth			
Selecting clothes Dressing self Grooming self Cleaning house Doing laundry Using telephone			
Taking medications as pre- scribed Handling money Handling public transportation Driving Using car or taxi service			

There are no "scores" or "passing grades" for this functional profile. It is primarily a guide for the health professional to use in evaluating the patient's functional ability.

The Fourth World

The phrase "fourth world" has been used to describe the life and environment of patients and relatives of patients with severe chronic illness. It's an apt description since it emphasizes the fact that illness—whether chronic or short-term—can suddenly transport any of us into a separate world far different from the one we have previously known. The adjustments that have to be made can be, and often are, frightening and traumatic.

When illness strikes, medical knowledge—represented by the physician and the art and science of medicine at his command—can be brought into play to combat the forces of disease and injury. Treatment can be initiated and carried out (see Part IV, The "The Gamut of Health Problems"). Beyond this, however, we enter the "fourth world" either as the patient or as the caregiver.

THE DEEPER ROLE OF THE CAREGIVER

None of us goes through life alone. True, some individuals are extremely reclusive, but for the vast majority of people life has no meaning unless there is daily contact with other human beings. Our first contacts, of course, are with our parents and other family members. As we grow older, the contacts expand to include friends, other relatives, schoolmates, colleagues in the workplace, and assorted friends, lovers, and enemies.

Of all of these, however, very few can lay claim to being the special caregiver in our life. He or she is a confidant, a friend, a comforter in time of need, an advisor, someone with whom we can share our innermost thoughts and our doubts and fears. Above all, this is someone we trust. This person is a significant force in our life.

Almost all of us have someone like this we can turn to—a wife or husband, brother or sister, lifelong friend or newly discovered companion. In good times and in good health, this person adds meaning to the joys and tribulations of daily living. And should we become sick or disabled, the need for the closeness and help of this special caregiving person becomes vital.

However, in the final analysis, each of us must make our own decisions as to what we really want and need and what is best for us. No one, not even the caregiver, can reach as deeply into our inner beings as we can ourselves. The caregiver can be there, however, to help clarify our thinking, to offer guidance, and to be supportive in reaching important decisions.

This is especially true in time of illness or injury, with resultant disability. Unless we have been reduced to a state where we can neither think nor reason, we have to control our own life and chart its course—with help, if necessary. This is where the caregiver comes in.

It's a unique role the caregiver must play—undertaking the responsibility for the shelter, caring and daily necessities of someone who is ill and disabled. And for those of us who someday will have to fill this role, or who now suddenly have it thrust upon them, it's important to know what's required of us.

BECOMING A CAREGIVER

It's happened to you. Someone close to you has had to turn to you for help in time of illness. You are needed. You are the caregiver. What can you do? The first thing is to define the role to yourself.

As a caregiver, you will become a manager, a consultant, and a collaborator. You will:

- obtain as much information as possible about the illness that has stricken the person who now needs your care so that you can provide knowledgeable care;
- realize the immediate emotional and physical and medical needs of the patient and how these needs might change in the future;
- evaluate as best you can how the patient will deal with the situation;
- assess your role as the caregiver so as to foster maximum independence in the patient;
- get the patient himself actively involved in the health care decisions that have to be made;
- recruit the support of others (family, friends, and medical and health professionals) to provide for the needs of the patient;
- take care of *yourself* so you'll continue to be able to provide the care that the patient needs.

It's obvious that you can't provide really good care if you're completely ignorant of the disease or illness that has stricken the person who will be in your care at home. Naturally you cannot be expected to delve deeply into the medical aspects of the problem, but you should make yourself as knowledgeable as possible about the illness or disease by consulting with the family physician, by reading available material in the library, and by contacting organizations concerned with the particular medical problem (arthritis, diabetes, or cancer, for example). Acquiring this knowledge should be an ongoing process for you. The more you learn and keep on learning, the better you'll be able to look after the needs of the one in your care.

Even though the cared-for individual may be very close to you, it's important to strive for a fresh and objective approach in evaluating not only how this person will deal with the situation but also what his immediate needs will be. Sit down and think things out calmly. Be aware that the patient's very closeness to you and the attachment you have to him may color your judgment and blind you to what has to be done.

It's also important to realize that the needs of the patient will probably change as time goes by. As far as changing medical needs are concerned, the physician will handle different medications or treatments. Other needs, especially emotional needs, will be up to you to handle. Your best way of dealing with this is by talking to the patient and, most important, listening to what he has to say. You'll then be able to provide for these needs and, in addition, allow the patient to maintain his independence.

None of us wants to lose control of our own life, and this becomes increasingly important to someone who has to depend on others for care. As the caregiver, you will have to be constantly aware of this aspect of your relationship with the cared-for individual. In attempting to help and provide care, it's easy to fall into the trap of doing too much, of taking over too completely the life of the sick or disabled person. This denies the patient his right and his need to feel in control of himself.

There's a real danger here of creating a passive patient, someone who becomes completely dependent upon you and the care you are providing. If this happens, the task will become even more difficult, and real harm can be done to the patient. By creating such a passive and fully care-dependent patient, you will initiate and perpetuate a cycle of unnatural dependency for both of you—unless or until one of three things happens.

First, the patient may awaken to what has been going on and then successfully wrest back control of his own life and thus restore his sense of self-esteem. This may not happen if the patient lacks motivation and the spirit to bring about a change because, over a period of time, he had been conditioned by you to feel so nurtured and cared for that change would not be desirable.

Second, the patient may die as passively as you have had him live, leaving a legacy of intermingled anger, reproach, relief, and guilt for you to contend with the rest of your life.

Finally, what may happen is that at some point you, as the caregiver, will realize that your role should be that of manager, not martyr, perhaps as a result of your own physical and mental exhaustion due to the way you have approached your responsibilities. Or illness may strike you also and make you realize you can't carry the responsibility all by yourself.

The task of providing home health care has to be shared by you, the patient, the health professionals and therapists, and concerned family and friends. Most of all, you must listen to the patient and what he has to tell you about his needs and desires. Then the next step is to get the support of others, mostly family and friends. And you must listen, also, to the advice of the professionals you call in—the physicians and specialists, the therapists, the nurses, and others. They have a vast collective reservoir of knowledge and experience on which to draw.

In short, it's a team effort, with the cared-for individual taking an active part in what is being done for him. This is the proven way to provide effective home health care.

Dealing with Stress

Preparing yourself for the role of caregiver for someone close to you requires that you get ready to deal with the stress that can be a part of everyday life in home health care.

When illness, injury, or accident places an individual in the position of requiring health care at home, this is decidedly a stress-producing situation.

First, the realization that a person's health has been affected to the extent that home care is required is a disruptive and traumatic experience. Next, the need for the individual to be cared for at home requires an adjustment in life style for both the caregiver and the patient, as well as for other family members and friends who may also be involved. The normal, everyday routine of daily living has been disrupted and changed, and in some cases will remain changed indefinitely. New worries and concerns have to be dealt with. Doctors, nurses, therapists, social workers, pharmacists—all the members of the home health care team—have now become a part of daily life. Attitudes will have to change. Plans for the future may have to be altered, perhaps even canceled. Roles may be completely switched around—in many cases the former breadwinner and major financial provider of the family has suddenly been relegated to a status of dependency on others.

Additionally, since the onset of chronic illness or disability often involves an aged parent or other relative moving in with the family, the potential for family tensions to develop and grow is inescapable. An elderly father, for example, sick and needing health care, is brought into his son's home. The son is no longer a child but a middle-aged man with a wife and with children of his own. At first, everyone tries to get along. They're all family. There's a bond here, a relationship formed in common roots and special memories. But then, gradually, strains in the relationship start to develop. Perhaps the old father still likes to smoke cigars, and the smell begins to permeate the house. Or he might criticize the behavior of the youngsters in the house and instruct them in what they should or should not do. He becomes very free with his advice and admonitions, much to the annoyance of all involved. Or his health could start to deteriorate badly, and the family would then have to contend with one crisis after the other, rushing him to the hospital, waiting agonizingly for the doctor's report on his condition, then bringing him home again, knowing that the pattern might soon be repeated.

Result? Stress—and often lots of it.

Guilt can be a part of the stress engendered in home health care. Both the caregiver and the patient can experience guilt and its resultant stress. The patient can feel guilty for having been the one to precipitate all this trouble by getting sick in the first place. The caregiver, in turn, can feel guilty for not being as good a caregiver as he or she would like to be.

Guilt feelings such as these should not be allowed to build until the stress reaches the crisis point. Below I've given you some guidelines for dealing with stress and minimizing its effects. These guidelines will also apply to stress caused by various other factors in home health care: fatigue on the part of the caregiver and patient; unreasoning anger at each other brought on by trivial events that get blown up out of proportion; marital discord (if one spouse is taking care of the other); and family tensions generated by worry over the patient (and perhaps over finances, too).

All of these stress-producing factors can result in guilt feelings on the part of all concerned—thus bringing everything back full circle.

Since stress cannot be banished from our lives, and distress can and does move in at times of crisis and ill health, here are a few suggestions and guidelines that have been found effective in helping to keep the stresses of home health care under control.

Work it off. Anger, frustration, and worry can build. These emotional stresses can be reduced by blowing off some steam through physical exercise. Running, walking, swimming, dancing, and gardening all provide a physical outlet for stress. Regular exercise on a daily basis, or at least three or four times a week, will help release the "energy" of pent-up distress.

Just how much physical exercise either the caregiver or the patient can undertake will depend on their physical condition, as well as on the degree of disability of the patient. The caregiver may be elderly; the patient may be arthritic or even in a wheelchair. Some form of exercise usually is possible. Consult the doctor or a physical therapist if in doubt.

Talk about it. By sharing our worries with a trusted friend, relative, clergyman, or counselor we may gain a new perspective on the situation. At the very least, the "ear" of a friend helps us to feel we are not alone in our distress—we have the support and interest of another person. If there is no one to talk to—or if worries and destructive feelings are getting too tight a grip on your thoughts—you might want to talk with a professional "ear." A social worker, or psychiatrist may be able to provide the needed listening along with trained and professional assistance to help you cope more productively with stress.

Communicating and expressing feelings is an excellent coping mechanism for dealing with stress. Talking about a problem with a good counselor is a course of action open to both caregiver and patient, and there should be no hesitancy about using this means of reducing the effects of stress.

Avoid alcohol and drugs. Tranquilizers and alcohol can numb or mask the symptoms of stress, offering some people relief from the pain of stress. Drugs or alcohol do nothing to help you deal with stress itself, however, and they may become habit-forming, adding to the problem. The decision to medicate has to be a professional one. If you feel that drugs will help, then talk it over with your doctor. Do not attempt taking drugs on your own.

The caregiver will usually have greater access to drugs and alcohol than the patient, simply because the caregiver may have greater mobility and can get outside more. Nevertheless, the patient can, if he so wishes, also develop contacts for getting drugs or alcohol. In neither case would this be a wise course to take.

Take care of yourself. Proper rest and sleep, good eating habits, and recreation all contribute to good health and to feeling good and will help provide the reserves of strength needed for dealing with stress. Some things may be beyond an individual's power to change—the illness that brought about the need for home health care, for example— but the caregiver and the patient each have the power to take good care of themselves.

The stress of caring for someone at home can create fears and resentments that should not be suppressed and allowed to smolder until they finally erupt, doing great emotional damage. The same holds true, of course, for the patient's inner feelings. Apprehensions, resentments, and just plain anger at fate should not be allowed to go unrelieved. The two people most intimately concerned in home health care—the caregiver and the person being cared for—are now in a position where they will have to interact with each other in unfamiliar roles on a daily basis. Tensions can build rapidly between them, bringing on emotional and physiological problems that can become very serious if not dealt with promptly and honestly.

Talk to each other. As simple as it sounds, this is often all it takes. Instead of waiting for an emotional explosion to occur, make it a point to spend some time just talking things over and being open and forth-coming about your feelings. Everything will not be resolved at the moment, nor will all be sweetness and light, but at least you will not have allowed inner tensions to take root deep inside you until they become dangerously painful to confront.

Your social worker has had much experience with people in simi-lar situations and can help you greatly in dealing with stress. If the stress is too much for you to handle on your own, don't hesitate to call on the social worker for assistance. Talk things over with her. Her insights and expertise in the matter of coping with stress will be of real value to you, whether you are the caregiver or the patient. Moreover, if the problem is severe, the social worker can bring in other profes-sionals—a psychotherapist, if necessary—to provide the additional help you may need.

While stress cannot—and should not—be eliminated from your life, there's no need for you to suffer from it unduly.

Setting up the Home

The anticipated day has finally arrived. The patient is being dis-charged from the hospital and coming home to you. You are going to be the care provider for someone close to you who will be looking to you for health care from now on. And it hits you. You haven't made any real preparations. The spare bedroom is there, and you've seen to it that it's clean and that fresh linen is on the bed and some colorful flowers are on the nightstand—but that's about all.

What are you going to do now? A dozen thoughts flash through your mind in a few seconds. What about the bathroom? Can the patient use it without difficulty? And what about meals? Can the patient maneuver down the stairs to the kitchen. And what about . . .?

This, of course, is exactly the situation you must avoid. As a mature and sensible person who has undertaken the role of care provider, you will make proper preparations for the big homecoming. What exactly, are "proper preparations"? This will depend entirely on what sort of disability the patient has.

Regardless of the disability, though, there are three fundamental conditions you must provide for home health care: accessibility, safety, and convenience. These three requirements form the bedrock on which to build the foundation of home care for the patient.

Let's assume, for the sake of discussion, that the patient has Par-kinson's disease and has been at the hospital for tests and examina-tions to determine the efficacy of a combined program of drug therapy, counseling, and physical therapy. His hand tremors have increased, his muscles are stiffening, and he's having trouble moving around. He's mentally alert and has a good emotional attitude, and the health care you'll be providing for him at home will help him manage his disease.

What about the first requirement? Just how accessible have you made the home for the patient? Will he be able to move about, even with his disability? Will he be able to use the bathroom? What about the stairs? Is the telephone where he can get to it? Where will he eat? The list can go on and on.

The same holds true for safety—there's much to take into consideration. What may be commonplace to you and to others who aren't disabled—a flight of stairs, for example, or a balky door—can be a genuine threat to the patient. The home in which you are going to provide health care has to be made safe.

It stands to reason also that no matter how accessible and safe certain areas of the home may be, if they aren't convenient for the patient to use, he can easily become frustrated and depressed, and his ability to manage his disease will be hampered.

What do you need to make your home accessible, safe, and convenient? The answer to this question will vary with the individual concerned and the type and extent of any disability. Also, the type of home you have—a house, an apartment, how many floors, and so on—has to be taken into consideration, as well as whether any structural changes, if required, would be feasible. Before you make any radical changes—or any large investment in devices or equipment, consult an occupational therapist, the health professional specially trained to plan and organize the home to promote the highest level of function possible for a patient.

The suggestions that follow are included to make you aware of the possibilities. A trained occupational therapist will be able to provide you with specific recommendations.

Setting up the Bathroom

"The bathroom is one of the most difficult rooms for disabled people. I bet if you did a study of the elderly living alone you would find a large proportion who don't take baths. They sponge themselves off."

These are the words of an occupational therapist, a health professional concerned with helping people function in a normal environment despite disabling handicaps, and her statement echoes the findings of all who have tried to cope with the problems bathrooms create for the disabled. It's safe to say that the bathroom could be the most dangerous room in a home, especially for someone who cannot move around very well.

Difficulties with the bathroom for the disabled, the elderly infirm, or anyone who doesn't have full mobility can present frightening and traumatic obstacles. Not only are bathrooms usually small and cramped and difficult for most of us to move around in, the very act of using the bathroom is, in our culture, considered to be highly intimate and personal and not for general discussion. Nevertheless, this is an aspect of daily living that cannot be avoided, and it deserves special consideration in getting the home ready for health care.

Don't be discouraged or start thinking you have to rebuild your entire bathroom when you begin preparations for making it safe, accessible, and convenient. You have to use your imagination and your common sense here. Stand in the bathroom and look around you at everything in there—the fixtures, the shelves, the light, the mirror, the cabinets—and visualize yourself as being unable to cope with any of these items because of a disability. Try simulating the disability yourself to see if you can figure a way around it.

How do you make a bathroom safe for use by the disabled? First, keep in mind that bigger is not necessarily better where bathrooms are concerned. It's a natural inclination to look at the cluttered, cramped bathroom and get the urge to open up all the areas and give the disabled person a pleasant, safe, modern place in which to perform all bathroom functions. Usually, this thought strikes when you realize that for a disabled person in a wheelchair the bathroom door will have to be widened. If this can't be done, then some other means will have to be found to allow the individual to get from the wheelchair into the bathroom.

Smallness, in itself, is not undesirable in bathrooms for the disabled. In fact, a completely rebuilt, huge, wide open bathroom might turn out to be a safety hazard. A disabled person sitting on the toilet should be able to reach the sink and the tub without having to lean and stretch dangerously. The less the individual has to maneuver, stretch, or strain, the safer the bathroom. So even if rebuilding the bathroom is not a problem for you, financially or otherwise, think twice before calling in the contractors.

It's not only wheelchairs that require a wider door. Someone using a walker or crutches would also have difficulty maneuvering through narrow bathroom doors in most homes. For some reason, building codes seem to allow bathrooms to be constructed with narrower doors (usually twenty-four inches) than the doors in the rest of the house (thirty-six inches wide). Not much can be done about this, however, if structural or financial considerations make it impossible to widen the bathroom door.

Even if you can't widen the bathroom door, you can make sure that the door opens and closes easily. This means that any towels hanging on the back of the door (a favorite spot for a towel rack) should be removed if they interfere in any way with the door movement. If you're setting up the bathroom for a disabled person before he gets home from the hospital, you'll have to try out the door movement yourself.

Once inside the door, look down at the floor. What kind of flooring is used? It is tile? If so, is it the slick, somewhat slippery kind? (A special non stick tile is available from local stores.) Is there a bathroom mat placed in such a way that the edge of it might trip an infirm person trying to get through the doorway? You'll have to make sure the floor surface is safe for the disabled person and that the bathroom mat is the type that will not slip or skid. The floor space in the typical bathroom may be small, but it has to be a major safety consideration in home health care.

Next check out the sink. The main precaution here is to make sure nothing is left on it that will present a hazard to the person using it. It's common practice in most bathrooms to leave a clutter of soaps, lotions, bottles, and other paraphernalia on the sink, especially if it has a wide counter top. An excess of items on the sink top presents too many opportunities for something to slip off, drop in the sink, or hit the floor (and if it's a glass bottle or an electric appliance such as a radio that could mean trouble), so it's best to keep the sink as uncluttered as possible. If the sink doesn't already have a fairly wide counter top you might consider installing one, since this will give the disabled person more room for maneuvering grooming aids (brush, comb, makeup, toothpaste, etc.).

The sink faucets may present a problem for a person with limited finger dexterity or gripping strength. Various types of faucet handles are available at the local hardware store. If a conventional handle will not solve the difficulty, extension handles of metal or plastic can be fabricated and installed without much trouble. Once again, ingenuity will be needed.

The tub or stall shower or tub-and-shower combination will require some adjustment, depending upon the type and extent of the individual's disability. Most important, provision should always be made for the disabled person to sit down. The amount of mobility the individual has determines how much assistance will be needed and whether or not bathing or showering is more desirable.

Let's start with the conventional bathtub. The first problem is how the individual with limited mobility will get over the high outside rim. A device known as a transfer bench resolves this difficulty. This is a long bench with rubber-tipped metal legs. One model places one end of the bench inside the tub and the other on the floor outside the tube. The seat can be made of any waterproof material that will allow easy sliding movement. The patient sits on the bench and, with or without assistance, as needed, lifts his legs over the edge of the tub and slides along the seat into the tub. It will take some practice, but users soon become adept at getting in and out of the tub.

Once in the tub, the process of bathing can begin. Soap and other necessary items should be near at hand, and for this purpose a shelf or a tub caddy can be used. Make sure it doesn't interfere with the person's movements or present an obstacle or safety hazard.

Grab bars and tub rails are a must, for obvious reasons. Use the ones that provide the greatest safety and convenience for the user.

The tub bottom should be covered with a rubber mat or have adhesive-backed safety strips placed strategically on the tub surface. Even though the user will be sitting down on a tub seat or bench, you have to provide the additional safety feature of a nonskid surface on the tub bottom.

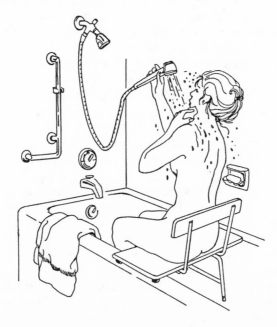

She's taking a tub shower safely—sitting on a tub/transfer bench, with safety rail in place, using a hand-held shower hose.

Some tub transfer benches are constructed in such a way that shower curtains can be pulled all the way across the tub even though the bench sits over the edge and extends outside the tub. Glass shower doors and glass doors enclosing the tub have to be removed and replaced with shower curtains. The danger to a disabled person presented by sliding glass doors in a bathtub should be self-evident.

If the tub or shower stall isn't already equipped with one, install a hand-held shower head on a flexible line. A great variety of these are available with various attachments and features. Plumbing connections are simple. The person sitting down will thus be able to shower and wash all areas of the body without strain or hazard.

If you have a stall shower, a nonskid stool can be placed inside for sitting down. Safety rails and grab bars are needed here also, as well as a mat on the floor of the stall. If you are able to do some remodeling in the bathroom, a roll-in shower that will accommodate a wheelchair might be considered—if the door has also been widened to allow the entrance of the chair.

If possible, install the kind of faucets that allow the temperature of the water to be set before the shower head is turned on. This will allow the user to regulate the temperature with little risk of suddenly being inundated with the spray of extremely hot or cold water. An additional safety feature that should be considered is using the type of faucets that maintain a set temperature and that will shut off automatically if the temperature of the water should suddenly rise. A disabled person cannot move quickly out of the way of scalding water should an accident occur.

As part of the general preparation of the bathroom for use by a disabled person, make sure the path to the tub or shower and all the other bathroom units are free and safe, no matter how small the room. Floor hampers should be removed and cleaning utensils stored away. Anything that can lie around loose or possibly be tripped over or form a barrier to a disabled person should be relocated or removed.

Next we come to the matter of the toilet. This is no place for false modesty. People use the toilet to urinate and move their bowels. These are natural daily functions, and for someone who's disabled they present many difficulties. Some of the more modern toilets are built very low to the floor, pleasing the hearts of decorators but raising havoc with the joints, muscles, and emotions of the disabled and infirm.

If the act of sitting down on the toilet seat and getting up afterward presents problems, there are devices to help overcome the difficulties. A portable toilet seat can be attached to raise the level of the seat, allowing the person to use the toilet without too much bending of the knees or lowering of the body. A variety of armrests and supports

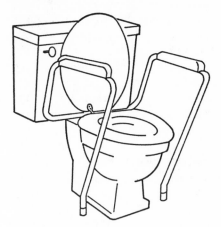

Rails mount around the toilet to help patients sit down and stand up safely.

A removable ring can raise the toilet seat up to six inches.

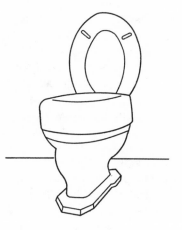

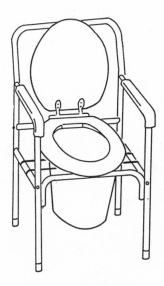

When access into the bathroom is difficult, a commode in the bedroom helps.

can be installed around the toilet to aid the user in getting up and down. Illustrated are examples of various devices that can enable the disabled individual to use the toilet with confidence and dignity. This aspect of bathroom use is very intimate and personal, and while someone might not object to being helped to bathe, using the toilet is another matter entirely. Every effort should be made to set things up so that the person can use the toilet alone and in privacy.

Sitting down in the shower or tub or on the toilet are not the only times a disabled person should be seated while in the bathroom. For some people standing at the sink, even with grab bars or other supports available, will be a tiring task or, in some cases, even impossible. If a wheelchair cannot be taken into the bathroom, a folding bridge chair can be brought in and placed in front of the sink.

The bathroom cabinet, which is usually over the sink, will be much too high for someone seated at the sink. Even standing and stretching up and over the sink might present a safety hazard. Medicines and other essentials can be placed in a lower cabinet to one side of the sink, or in any other convenient location.

If the bathroom cabinet is too high, the mirror will also be too high. A separate mirror on an extension arm or gooseneck can be installed at the proper level to allow use by the person seated at the sink.

Since the disabled person presumably will be alone in the bathroom with the door shut for varying periods of time, it's important to have some sort of signaling or calling device handy. A bell or buzzer or even a cordless phone will suffice. This is just another safeguard against any accidents or problems that might occur.

As mentioned before, if you have the services of an occupational therapist in caring for the disabled person, ask the therapist for advice about how to set up the bathroom, preferably before the person comes home from the hospital. The therapist is very familiar with all that can be done to make a bathroom fully usable by a disabled person. Also the therapist will help you set things up so you avoid any sort of "institutional" look in the bathroom. It will still be a place that the entire family can use.

A little thought and some creativity are all you need.

Setting up the Bedroom

It's been said that we spend about one-third of our lives in bed, sleeping or trying to get to sleep. A disabled person may spend more time there than that. Also, the physical action of getting in and out of bed, so ordinary for most of us, can in some instances take on the dimensions of an insurmountable task for the disabled.

It's not an absolute requirement to have a hospital bed installed in the bedroom for home health care. There's a tendency to rush out and buy or rent a hospital bed once it's been established that the person will require long-term or permanent home health care. This is a natural reaction, especially if someone has spent a lot of time in the hospital or is coming home in a weakened condition or with mobility limitations.

The advantages of a hospital bed are that the top or bottom can be lowered or raised to convenient levels. Also, the bed is built at a height that makes it easier to tend to the person while in bed. Unless the individual requires this sort of bed treatment, there's no need for a hospital bed at home. An ordinary bed, preferably the same one the disabled person always used, will usually do just fine. It will be familiar and comforting to the person just back from the hospital. Moreover, since it's built much closer to the floor than a hospital bed, it will be much easier to get in and out of. There'll be no need for the low stool at the side of the bed that hospital patients use.

Another good reason for not using a hospital bed at home is to encourage the person to resume as normal a life as possible, consistent with the limitations imposed by the disability. If there's a hospital bed in the home bedroom and other types of hospital furnishings throughout the house, the individual will continue to think of himself as being sick and needing the kind of twenty-four-hour care provided in a hospital setting.

Of course, in some cases a hospital bed—or at least a guardrail setup on the conventional bed—will be required at home. Hospital beds can be purchased or rented, whichever is most applicable or feasible, and special guardrails for attachment to a conventional bed can be obtained at a home care pharmacy or surgical supply dealer.

Since a disabled person may spend more time in bed than a well person, it's important to provide as much comfort, convenience, and safety as possible. Clean sheets are a prerequisite, and two or three comfortable pillows are just about mandatory. Also, if the person will want to spend some private time in the bedroom, a comfortable chair, preferably a recliner, can be purchased and placed there. It's best to let the person try out the chair or the recliner himself before making a final selection. Some recliners require a certain amount of arm strength to operate. Some have a lever on the side for extending the recliner, and others use a pushing motion. The person who will be using the recliner should be the one to test it out before it's placed in the bedroom.

If an ordinary chair is to be used instead of a recliner, make sure

An over-bed table offers bed-bound patients a convenient and sturdy surface.

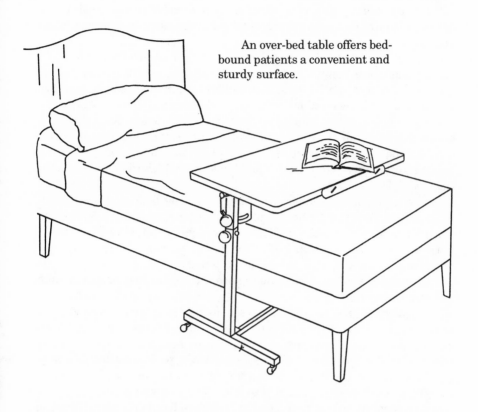

The bedside caddy holds personal items conveniently.

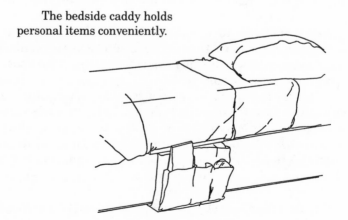

it's a chair the disabled individual can get in and out of without difficulty. If the person has to transfer from a wheelchair to a recliner or ordinary chair, test everything out first to be sure it can be accomplished.

Another good idea in the bedroom is an over-the-bed table or a side table or nightstand convenient to reach. If required, a small water pitcher (plastic, of course) and a glass can be kept handy on the side table, as well as facial tissues and other items, including medication. There are various types of bed caddies, bags, and other such devices that will make the bedroom a more comfortable and convenient place for the disabled person. Do not forget a simple wastebasket. Even a fully ambulatory person will need a wastebasket in which to dispose of used tissues and other items.

The main thing to bear in mind is that the bedroom is a special place to the individual who spends time there. The room should be as cheerful as you can make it. Take advantage of the window arrangement to bring in as much light as possible throughout the day. For nighttime, several lamps, well placed, will keep things cheery. If the person will be reading in bed, make sure the bed lamp is bright enough to avoid eyestrain.

Ensure the privacy of the person using the room. If you've ever been in a hospital, either as a patient or as a visitor, you know how disturbing it is to have people walking in and out as they please. Obviously, the hospital staff has much work to do and needs ready access to a patient's room, but there's no need to duplicate this situation at home. Privacy is one of the delights of being at home.

In planning the arrangement of furniture in a bedroom, as well as which items to purchase, be sure to take into consideration the safety factor. As with the bathroom, avoid anything lying around loose or in the path the person might use in going from one part of the bedroom to another. Consider also the person's range of motion. Is he sufficiently ambulatory to take care of all his needs in the bedroom without calling for assistance? Does he have sufficient use of his arms, hands, and fingers to reach for things and grasp them? How does his disability limit his reach, if at all?

In addition to evaluating reach, don't overlook the range of activities of the person using the bedroom. Is he in a wheelchair or can he walk around without difficulty? Will he be spending a lot of time in the bedroom? If so, what will he be doing? Watching TV? Reading? Writing letters? Telephoning friends? Running a small business from home? How much will he be moving around?

Sometimes a disabled person does not have a great deal of mobility and must remain mostly in one place in the room for long periods of time, either in a chair or in bed. If this is the case, make sure the person is placed where all or most of the items he'll need—books, magazines, tissues, telephone, TV remote control, etc.—will be within his reach. He'll be able to take care of himself to the fullest extent possible.

As with the bathroom arrangement, some sort of calling or signaling device should be close at hand. If this is a large house, an intercom system, if feasible, will allow the person in the bedroom to communicate with others in the house.

One of the most important and sometimes most neglected aspects of the bedroom is the mattress. Most people take a mattress and box spring for granted since they are not purchased frequently and usually last for years. In fact, many of us are not even aware of the need for a new mattress until the stuffing starts coming out of the old one. It's usually then that we realize how much we have become accustomed to the old mattress, even though it slopes dangerously at the edges.

There's a safety factor here that mustn't be overlooked. A soft, sloping mattress can be responsible for serious injury to an infirm person trying to get out of bed. The edge of the bed can suddenly give way, and the disabled individual slip or fall to the floor. If this is the case, consider purchasing a new, firm mattress. If a new mattress can't be immediately obtained, a board cut to the size of the mattress and placed between the mattress and the box spring will serve temporarily.

Depending on the type of disability involved, you may have to add additional devices and aids in the bedroom. It it's difficult for the person to sit up or shift around in bed, various bars and trapezelike arrangements can be suspended over the head of the bed. In cases where even the touch of a sheet on the person's feet is painful, there are methods for keeping the bedding off the person's feet, one of which is illustrated here.

If you have a motorized adjustable bed, it may prove useful in helping the disabled person rest more comfortably or in a position that has therapeutic value. If a motorized bed is out of the question, various wedges and foam inserts can be manually inserted to bring about the same effect.

No matter what the requirement, there is usually someway to assist the disabled person. As in many other aspects of setting up the house for the home health care, imagination and ingenuity are needed. Again, consult the occupational therapist treating the patient, if there is one.

A word of caution here. In attempting to set up the bedroom for its most effective use, be careful all your arrangements don't backfire on you. It may turn out that all the aids, devices, and special arrangements will encourage the person to stay in the bedroom more than necessary or, in extreme cases, seldom leave the bed itself. One way to

A trapeze can be used to help the patient move around in bed. Note that it can only be attached to a hospital bed.

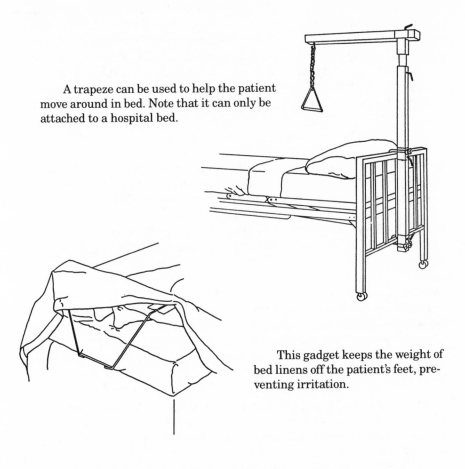

This gadget keeps the weight of bed linens off the patient's feet, preventing irritation.

Wedges can be used to elevate the head or the feet.

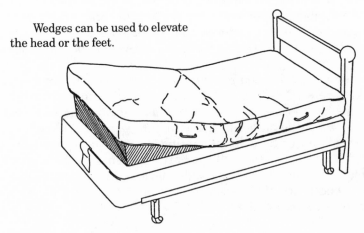

avoid this is to make sure the disabled person gets dressed in street clothes every day and that, whenever possible, you bring him out of the bedroom. It's unhealthy for anyone to spend too much time in bed. The lungs can fill with fluid, and bodily functions generally become sluggish.

A New Look at the Kitchen

Next to the bathroom, the kitchen can be the most dangerous room in the house. The reasons for this are obvious—electricity, gas, appliances, heat, fire, and flame are all present there, to say nothing of cabinet doors that can swing open, knives that can be left lying about, and many other hazards. As the caregiver you should step back and take a "new look" at the kitchen. Try to see it through the eyes—and with the fears—of the disabled person at home.

In setting up the kitchen, you will have to use imagination and ingenuity. It's an important room, and the disabled person should not be denied the use of it. The kitchen is often the hub of household activities and represents happy memories for many people. There's no reason why it should not continue this way, regardless of disability or limitations on the person who finds enjoyment in the kitchen.

Two possible uses of the kitchen are involved. The individual may only eat there, or he or she may actually prepare meals in this room. In either case, safety has to be the primary consideration.

If the kitchen is to be used only for eating, the convenience and ease of sitting at the table will be the main concern. If the individual is in a wheelchair, room must be made in the kitchen to maneuver the chair and the table must be the right height to allow the chair to move in underneath.

If the person has some degree of mobility, the path to the table must be clear, the chair conveniently placed and sturdy enough to provide support if the person grips the back or arm of the chair as an aid when sitting down.

One of the first things that must be done in setting up the kitchen is to check the range of mobility and the reach of the disabled person. We'll assume here that this person may want to cook occasionally and may eat in the kitchen there as well.

To check mobility and reach, have the disabled person present in the kitchen. If this person is in a wheelchair, he or she can be positioned at various points in the kitchen and attempt to maneuver around and to reach for things. In this way you'll be able to determine what has to be changed and what adjustments the person will have to make.

Bear in mind that unless you are going to tear the kitchen apart and completely rebuild it, the process of setting up the kitchen will take time. Certain changes and improvements can be accomplished quickly—moving some items around in a cabinet to make them easier to reach, for example—but most others will have to come after you determine what's needed in the way of alterations and enabling devices.

Lighting is important, but this shouldn't present a problem. Most kitchens are well lit with ceiling fixtures and fluorescent lights. About all that will be needed in this respect is to make sure the light switches are conveniently situated and have well-secured safety plates. If the disabled person cannot easily reach the light switch from the wheelchair, a simple device, such as the one illustrated, can be used. It's merely a rod on a swivel suspended from the switch, allowing the person in the wheelchair to activate the switch from a lower position.

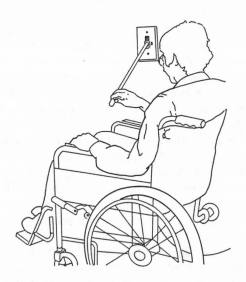

This adaptation to a light switch permits a person in a wheelchair to control the lights.

A sufficient number of electric outlets should be provided, both for convenience and for safety in using electrical appliances. All outlets should be electrically grounded to avoid the possibility of electric shock. If your kitchen isn't already so equipped, an electrician can be called in to make the necessary installations.

Even if the disabled person is not going to be in a wheelchair, it's likely that he or she will want to sit down as much as possible when working in the kitchen. Using either the wheelchair, chair, or stool the person will be sitting on, check the space under the counter. The counter should be high enough to allow knee room underneath and, at the same time, be low enough so the person can work comfortably at the counter. In setting up this type of counter space, keep in mind that other members of the family will be using the kitchen also.

Knee room should also be provided under the sink. If possible, lower the sink to a convenient height for use by the disabled person and remove doors under the sink to allow for knee room underneath. Plumbing should be moved out of the way and pipes carrying hot water either relocated or covered with insulation to avoid the possibility of burns. If sink alterations of this nature are not possible, see if the person can work at the sink on a raised seat or chair. Experiment with various techniques and positions and minor alterations. Keep safety uppermost in mind, but do not overlook accessibility and convenience. Illustrated is an ideal sink setup for a disabled person.

A faucet that can swivel back and forth and a spray head on a flexible hose are features that, if not already on the sink, a plumber can easily install. If the disabled person cannot reach the faucets, an extension rod with a faucet-gripping device at the end can be purchased or improvised.

A rubber mat placed in the bottom of the sink will provide a safeguard against dish breakage if the disabled person doesn't have good gripping strength. If the person has full use of only one hand, a small brush can be fastened to a block and placed in the sink so that glasses or dishes can be cleaned by rubbing against the brush. Keep soap, detergent, brushes, and all other frequently used utensils and materials within easy reach.

The stove presents a challenge. The best type of stove is an electric cooktop with burners placed in a single row across the front rather than one behind the other. If you can't replace your present stove, you'll have to adapt it for efficient and effective use by the disabled person. A well-placed mirror can help the person see inside the pots on the stove. Gas ranges may be a bit more difficult to handle than an electric stove, but it can be done. Where a gas oven has to be lit and the person cannot bend down to use the match, obtain long fireplace matches, sold in gift shops, and use them for lighting the oven.

No matter how you alter or adapt your stove, you'll have to be conscious of the importance of safety. Using empty pots and pans and an unlit stove, have the disabled person practice moving everything around. Ideally, the person should not have to reach over or behind

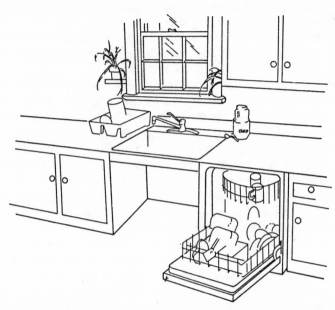

This "ideal" sink provides room for a wheelchair or
stool with ample leg room to sit at the sink.

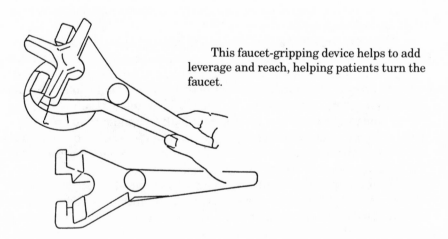

This faucet-gripping device helps to add
leverage and reach, helping patients turn the
faucet.

any pot or pan on the stove. If this is not possible, because of the layout of the burners, then meal preparation will have to be planned so that the back burners either are not used or are used in such a way that pots on them will not have to be handled too frequently.

Spend a lot of time with the disabled person at the stove until methods, techniques, and movements are perfected to the point where the stove can be used safely and efficiently.

A side-by-side refrigerator is the best for use by a disabled person. The doors open outward from the center, and the entire contents of the refrigerator and freezer compartments are in view and usually fully accessible. Some "practice runs" will quickly establish how many of the items can be reached and which have to be moved to more convenient locations on the shelves.

There are many ways in which a kitchen can be set up to be functional for a disabled person. Here are some methods and devices that have proved helpful to others:

- Use lazy Susans wherever possible. These are excellent devices for enabling a disabled person to reach a great variety of items with a minimum of effort.
- A toaster oven or a microwave oven can be used instead of the conventional oven, or in conjunction with it, for added convenience in food preparation.
- Reaching devices, such as shown on page 134 can be used to reach for and grasp light objects that are on high shelves or too far back for the person to reach. Keep in mind that these tonglike devices have limited use, especially for heavy or awkward objects.
- Sliding racks and shelves should be used wherever they can be conveniently located. These allow many items or utensils to be pulled out for easy accessibility and are almost a necessity where the person cannot bend down or squat to reach into the backs of cabinets.
- Narrow shelves are another convenience. They allow storing of cans and bottles and other essential items in a row so there's no need to reach in back. A bar in front of the shelf keeps the items from falling off.
- Pegboard panels allow for convenient storage of a variety of items, especially pots and pans. There are many pegboard fixtures and holders that can be used, and the housewares section of your local store will have them available.

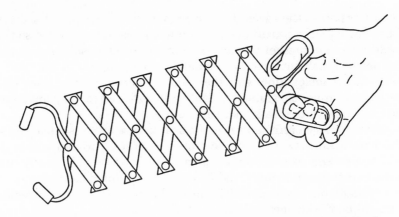

Reaching devices like these help pick up difficult-to-reach items from high or low places.

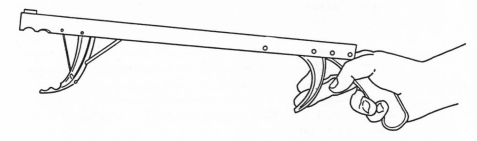

- Handle loops can be installed on refrigerator doors, cabinet drawers, closets, or any other place where the person would have difficulty grasping handles or knobs.

Living in the Living Room

A patient returning from the hospital may look forward to coming home, but at the same time he or she is often fearful of leaving the security represented by the hospital and the special care that was received there. This is especially true when the illness has been severe and the recovery slow. Coming home can be frightening as well as joyful.

To counteract this fear, some caregivers try to set up a substitute hospital room in their living room. It's an understandable reaction, but it should not be allowed to dominate the living and sleeping arrangements in the home.

Sometimes the returning patient doesn't want to feel isolated by being relegated to an upstairs bedroom. The living room downstairs is where the family gathers, and so a bed in the living room seems like the only way to join in with the family.

Still, as undesirable as it may be, there will be times when there is no alternative to putting a bed in the living room. A good example of this is when the disabled person is coming to live in someone else's home (a son's or daughter's house, for example) and there is no spare bedroom. In other cases, the stairs may present an insurmountable problem for the patient and it isn't possible, for financial or other reasons, to install a stair lift.

If the living room must be converted into a bedroom, then consider curtaining off the portion of the room for this purpose. When privacy is needed, the curtains can be drawn. At other times the curtains will be open and the disabled person will be a part of the family activity in the living room. The same effect can be accomplished with screens. Imagination and adaptability will have to be brought into full play here.

If there is a bedroom upstairs and the disabled person cannot use this room because of the stair problem, which would isolate him from the rest of the house, perhaps the upstairs bedroom can be converted into a den for use by the family instead of the living room.

In any use of the living room as a bedroom, you have to consider the rights of all the family. The disabled person has a right not to be isolated from family activities, but at the same time he also has the right to privacy and dignity. The other family members have the right to continue their lives as normally as possible. Compromises will have to be made, but the main thing to keep in mind is that the disabled person should be fully participatory in the family routine and daily living.

If it doesn't have to be used as a bedroom, the living room should remain as much as possible the way it always has been—with the exception that it's made accessible, safe, and convenient for the disabled person. Obviously, hazardous furniture should be moved out of the way, and if a wheelchair is to be used, room should be made for maneuvering. If the disabled person does not use a wheelchair but has limited mobility, one chair or recliner that the person can get in and out of comfortably should be kept for his exclusive use. The cared-for individual must feel, and know, that the living room, the place where the family congregates, is as much a room for his use as for the rest of the family.

II

Daily Living

5

Living Each Day

WE ARE EACH unique in the ways we have learned to live, love, work, and play. Our ability to handle the everyday stress of life—including the distress of pain—depends upon our own set of inner responses. Thus, each of us approaches the aftermath of an acute illness or the prospect of long-term or permanent disability in a unique, personal manner. Whether we are the patient or the caregiver, our reactions to the particular set of circumstances that must be faced because of an illness will always be our own.

This chapter looks at three types of daily living situations that will involve individual reactions and responses:

- Recovery of health from an acute illness following a hospital stay.
- Readjustment following an illness with an acute or rapid onset—a stroke or an amputation, for example—with its changes in physical or functional ability and its impact on living patterns.
- Adjustment to the changes—sometimes slow, sometimes rapid—that can result from a progressive disease

Coping with home care following an acute but curable illness involves a special frame of mind. Plans and routines can be suspended for a while in order to assist a wife or husband, mother or father, sister or brother for a relatively brief and finite period of time. Business travel often can be postponed; social commitments can be delayed. This state of "suspended animation" can work for a while, but the need to return to normalcy inevitably sets in when life as it is usually lived is delayed too long. Unless the patient's recovery is completed within a reasonable period of time, those involved with caring for the patient will find it necessary to make some changes to adopt a less disruptive and invasive course of action.

A home health care plan designed to deal with the problems of either a progressive illness or the acute onset of an illness with long-term effects on life style and living patterns will require a series of adjustments and readjustments. The needs of the patient must be considered—his support system, his home living situation, his financial situation, and his physical, emotional, and mental condition.

This chapter offers guidelines, suggestions, and examples to help both patients and caregivers. However, there is no absolutely right or wrong way to organize for living each day. With the patient as a partner in the decision-making process, the "right" way is the approach that provides the best solutions for a set of given circumstances—and which "feels" right for both the patient and the caregiver.

The team of health care specialists recruited to assist in providing effective home care for the patient can do much to point out methods, approaches, and procedures that have worked for others in the past. However, as many an experienced and competent therapist has discovered, the best solutions to many of the problems of day-to-day activities are the solutions the patients have discovered themselves and subsequently taught to their therapists.

A portion of this chapter includes tips and suggestions for improving functional ability. Obviously, because of the wide range of abilities and disabilities, not all the suggestions offered here will apply to everyone.

Acute Onset—Expected Recovery

Patients are now going home from the hospital "sooner and sicker" to continue recovery and recuperation at home. Intravenous tubes may still be in place; a respirator may be operating; major surgery may have been undergone; a cancer may have been diagnosed and chemotherapy may be on the horizon.

Orchestrating high quality health care in a home environment can be terrifying, yet rewarding—terrifying because, instrusive as they may be, nurses, orderlies, nurse's aides, and other hospital personnel create a sense of security for the patient in a hospital. These people are familiar with the sometimes complex equipment; they know what to do in emergencies; and when professionally competent they handle themselves and the patients with quiet authority. They can be coolly objective as they care for the patient and, when necessary, urge and cajole him to turn in bed to avoid pressure sores, to cough and clear his lungs, and to dress so he'll feel more like himself and less like a dependent patient.

When the patient does go home, spouses, adult sons or daughters, and other relatives who have not had previous experience with prolonged illness may feel more than a twinge of panic. Despite the fact that home health nurses and aides may have been ordered, the family caregivers realize that the ultimate responsibility for the patient is theirs—and this can be a decidedly uncomfortable realization.

The discomfort is often heightened because it is difficult for a family member who has taken on the role of caregiver to be objective about this person, the patient, who may be a mother or father or a sister or brother. If, for example, you are the caregiver and the patient is your mother, you will find that, unlike the health professionals who met your mother only as a patient in the hospital after the onset of her illness, you have a clear memory of what she was like before illness struck. Chances are mother was a healthy and independent individual, and now, while you are trying to cope with the fact that your mother has an illness and that for a while at least your life will change as you help her manage, you are expected to tune in to the procedures of health care and learn about the "bells and whistles" that operate the imposing health care equipment.

Home health care for the more acute illnesses usually means mobilizing a team of health care professionals. The services of nurses, physical and occupational therapists, home health aides, and other team members ideally should be arranged for prior to the patient's discharge from the hospital. You, as the caregiver, know that the atmosphere at home will be a lot more pleasant than the intrusive and impersonal environment of the hospital. Besides, it shouldn't be for long. In time, mother will be up and around. The surgical wound will heal or the chemotherapy will be completed or the last of the dressings will have been removed—and mother will improve more readily because her care has continued at home. There's a measure of comfort and accomplishment and a rewarding feeling for you because of your involvement in orchestrating the care.

Managing Continuity of Care

The seriously ill patient recuperating at home may require the re-creation of certain elements of the hospital situation. As has been mentioned, by the time the patient goes home, arrangements should have been made for home nursing or home health aides and the appropriate equipment and therapies. If possible, time the day of discharge from the hospital to coincide with the initiation of the support services. It's easier on the caregiver and better for the patient. Often, families will insist on taking a patient home on a Friday, in time for the weekend, under the impression that because most family members are available on weekends, they will be able to assist more readily with caring for the patient during the first few days at home. There's some truth in this, of course, but unless arrangements can be made to begin home health aide services on the Friday or Saturday, you and your recently released patient may be left to fend for yourselves until Monday or Tuesday of the following week—despite the available assistance of one or more untrained family members.

Many home health agencies require a nurse's home visit prior to providing any other assistance. After the nurse has completed her evaluation, the order for a home health aide may be written. At many hospitals this process can be begun while the patient is still in the hospital; however, there are times when, for one reason or another, this preliminary nurse's evaluation has to be delayed until after discharge. Be sure to check with the discharge planner, and remember to ask which days are better for hospital discharge in order to assure continuity of care.

A clear, concise plan of action and treatment has to be created for anyone on home health care. In the hospital, the treatment plan is written by the doctor and entered in the patient's medical record. For home health care, the home health nurse-coordinator is usually responsible for preparing the treatment plan and submitting it to the physician for approval.

The treatment plan can be a very helpful document. As you and the nurse-coordinator talk through the various steps outlined in the plan, be certain you understand each element. Make sure you note down who will perform each of the outlined treatments and when and at what intervals it will be done.

Forms and formats will vary, but the nurse's treatment plan will probably include these items:

- patient's name and age, the diagnosis, and the physician's name;
- treatment requirements, such as IV (intravenous) catheter care, parenteral or enteral nutrition (special feeding techniques), dressing changes, decubitus (bedsore) prevention, urinary catheter care, respiratory therapy, speech therapy, occupational therapy, or physical therapy;
- personnel requirements and a recommended number of visits per week by the various health professionals. Personnel requirements will vary, but they may include visits by a registered nurse, rehabilitation therapists, and home health aides;
- medical support equipment and supplies and medications necessary for treatment;

- requirements for special health care services, such as toileting assistance, dressing assistance, and other personal care. Also, incidental household services, such as meal preparation, shopping, and light housekeeping.

It may help if you rewrite the formal treatment plan in a format that is easier to follow (see chart).

You the caregiver are the manager of the home health care arrangements. Knowing who is responsible for accomplishing each part of the plan, when it is to be done, what is to be done, and where it is to

TREATMENT PLAN

Personal care	How?	When? How often?	By whom?
Brush teeth			
Wash			
Bath			
Toilet			
Dress			
Hair care			

Measuring vital signs

Temperature			
Pulse			
Blood pressure			

Medications schedule

Mealtimes / special diet

be done, will help clarify the tasks and plan for and coordinate the patient's health care. With the physical and medical care under control, you are free to address the emotional and social needs of the patient.

Tracking Progress

The hospital chart functions as the internal communications link and medical record document for a hospitalized patient. Nursing notes, physicians's orders, medications, laboratory test results, and progress notes are all recorded in the daily records of the hospital chart. Each member of the team of health professionals is then able to check the chart to find out what has happened to the patient since his last visit. Doctors find out if the tests they had ordered the previous day have been completed, and therapists learn of changes in the medications schedule—information that may, for example, change the goals of a speech therapy session. (If the pain medication has been increased significantly and the patient seems drowsy, this is not the time for an evaluation.)

The nursing notes are one of the more informative sections of the hospital chart. Here, the nurses record the completion of tasks requested by the doctor and note the patient's comments, feelings, or reactions to the illness or treatments. Armed with this insight, members of the health care team provide for continuity of care during the patient's hospital stay.

A health care chart is even more valuable for someone on home health care. Members of the home health care team can better help each other help the patient by carefully noting any and all procedures, medications, therapy, and progress for the patient. Changes in therapy and follow-up care can be documented in the home health care chart as a reminder to the personal health aides or the family. The aides and the family members, by carefully noting the patient's physical, emotional, and spiritual progress, can provide the nurse or doctor with vital information for monitoring care. Days or even weeks may pass between visits to (or by) a doctor. The chart works as a far more accurate picture of day-by-day progress than any informal verbal description by family members or health aides.

A home health care chart, although not a standardized document (as are many of the charts and documents used in a hospital), should be made up by the home care nurse or the physician and explained to the caregiver and the health aides so each item will be understood and the information the nurse or physician requires can be properly recorded. (See the charts on the next three pages.)

The potential benefits of health care at home are multiplied by addressing the patient's spiritual, emotional, and social needs. Articles in medical journals and in consumer magazines have documented the power of the human spirit in combatting or controlling illness. Whether you label it the will to live or consider it the active participation of the patient in the treatment of his illness, there's little doubt that the mind can exert strong health-promoting medicine.

In his book, *Anatomy of an Illness* (W. W. Norton & Co., 1979), Norman Cousins describes the action plan he and his doctor developed

WEEKLY RECORD OF ACTIVITY AND TREATMENTS

Week beginning _____

Activity / Treatments	Sun.				Mon.	Tue.	Wed.	Thurs.	Fri.	Sat.
	AM	N	PM	BT						
Exercise										
Range of motion										
Skin care										

Comments (Note changes in feelings and appearance.)

Sun. _____

Mon. _____

Tue. _____

Wed. _____

Thurs. _____

Fri. _____

Sat. _____

to wage a successful fight against a crippling illness. The plan capital-
ized on the powerful impact the mind can have on the body. It mobilized the positive emotions of laughter and hope as weapons in his war
against the disease that had paralyzed his body.

Mr. Cousins moved out of the hospital to a hotel, where the inter-

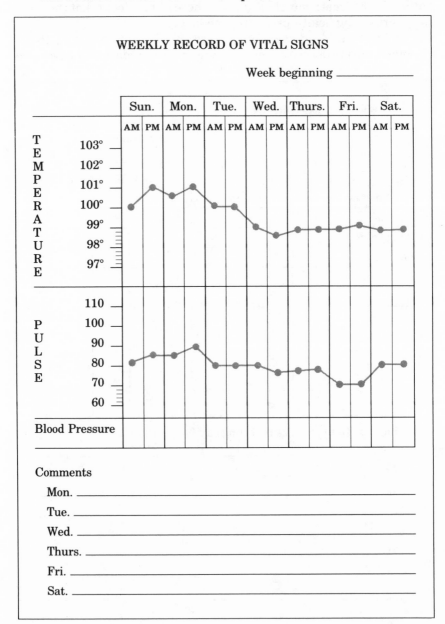

ruptions that are part of a hospital stay would be minimized. The new health care setting represented an environment over which he had some control. He slept when he wished, bathed when he wished, and ate his meals on his own schedule. Laughter, he felt, would work as "good medicine"—and he found the way and the means to laugh each day. Reruns of old "Candid Camera" shows and Marx Brothers movies worked as laugh inducers. Laughter, he found, reduced the pain and had a tranquilizing effect that permitted him to sleep.

According to Cousins—and this has been confirmed by other literature—his active participation in developing the medical treatment plan, the strong partnership he developed with his doctor, and his own belief

DAILY RECORD OF FLUIDS

Date _____

	Intake	Output
6 AM		
7 AM		
8 AM		
9 AM		
10 AM		
11 AM		
12 noon		
1 PM		
2 PM		
3 PM		
4 PM		
5 PM		
6 PM		
7 PM		
8 PM		
9 PM		
10 PM		
11 PM		
12 midnight		
Total		

in the positive results that could be anticipated worked to mobilize inner resources to reach his goal: the return of health and his return to work. The discouragement and depression he had experienced early in his illness were related to his expectation that his doctor would fix

WHAT I SHOULD BE PREPARED TO TELL THE DOCTOR

The following are the kinds of questions that your doctor may ask on the first visit. Write down your answers ahead of time. Take them with you for a quick reference.

1) Why are you here?

2) Where is the pain? When did it begin? When does it occur (night, day, all the time)? What relieves it? What aggravates it?

3) What medication do you take and why, how much, how often? Does the medication help? Bring container with you.

4) What do you do for daily exercise? Do you have pain upon or after exercising? Where?

5) Have you been hospitalized? When? For what?

6) Have you had any operations (surgery)? When? What?

7) Do you have any allergies?

8) Are there any diseases or illnesses that seem to run in your family?

9) Check any of the following conditions you have or have had:

EARS • NOSE • THROAT • DENTAL • EYES

___ Hearing aid
___ Ringing in ears
___ Nose bleeds
___ Sinus problems
___ Hoarseness
___ Bleeding gums
___ Blurring / watering eyes
___ Glaucoma
___ Cataracts
___ Glasses / contacts
___ Dentures
Other_____
_____

RESPIRATORY (LUNGS)

___ Cough

___ Blood expectoration
___ Asthma
___ Pneumonia
___ TB
___ Shortness of breath
___ Bronchitis
___ Emphysema
___ Uses oxygen
___ Pleurisy
Other_____
_____

CARDIOVASCULAR (HEART AND CIRCULATION)

___ Chest pain
___ Palpitations
___ Edema (swollen feet)

___ Angina
___ High blood pressure
___ Stroke
___ Heart attack
___ Irregular heartbeat
___ Pacemaker
___ Tingling extremities
___ Cold extremities
___ Anemia
   Other _____

MUSCULOSKELETAL
___ Deformities / handicaps
___ Fractures
___ Amputations
___ Paralysis
___ Tremors
___ Arthritis
___ Numbness
___ Joints swollen
___ Stiffness
___ Backaches
   Other _____

SKIN
___ Itching
___ Rash
___ Lesions / growths
___ Sores / decubiti
___ Wounds
___ Dressing
   Other _____

STOMACH • INTESTINAL •
ABDOMINAL
___ Indigestion
___ Nausea / vomiting
___ Gas / heartburn
___ Ulcers

___ Hernia
___ Masses
___ Change in bowel habits
___ Rectal bleeding
___ Hemorrhoids
___ Illeostomy / colostomy
___ Tubes / drains
___ Swollen abdomen
___ Gall bladder problems
   Other _____

URINARY KIDNEY
___ Frequent urination
___ Blood in urine
___ Incontinence
___ Burning
___ Dribbling
___ Infections
___ Frequent urination at night
___ Kidney disease
___ Bladder disease
___ Foley catheter
___ Prostate disease
___ Ileo conduit
   Other _____

ENDOCRINE
___ Thyroid problems
___ Diabetes
___ Overweight
___ Underweight
   Other _____

REPRODUCTIVE (FEMALE)
___ Breast lumps
___ Hysterectomy
___ D / C
___ Vaginal discharge
   Other _____

FUNCTIONAL SUMMARY

Status before *and* after *Illness*

ACTIVITY	NO ASSISTANCE NECESSARY		NEED ASSISTANCE		UNABLE TO DO AT ALL	
	before	after	before	after	before	after
Dressing						
Bathing						
Transfers						
Walking						
Bed mobility						

his body as though it were an automobile that needed repair. He says of his experience, "But then I realized that a human being is not a machine—and only a human being has a built-in mechanism for repairing itself, for ministering to its own needs, and for comprehending what is happening to it. The regenerative and restorative force in human beings is at the core of human uniqueness."

While few people afford rehabilitation therapy in a hotel room with reruns of old TV shows and famous movie comedies, the example set by Norman Cousins can be a guide for all to follow. The same spirit and drive and energy that Mr. Cousins activated in himself exists within each of us. With his creative energies and innovative approach, he was able to develop his own program and engage the assistance of others to help make it happen. For other patients, this drive and spirit may need to be sparked. While it is not within the power of one person to give another the spirit and recuperative will to live, a caregiver can create an environment and provide the means to encourage that spirit to be ignited, cultivated, and mobilized. Some patients may find that a visit from a priest, rabbi, minister, or other spiritual advisor will help in this respect. If so, as the caregiver you can help arrange such a visit—but only, of course, after talking it over with the patient first.

Tips to Consider

Surround your patient with the things and people that promote good feelings. Involve him in all planning. Within the framework of reason and medical approval, serve his favorite foods, set up the bedroom or other area with the hobbies, books, music, and recreation he likes. Ask him whom he would enjoy visiting and whom he would rather avoid. Find the ways and means to laugh. For Mr. Cousins it was old movies, but for others it may be reading and sharing anecdotes and funny stories found in the writings of Thurber or Eastman, or watching reruns of "Taxi" or "The Carol Burnett Show" on television.

Involve the cared-for individual in creating and declaring short-term and longer-term goals, and work with him to help reach these goals. In some cases, the goals may relate to progress in recovery from the acute illness. In others, the goal may be to join others for a meal in the dining room, or to eat out at a local restaurant, or visit a local park or store. With a goal firmly visualized, conscious and subconscious energies are mobilized to realize that goal. The enjoyment and sense of accomplishment at its attainment help to encourage the creation of new goals.

Identify and use "good" time. Some of us are morning people. After a night's sleep we wake up quickly and start each day with high energy. Others are night people. They awaken slowly, and their alertness and energy seem to build as the day progresses. While the energy cycle may vary in times of ill health, there's no question that it exists. Also, there are energy cycles throughout each twenty-four-hour period. It's expressed in the peaks and valleys of energy and fatigue we experience—from alertness and accuracy to sleepiness and slower reaction time. You can help assure a tailored treatment plan by identifying the "good" and "bad" times for the person on home health care. Moreover, it you are aware of his priorities and goals, you may be able to help him conserve energy at one time of the day for a more enjoyable "expenditure" later in the day.

Good time activities depend on the preferences and the personality of the individual. Higher energy periods may be used to teach and practice rehabilitation techniques. Visits from friends, relatives, and neighbors can be planned for good times during the day. Phone conversations, work from the office, reading, cooking, sewing, card playing, stamp collecting, writing, walking, and other forms of exercise are good time activies. The treatment plan, visits from therapists, medication schedules, meals, naps, etc., can be planned around the patient's energy cycle. Discuss the plan for "good time" and "rest time" activities with the advice and involvement of the patient. No one knows better how he feels than the person himself. Involving him in noting his own peaks and valleys of performance and energy will encourage his active participation in planning his treatment and his rest schedule.

Of course, no schedule must be adhered to rigidly; flexibility is important. There will be times when it's advantageous to go off schedule to help relieve boredom. The patient himself will be the best judge of this, but you, as the caregiver, also must be alert to any preliminary signs of boredom or restlessness in the patient. If you see such signs, do not wait for it to come to a head, but instead talk it over with the patient. If the two of you realize that a brief respite from the schedule will be helpful, then by all means go ahead and take it. Both you and the patient will be the better off for it.

Unlike a hospital or other health care institution, where the routines and regimens are implemented to best suit the scheduling problems and needs of the staff, the home care schedule can, and should, mesh with the individual's wishes, energy cycle, and other needs. He may be able to participate in household activities: joining the family for supper in the dining room, watching television with others, visiting with family and friends as they return from work. Weather permitting, and with the nurse's (or doctor's) approval, some part of each day can be spent out of doors, whether in a wheelchair, sitting on a porch chair, or taking a walk. With the ability to take cat naps as needed and with therapy and other treatments scheduled to accommodate the more enjoyable social and recreational interludes in the day, the person on home health care will enjoy a better quality of caring than would be possible in a hospital. It is this independence and participation on the road to wellness that seems to make a measurable difference in the speed and course of recovery.

An Amended State of Wellness

On Monday morning Carol was greeted at the door by Sara King, George King's wife. Carol, an experienced occupational therapist, was the first member of the home care team to call on George. Three weeks earlier, George had been hospitalized after suffering a mild stroke. When he had been discharged from the hospital the previous Friday, the nurses and doctors involved in his care were quite happy about the progress he had made during his hospital stay. Although his communication skills were poor (he remained silent most of the time) it was determined this was not due to his stroke but to a long history of manic-depressive behavior.

Carol had read the discharge summary on George's hospital chart and had learned that George's left arm was weakened and his balance was described as "unsafe." The discharge planning team had ordered a part-time home health aide for a few weeks to assist George with some personal care and help him and his wife readjust to being at home. The consultive services of a physical therapist (PT) and an occupational therapist (OT) had also been ordered. The PT's task was to set up a home exercise program for George to maintain range of motion in his affected arm and build strength and better balance control. Carol's job as OT was to evaluate George's ability to manage his own physical and personal care and to help him maximize his functional abilities in the activities of daily living.

On that Monday morning, Carol found that in the three short days George had been home, quite a number of changes had already been made in their living patterns and in the setup of his split-level home. The living room had been converted into a hospital bedroom. Carol's inner voice wanted to ask who had ordered the probably unnecessary hospital bed, but years of experience had taught her to hold her tongue, especially during the first visit. George was unshaven, in his pajamas, and in bed. A half-eaten tray of food rested on the coffee table nearby.

During the first visit, Carol found that George had spent the entire three days in the hospital bed in his living room. He had used the guest bathroom on the main floor to wash and use the toilet—but had not ventured up the six steps to the bedroom level of his home. Sara was exhausted from catering to George.

Carol helped George get out of bed and asked him to walk around the room. After some initial unsteadiness, George demonstrated he was able to walk around the living room without losing his balance. Next, Carol tested George on the steps. He was wobbly and frightened, but she knew he would be able to go up and down the steps at least once a day. The upstairs bathroom was next. Here, Carol met more resistance. George had had his stroke in this bathroom and didn't feel too comfortable about reentering it. A quick look inside told Carol that a folding chair in front of the sink would help, and a goose-necked mirror would permit him to shave while sitting down.

Carol helped George set up the bathroom. He had no problem sitting on the toilet or standing up from a seated position on the toilet seat. However, the bathtub-shower combination did pose some real problems for George. Two years earlier he had had sliding glass doors installed to enclose the tub. While the doors did permit a nice steamy shower, they now posed a safety hazard for George. It would be much safer for George to take a shower sitting down, and with George's intermittent balance problem, a tub bench and grab bars were a real necessity. When Carol suggested they consider removing the doors, George and Sara declined, insisting that in a few weeks, when he would be "all better," it wouldn't be necessary.

Carol knew that although some further improvement could be expected, the glass tub enclosure would still present an unsafe obstacle. In time George and Sarah would realize that he would be operating from an amended baseline of wellness—a state in which he would slowly be getting well, but without full return of all his abilities for a long time, or perhaps not at all. His balance could be unsure for months, although physical and functional ability might return to his left arm. Sarah asked if they could rent a tub bench that would work in their tub—to tide them over until George got "back to himself." Carol gave them the name and manufacturer of a suitable tub bench.

Carol's years as a therapist had taught her that readjustment takes time. Forcing patients to modify or change things too dramatically before they're ready to make those changes is a mistake. Sara and George needed time to establish new routines. George probably would not return to his job as an estimator, Carol guessed, and he might have to take early retirement, or he could find another less demanding job—but those decisions did not have to be made right at the moment.

The "right this minute" actions and decisions for George and Sarah should relate to resuming healthy living patterns. Primarily, that meant no hospital bed; it simply was not needed. George had to learn to function to the best of his ability with whatever residual disability he had.

Carol wrote down a series of suggestions and tips for Sara and George and for the home health aide expected later in the day, then made an appointment for the following week. "And George," she said as she was leaving, "I want to see you in street clothes next Monday, not your pajamas."

The guidelines Carol gave to George and his wife could apply to most people recovering from an illness in which there had been a change of functional and physical ability. Basically, Carol suggested that George should pursue healthy behavior, with as much immediate independence as possible. With the assistance of an OT or a home health aide, if necessary, George and Sara should institute as much normalcy in their living situation as possible. That meant George should eat in the kitchen or dining room, sleep in the bedroom, and use at least some of the furniture already in the home. Shaving, washing, and dressing each day would promote a greater feeling of well-being. Staying in bed all day would weaken the body and promote depression.

The sense of self-esteem and self-worth that results from being able to take care of oneself is important. This does not necessarily mean that the person does absolutely everything for himself each day. Once he realizes he is and can be self-sufficient in dressing or bathing, for example, he may choose not to do some routine chores at times, mainly to conserve energy or to allow someone else to complete the task more quickly.

For George to be independent, he had to be taught to select his own clothing from his closet or bureau. Initially, he could not use the bottom drawer because he would have fallen over. By bringing a chair over to his dresser, he was then able to sit down and select the socks and shorts he wanted to wear. The problem was solved. George might not do this task each day (probably his wife would frequently select his clothes), but he would know that it was within his own ability. He would not have to sit and wait for Sara in order to get dressed.

Goals Are Important

Whether you are six or sixty, ill or well or somewhere in between, you are living in a goal-oriented society. Today, you may be seeing the results of what happened in your life yesterday. Your thoughts and dreams for tomorrow form the basis for your goals, plans, and actions today. Hobbies and other enjoyable activities result in a sense of accomplishment, health, and well-being. Whether it's through gardening, cooking, stamp collecting, painting, reading, or writing, each day will have more meaning if there is a sense of purpose upon arising and a sense of accomplishment at the end of the day. Social exchange, with visits to and from friends and relatives, and perhaps rejoining a community center and attending concerts and social functions, are all part of getting on with living.

Recreational and diversional activities work well as a refreshing outlet for the patient. The good feelings engendered can flow over to help with the recovery process. The particular activities will vary with each individual, but whatever the choices, they should be a source of pleasure and enjoyment for the patient.

If television is one of the choices, be assured that there's nothing wrong with watching television, either in the daytime or at night. If this is a form of relaxation and recreation for the patient, by all means encourage him to go ahead with it. Be aware, though, of the danger always lurking in the background where TV is concerned—it's very easy to let it take over your life. Having to stay at home for days or weeks or months can wreak a lot of damage on the human spirit. Television far too often provides a seemingly easy way of handling the depression that can set in with the patient.

The problem arises when TV watching becomes an end in itself—a daily habit that allows the patient no time to explore all the other ways the quality of life can be improved in a home health care situation.

For example, if the patient has full use of his or her hands, he or she can write, draw, paint, sculpt, knit, play chess or checkers with a friend, to name only a few possible activities. In fact, all these things, and more, can be done without full use of the hands.

There's always the telephone. It's the patient's link with the outside world, with friends, relatives, and even strangers. If the patient wishes, the phone can be used to make daily calls to some truly housebound people, giving them the same contact with others that the patient himself may need. The telephone can be a source of pleasure for both the patient and those whom he contacts.

Hobbies? Almost all of them can be followed. Photography, for example, offers the opportunity for the expression of inner emotions and the person's unique view of the world around him, the same as painting or the other visual arts. Depending on the degree of the disability, almost all types of photographic equipment can be used in pursuit of this hobby. Being confined to home should not restrict the patient's photographic interest. For example, a recent book by a woman photographer consists only of photographs taken over the years from a window in her apartment overlooking Central Park in New York City. The photographs have received high praise—and the photographer was not disabled or confined to home in any way. She saw the potential in photographs from her window, and made the most of it.

If the patient is able to move about and get outdoors, gardening offers still another means of recreation and relaxation. If mobility is restricted, there are still many opportunities for indoor gardening.

Billiards, woodworking, indoor shuffleboard, swimming, playing a musical instrument, singing—all of these and many others are activities the patient can engage in. There's freedom here—freedom to pick and choose, freedom to enjoy, but most of all, freedom for the patient to improve and sustain the quality of life.

Some people seek to participate in group activities; others are loners. If the loners were more socially oriented prior to the onset of illness, the quest for isolation, brought on by initial depression, may be short-lived, especially if there is encouragement from friends and others to rejoin groups and take part in social activities.

The person on home health care should select activities that are within his or her physical and functional ability. If any activity poses a problem—for example, starting or revitalizing a coin or stamp collection, despite a decline in vision—this activity may be shared with friends as they visit. The activity works as a focus of conversation (rather than the medical problem), and guest and patient enjoy a purposeful activity together. The choices are many, from crafts and art to music, games, literature, and domestic activities. There are many outside resources that will provide learning as well as companionship—schools, libraries, museums, concerts, and specialized classes at the local community center, such as cooking or drawing and painting. (See the Appendix for more suggestions.)

Conserve Energy and Plan Ahead

Good planning can make all the difference between mere survival and an enjoyable and enriching life—whatever the patient's age and whatever the abilities or disabilities.

Pat Kaye, for example, loved to entertain. She had always enjoyed the laughter and the talk that flowed during a dinner party or tea in her home. A year ago, Pat tripped and fell outside a local supermarket. Although she did not break a hip or a leg in the fall, it did result in a hairline fracture in an ankle. There's a limit now to the amount of walking and standing she is able to tolerate before the pain becomes so unbearable that strong medication is necessary. The medication has the undesirable side effect of making her drowsy.

Her first dinner party following the accident showed her how to cope with her disability and become a better planner. While shopping and food preparation were kept to a minimum (it was a potluck supper and each of the guests brought a prepared dish), organizing for the party proved to be quite a challenge. Pat never realized just how many trips she routinely made between the cupboard and the dining room table just to set the table. First the plates, then the glasses (only two or three at a time), then the silverware and serving pieces. Although the dining table was just fifteen feet from the kitchen cupboard, she must have walked the equivalent of two or three city blocks just to set the table and prepare for the party. By the time her guests arrived she was exhausted, and she promised herself she would do it differently next time.

Her next dinner party was far more enjoyable. Although her strength and endurance had not changed, her approach to the tasks at hand was considerably different. A decorative tea cart on wheels that had been gathering dust in a corner of the dining room for years now became a most helpful aid. With one well-planned trip, all the dishware, glasses, and serving pieces were tranported from the kitchen cupboard to the dining table on the cart. By rolling the cart around the table, each place setting was arranged without difficulty. The entire process was completed with one trip around the table. Pat also realized that the table could be set earlier in the day, or even the day before, to allow adequate time to rest.

It's helpful for all of us to plan ahead and conserve energy, but the finite energy reserves following an illness demand that more attention be paid to how the day's supply of energy is spent. If this one-day supply of energy were likened to a cupful of water, consider the following: Over the course of the day, the cupful of energy is dipped into and spent on a variety of physical and emotional activities. Washing, dressing, and shaving may use up more energy for some people than others. Argument, conflict, and stress soak up their share. Unless the cup is replenished by rest and relaxation, there may not be enough energy available to participate in a full day's activities. With only one cupful of energy available each day, careful planning helps conserve and spend energy efficiently. As Pat Kaye discovered, there are numerous techniques and devices to help maximize function and efficiency. (See "Tips for Daily Living," pages 166–191.)

In order to conserve energy, you need to plan ahead, to list all the things you want to do, set priorities, plan for rest and recreation, and delegate the chores or tasks that others can do for you. By discussing these chores, tasks, and priorities, both the caregiver and the patient will be working toward achieving a higher energy level and a more enjoyable day. If this sounds like the teachings of a compulsive list-maker, your're right. But I believe that planning and scheduling are helpful as new habits and new circumstances are encountered. Using lists directs attention to situations and activities that are so routine we pay little attention to them. By thinking through a day's activities, the patient and caregiver together may learn, for example, that the patient stands up in many situations when he could be sitting down. Or they may see that gardening and photography, two hobbies that the patient particularly wants to enjoy, usually have been started in the late afternoon, when the patient is too tired to enjoy them properly.

The patient and the caregiver should try preparing a workable time plan, listing the chores and activities that must be done and being sure to include those special activities that the patient *wants* to do. Give some thought to the patient's energy cycle (and the caregiver's, too!), and then create a schedule for the next few days that includes enjoyment and recreation time. Be sure to allow for rest periods after each major task. Follow the plan, and adjust it as it becomes apparent where it did and did not work.

It's not easy to change routines and habits that have taken a lifetime to develop. However, simple changes now can make a considerable difference in the quality of the patient's living situation, enabling him to pursue his favorite activities.

A Perspective on Chronic Illness

There are few things more profoundly disturbing than discovering that someone you love and care about has a problem that will not go away. It can happen when you see a parent or an elderly relative show the increasing effects of advancing age by becoming less active and more forgetful. It can happen when a brother or a wife begins to have the complications of diabetes that you had known about only through books or stories about others in the family. And it can happen when there's been a diagnosis of some progressive incurable disease. Whether the illness may ultimately immobilize the body, as can happen with the motor neuron disease amyotrophic lateral sclerosis (ALS—"Lou Gehrig's disease") or destroy the mind, as can happen with Alzheimer's disease, learning the diagnosis of an illness and possible course of an illness can be devastating. The outcome of an illness is usually impossible to predict. The fantasy of what may happen can actually be more debilitating than the disease itself.

Dwelling on all the possible problems of the future can be nonproductive, and trying to identify solutions for problems that have not as yet occurred can waste considerable emotional energy.

On the other hand, some patients do feel that the diagnosis of a progressive or chronic illness, such as Parkinson's disease, now gives them license to make unreasonable demands on other family members. Previously they may have tried unsuccessfully to manipulate a family member to do things for them, and they now seek to cultivate guilt feelings in the family member to achieve the desired response. Dr. I. S. Cooper, in, *Living with Chronic Neurologic Disease*, describes the case of a woman who suffered from a moderately advanced stage of parkinsonism. Although she was able to manage with minimal assistance, she used her early symptoms literally to terrorize her adult children into doing things for her and taking care of her. In fact, one of her sons moved his entire family into his mother's home to be better able to care for her. The result was that the entire expanded family was manipulated into becoming locked into her illness. The more she infiltrated their lives—and the more they did for her—the more incapacitated and dependent she became, further imprisoning them.

There needs to be an objective assessment of what is appropriate behavior in this kind of situation. There has to be a balance between compassion and common sense. The mere announcement of a potentially progressive illness is not necessarily a death decree. As Jacob Javits, himself an ALS sufferer, stated in May 1984 to an audience of physicians and other health professions, "We are all terminal—we all die sometime—so why should a terminal illness be different from terminal life? There is no difference."

Most chronic illnesses evolve and progress over time. The diagnosis of Alzheimer's may be made years before any real incapacity becomes evident, and the knowledge that someone we care for has Parkinson's disease does not demand that we abandon our own lives and devote it to taking care of that person. What, then, is a reasonable course of action? The primary requirement is that, although you are actively concerned and involved in what has happened, you must still leave adequate room for the individual to take responsibility for himself.

Learn all you can about the illness or condition. Armed with knowledge of available treatments, therapeutic alternatives, and the short-term and long-term outlook, you may be able to deal with the situation more objectively. Consider the personality and physical and emotional strengths of the person being cared for, and try to identify resources and support groups that will build on and reinforce these strengths. Avoid trying to do too much. Any excessive efforts on your part as the caregiver may deny the patient's individuality. By encouraging independence and self-sufficiency, you are helping to maintain and build the all important sense of self-worth and self-esteem. Loss of independence results in feelings of depression and despair. Provide information about resources if it is requested, but acknowledge that this individual is an adult and must make the ultimate decision to pursue any course of action on his own. It is, after all, his life—and he does have the right to handle it in his own way. Imposing your will— and winning—may result in damaging any real sense of independence the patient may have.

Balance your responsibilities as a caregiver with the other priorities in your life and with the reality of the physical and emotional conditions that exist in the situation. While there may well become a time when your active involvement is essential, there's no need to abandon your life and your priorities every moment of each day. Use the informational and self-help support resources that are available. There is much to be learned from others who have gone (or are going) through a similar situation. And many of the support groups that do exist welcome family members as well as patients. Most important, be sure to take care of yourself! Plan for and *do* the things that make you feel good about yourself. The better you feel about yourself and the stronger and healthier you are, the better able you will be to pitch in and be of assistance to someone you love.

Learning to Cope: Day by Day

Imagine the frustration of staring into a well-stocked refrigerator only to see that each of the containers is sealed. If you are thirsty and you have one good hand (the other hand, may have been weakened by a stroke, for example) are you destined to wait until someone returns home to uncork or unscrew the wanted thirst quencher? That's foolish! There are tricks of the trade and gadgets specially designed to help those who have been disabled by illness.

A list of equipment and some major suppliers can be found in the Appendix. You may want to order their catalogs and experiment on your own, or you may find it more efficient to ask the occupational therapist to do an activities of daily living (ADL) evaluation. Your local hospital's rehabilitation department or the American Occupational Therapy Association should be able to suggest a choice of licensed therapists. If the local pharmacist has a home health care department, he may be able to help. He certainly should be able to put you in touch with occupational therapists in your community.

According to Ann Goldberg, an occupational therapist on Long Island's North Shore, "Everyone has a right to know that they can function independently. And most people can learn to use all the resources available to them more efficiently."

Calling in an OT for advice and consultation and to provide tips and guidance can make a world of difference for the patient between depressing dependence and energizing independence. The OT's professional fee at this point is an investment in expertise and can save many times the cost of the fee in purchases you might make on your own that could turn out to be ineffective or useless. Most OTs have a solid familiarity with the gadgets and equipment available to assist the home health care patient in maintaining greater freedom and independence. Also, the OT will know when a homemade substitute will work just as well or better than a manufactured item—an important consideration when you are trying to keep costs down.

At the end of this chapter you will find tables with "Tips for Daily Living." It is here, too, that consultation with an OT will be helpful. The tables list many special devices and aids for use in helping the home health care patient accomplish many of the various tasks encountered during the course of a day. The OT can advise you as to the feasibility of purchasing some of these aids, especially if the disability suffered by the patient will be relatively brief.

For short-term use of any of these aids, it would be a good idea to check with your physician or therapist concerning possible sources where you may obtain some of the aids either on loan or at reduced costs. You can also contact the local chapters of appropriate support groups and associations (Multiple Sclerosis Society, Arthritis Foundation, etc.), who may also be able to help (see the Appendix).

Unfortunately, gadgets, devices, and other aids that are not medically necessary, even though they improve the quality of life for the patient, are not covered by Medicare. Although it's unlikely that other third-party payers will cover such items, be sure to check any private health insurance policy the patient has to see whether coverage might be provided for certain aids or devices.

Many of the devices listed in the table can be made at home out of materials and items already in the home or that can be purchased for nominal sums at local discount stores. Ingenuity will pay dividends here.

There is, of course, more to home health care than carefully following a medical treatment plan for the patient—making sure that medications are taken at the proper time in the prescribed dosage, changing wound dressings, keeping required records, charting progress for the nurse or physician, and all the other details the caregiver has to keep in mind. Above and beyond all this is the matter of daily living. The patient and the caregiver have to work together to maintain a good quality of life for the patient, and this means setting things up so the patient can be as independent as possible, despite any handicaps or disabilities.

MANAGING DAILY ACTIVITIES WITH ONE HAND

No matter what the cause of the disability, the patient with the ability to use only one hand will have difficulties with tasks that previously had been performed with two hands. The difficulties need not all be insurmountable, though. The human mind and body can make remarkable adjustments over a period of time to compensate for a disabling condition. Also, occupational therapists, researchers, inventors, medical professionals, and many others, including everyday people with no particular previous training, have managed to devise various techniques and special aids to assist an individual in performing one-handed activities. The tables at the end of the chapter show how it can be done.

MANAGING WITH LIMITED FLEXIBILITY
AND REACH

The tips offered in the tables below address basic tasks that are of special importance to people who use ambulation aids. Because one or both hands are occupied with holding or maneuvering the cane or crutches, carrying items can be troublesome. The right technique and/or assistive aid will help to accomplish the task safely and efficiently. ing your hair may now become exhausting, painful, and difficult. People living each day in a restricting brace because of severe back problems, or in a cast or traction device, will welcome the assistance provided by the right technique or device. Because of the range of problems and equipment available, the suggestions offered in the tables below for coping with limited flexibility and reach will not apply to everyone in all situations. A physical therapist or occupational therapist can aid in identifying which self-help device is most appropriate for the patient.

MOVING ABOUT WITH AMBULATION AIDS

Canes, crutches, and walkers are manufactured in an astounding variety of models and styles. Once the physician has prescribed an aid and the physical therapist has selected the aid that works best for the patient, it is often further modified for a custom fit. Although the selection of the right ambulation aid depends on the patient's abilities and disability, the therapist can also help the patient get the most effective use from various aids. For example, a cane may provide the modest support needed most of the time, but a walker will be an absolute necessity for long walks, during which the patient may tire.

In some circumstances, a wheelchair may be the better choice. The physical therapist will consider the patient's functional needs and home and work environment. The right ambulation aid not only helps the patient "get from here to there," it also offers ease, efficiency, and safety to allow the patient to function independently.

The tips offered in the tables below address basic tasks that are of special importance to people who use ambulation aids. Because one or both hands are occupied with holding or maneuvering the cane or crutches, carrying items can be troublesome. The right technique and/or assistive aid will help to accomplish the task safely and efficiently.

People with leg impairments should seek to do as much as possible from a seated position so as to rest the legs while leaving the hands free. However, this may mean that often repeated sit-down and stand-up motions may call for special attention.

In addition, moving about with an ambulation aid means that extra energy is expended. Energy conservation is a must in order to avoid falls or accidents that are the result of walking about while overtired. If the cane, crutch, or other ambulation aid is needed for assistance while the patient is attempting to move around, easy access to the aid must be assured at all time.

USING A WHEELCHAIR

Whether you are renting or buying a wheelchair, it is most important to obtain professional assistance to assure that it is properly selected and fitted. Wheelchairs come in all sizes and shapes, in varying styles and widths, and with different types of wheels, brakes, and accessories. Consulting a trained rehabilitation therapist is essential for safe wheelchair operation and use, proper positioning, and patient comfort. The rehabilitation therapist considers the abilities and disabilities of the individual, the home and work environment, and other life style considerations. When his evaluation has been completed, the therapist may select and recommend any of the following:

a motorized chair
a one-hand-driven chair
a lightweight chair, easily folda-
    ble, to place in the car
knobs added to the wheels to
    make propelling the chair
    easier
adjustable/removable leg rests
removable arm rests to permit
    easy sliding transfers

recessed, desk-height arm rests
    to slide under a table or desk
foam or gel cushions for comfort
    and to prevent skin break-
    down and pressure sores
thick cushions to raise the person
    higher in the chair
harnesses and safety straps
special brakes

Once the right chair is selected and modified to meet the special needs of its user, it should be maintained in good working order.

In using a wheelchair, accessibility is a key consideration. Can all rooms in the house, including the bathroom, be entered in the wheelchair? This means wide doorways, adequate room to turn and move around, few stair steps (preferably none at all), and smooth, uncarpeted floors.

Are all activities doable from the wheelchair? Are countertops too high? Are faucets easy to reach? Do closet doors and cupboards get in the way?

The need to use the wheelchair in the bathroom will depend on the abilities and disability of the person involved. Someone with a spinal cord injury may need to use the chair to enter the bathroom and transfer to the toilet or to a tub bench. Most certainly, the wise and practical guidance of an occupational therapist is essential here. The series of activities of daily living—washing, dressing, food preparation, food serving, cleanup, housekeeping chores, recreational activities—all should be evaluated on an individual basis by the occupational therapist, who will then be able to provide recommendations that will help the patient to be as independent as possible.

Once again, the suggestions offered here and in the tables below do not apply to everyone or in all situations, but are noted here to spark your imagination and to suggest alternatives for consideration.

THE BEDBOUND PATIENT

When a nurse or therapist talks with you about helping a person confined to bed, the first question they usually ask is: Are you sure the patient can't get out of bed and into a chair, even for a short time each day?

Today, even in acute care hospitals, patients are encouraged, cajoled, and even carried out of bed for at least a short period of time. Post-surgical patients are up and walking within days, and poststroke patients spend time out of bed reclining or sitting in a chair. Health professionals agree that it is physically and psychologically debilitating to remain in bed all day, every day. Blood circulation is hampered. Also, there is concern about skin breakdown (pressure sores), which can result from continuous pressure exerted on the skin by the bony areas of the body pressing the skin against the mattress and cutting off circulation (see Chapter 10, "Pressure Sores").

Some circumstances, however, demand that the patient remain in bed. A person in traction or on bed rest for weeks or even months because of back injury will be "bedbound" for an extended period of time. Also, the very ill and debilitated patient—perhaps on chemotherapy or recovering from a major medical crisis—will be confined to bed.

Although it is assumed that a completely paralyzed patient, confined to bed, will be cared for by health professionals (or by trained family members), there are tips to be found in the tables below that may suggest alternatives to the caregiver. Other patients on bed rest will feel better when the means to be as independent as possible are provided. Of course, this depends on the age, illness, abilities, and disability of the individual.

Priorities play an important role here. For people with reduced stamina, it may make better sense to provide considerable assistance with many of the routine tasks of washing and grooming so that whatever energy the patient has can be devoted to social exchanges, hobbies, and other enjoyable activities.

In many situations, people do feel better about themselves when they can actively participate in their own self-care. Providing such opportunites for the bedbound individual requires patience and understanding.

In the following tables the tasks of daily living for the home care patient have been broken down for convenience and easy reference into seven major categories:

> *Table* 9. GROOMING AND PERSONAL CARE
> *Table* 10. DRESSING
> *Table* 11. FOOD PREPARATION
> *Table* 12. EATING AND DRINKING
> *Table* 13. HOUSEHOLD CHORES
> *Table* 14. SPORTS AND RECREATION
> *Table* 15. GENERAL ACTIVITIES

In essence, the tables provide "recipes for independence" that have worked well in the past for many patients. Use them as guides to help you reach the goal of greater freedom and independence for the home health care patient.

Table 9 ■ TIPS FOR DAILY LIVING: GROOMING AND PERSONAL CARE†

Technique	*Special aids*	*Disability**
WASHING HANDS		
Wear a terry cloth mitt over the impaired hand. By rubbing the good hand over the terry-covered hand, you will be able to scrub the functioning hand.	Terry cloth mitt	A
Use a long-handled sponge to help reach hard-to-reach areas.	Long-handled sponge	A B
Wear soap on a rope around your neck to eliminate the hazards of dropping the soap.	Soap on a rope	A B C D
Use a suction-mounted nail brush to clean nails.	Suction-mounted nail brush	A B
Use a water-filled basin with a wash mitt. Some commercially available mitts have a pocket in the palm to hold soap.	Mitt with soap pocket	E
BRUSHING TEETH		
Hold toothpaste tube between knees to stabilize it while unscrewing cap with good hand. Place toothbrush on sink top with bristles up. Use good hand to guide toothpaste onto brush.		A
Use battery-operated toothbrush (and basin of water if bed-bound).	Battery-operated toothbrush	A B E
Use a toothbrush with a jointed handle extension to minimize arm movement.	Toothbrush with jointed handle extension	A B E

† If the patient cannot stand at the sink when performing any of the grooming and personal care activities (brushing teeth, shaving, etc.), a straight chair or a wheelchair can be placed at the sink. A lowered sink, if structurally and financially feasible, will help.

*Disability key:

A	One-handed	**C**	With ambulation aids	**E**	Bed-bound
B	Limited reach	**D**	Using wheelchair		

(Table 9 continued)

Technique	Special aids	Disability*
FLOSSING TEETH		
Use dental floss aid designed for one-hand use.	One-hand dental floss aid	A B E
DENTURE CLEANING		
Use suction-mounted denture brush.	Suction-mounted denture brush	A B
SHAVING		
Use a soap dish or suction holder to hold the shaving cream. Dab on cream with the good hand, then rinse hand under tap. Use razor carefully. If grasp is weak, a built-up handle may help	Suction-mounted soap holder	A B
Use a razor with a jointed handle extension to minimize arm movement	Razor with jointed handle extension	A B E
Use an electric or battery-operated razor. If grasp is weak, a razor holder may help. Mount an electric or battery-powered razor on a gooseneck arm, and shave by moving face against razor	Gooseneck mount	A B C D E
Use roll-on deodorant bottles to hold and apply aftershave lotion		
Sitting down may make a world of difference. Rest elbows on table or sink	Mirror or extension mirror that tilts	B C D
APPLYING MAKEUP		
Use a mirror mounted at a convenient height on the wall, or a gooseneck-mounted mirror that can be positioned for easy visibility	Gooseneck mount	A B D E

(Table 9 continued)

Technique	Special aids	Disability*
HAIR GROOMING		
Use a comb or brush with a jointed extension handle to minimize arm movement	Comb or brush with jointed extension handle	A B E
A large-handled comb and brush may be easier to use. You can buy these ready-made or make your own by using foam hair rollers on the handles	Large-handled comb and brush	A B E
Use a wall-mounted holder for the hair dryer to dry the hair while styling it with the functional hand	Wall-mounted hair dryer holder	A B
Try clip-on or velcro curlers to set the hair		B C D E
Choose a short, simple, easy-to-care-for hair style		A B C D E
Keep shampoo in applicator bottles. Use old liquid soap bottles that have an easy pop-up spout		A B C D E
Shampoo sitting down in the shower or tub. Assemble all rinses, soaps, etc., before turning on the shower		A B C D
Use a molded plastic rinse tray with a comfortable neck rest to wash and rinse hair. There's also a shampoo tray available with an inflatable ring and a large drain tube to carry rinse water into a pail. (The patient will need assistance here.)	Plastic shampoo rinse tray or inflatable shampoo kit	B D E
GENERAL GROOMING		
Keep all grooming aids in easy reach in a carry-all that sits securely on the bed, bedside table, or tray table	Carry-all	A B C D E

(Table 9 continued)

Technique	Special aids	Disability*
Use an extension-handle holder— a long handle with a pocket for holding a variety of grooming aids	Extension-handle holder	A B C D E
If grasp is poor, build up the handle of the extender with adhesive tape or a foam roller	Various grooming aids (comb, brush, etc.) with built-up and enlarged handles are available commercially	A B C D E
Use a cuff-handle extension device, which is fastened to a cuff that fits over the palm of the hand, eliminating the need to grasp the object	Cuff-handle extension	A B E
Use a tray table with a mirror attachment as an aid in grooming	Tray table with mirror	A B C D E
A flexible-mount mirror mounted on a side table can be positioned for best visibility wherever the patient is seated	Side table with flexible-mount mirror	A B C D E

TOILETING

Technique	Special aids	Disability*
There are hygiene aids of varying lengths, adjustable to varying angles, to help people with limited arm motion cleanse themselves after eliminating	Toileting hygiene aid	A B E
Toilet paper held in tongs can be used if the patient has some flexibility and motion	Toilet paper tongs	A B E

(Continued on next page)

Disability key:

A	One-handed	C	With ambulation aids	E	Bed-bound
B	Limited reach	D	Using wheelchair		

(Table 9 continued)

Technique	Special aids	Disability*
Toilets can be equipped with a bidet seat, enabling the person to wash himself with a stream of water. There are electrically equipped bidet seats that will also dry with a stream of warm air	Bidet seats (some use water from a pitcher, which flows into the bidet by gravity)	A B C D
A multipurpose commode chair on wheels can help. Without its cushion, the chair can be rolled to straddle most toilets. It's narrower than many wheelchairs and may fit through bathroom doors	Multipurpose commode chair	A B C D E
Use a raised toilet seat to help a person who has difficulty sitting or standing. Depending on the model, the toilet seat can be raised 4–8 inches higher	Raised toilet seat (both portable and permanently installed models are available)	A B C D
Grab bars mounted near the toilet can be a real help. For best results, they must be positioned properly and offer sturdy, secure support. Consult a trained rehabilitation therapist to help select the safest and easiest-to-use equipment. If possible, test out a few models before selecting	Grab bars are available in numerous styles and sizes	A B C D
A bedside commode chair is usually preferred to a bedpan. Toilet tissue can be mounted on the commode or kept within easy reach	Bedside commode	E

WASHING, BATHING, SHOWERING

Long-handled sponges help in hard-to-reach areas. If there is a hinge in the handle, the angle can be changed to scrub the	Long-handled sponge	A B C D

(Table 9 continued)

Technique	Special aids	Disability*
back with a minimum of shoulder movement		
If there is limited movement and flexibility, feet can be washed with a washcloth held in a pair of tongs or wrapped around a long rod	Tongs to hold wash-cloth	A B C D
Hang soap-on-a-rope around the neck for handy use and easy retrieval	Soap-on-a-rope	A B C D E
A hand-held shower head helps you enjoy the shower safely, sitting down. Many types are available	Hand-held shower head	A B C D
Use a tub bench in the bathtub. Select it carefully. The right tub bench—right height and safest and easiest to use—is essential for safe seating in the tub. If possible, consult an occupational therapist	Tub bench	A B C D
Use a sliding board to transfer from a straight chair or a wheelchair to the tub bench. Lubricating the sliding board allows smoother transfer when the person is wet and nude. Try using a body lotion. Professional guidance will help here also	Sliding board	C D
Well-placed grab bars are essential for safety in the tub or shower	Grab bars	A B C D
If the person is bedbound but can sit up in bed, a water-filled basin can be used		E

Disability key:

A	One-handed	**C**	With ambulation aids	**E**	Bed-bound
B	Limited reach	**D**	Using wheelchair		

Table 10 ■ TIPS FOR DAILY LIVING: DRESSING

Technique	Special aids	Disability*
DRESSING		
Easy-care fabrics, knits, and stretchable fabrics are elastic and easier to manage. Loose-fitting clothing is easier to get on. If shoulder mobility is limited, use blouses or shirts with wider armholes for easier slipping on		ABCDE
Wear clothing that can be buttoned or zipped up the front. If arm flexibility is not a problem, a pullover can be worn. If buttons or zippers present difficulties, replace them with Velcro closures. (Remember, the Velcro fastener must be closed when laundering or it will catch on the other clothing and also collect lint.)	Velcro fasteners	ABCDE
When dressing, slip weakened arm into sleeve first, then stronger arm		AB
Use elastic thread or a button extender to allow neckline and cuff fastenings to be closed before dressing. When clothing is slipped on, fastenings will stretch and then close after garment is on	Elastic thread and button extender	ABCDE
Button hooks can help in looping buttons through buttonholes	Button hook	ABDE
Use elastic at waistbands on skirts and pants rather than back or side buttons		ABCD

Disability key:

A One-handed	**C** With ambulation aids	**E** Bed-bound
B Limited reach	**D** Using wheelchair	

Table 10 (continued)

Technique	Special aids	Disability*
Jumpers, wraparound skirts, and slacks with front closures are easier for many people		ABCD
Front-closing bras are easier to put on. A stretch elastic bra can be fastened in front, then slipped around in back. Velcro closures can be used to replace bra hooks	Velcro fasteners	ABCDE
Neckties can be left loosely tied, then slipped over the head and tightened. Or a tie can be knotted around a loop of elastic, which can then be slipped around the neck and hidden under the collar		AB
Wheelchair skirts, long in front and short in back, may be more comfortable.		D
Loops can be added to a zipper to help pull it		AB
If there is limited arm motion, or if bending is a problem, use a dressing hook to help pull on and remove clothing. A dressing hook can be purchased, or you can make one from a dowel rod and a cup hook, which can be found at any community hardware store. If desired, you can use special china cup hooks that have a spring-clip "holder" on the hook, which closes after the hook is engaged. This will keep a zipper or a skirt loop from slipping out of the hook. Two dressing hooks can be used to latch on to loops on each side of a skirt or pair of pants to help pull up the garment	Dressing hooks or cup hooks and dowel rods	ABCD

Table 10 (continued)

Technique	Special aids	Disability*
Stocking and sock helpers (similar to dressing hooks) are an aid in putting on socks, stockings, and pantyhose. They are available in many styles	Stocking helpers	A B C D E
Slip-on shoes (loafers) or shoes with permanently tied elastic laces will make putting on shoes easier. Make sure the laces are not too tight as this can cause swelling of the feet. (If you have circulation problems, check with your doctor before using elastic laces.)	Elastic laces	A B C D
Use a long-handled shoe horn to help put on shoes	Long-handled shoe horn	A B C D
Use a boot jack to help remove shoes from a standing or seated position	Boot jack	A B C D
Rain ponchos offer good protection in rain	Rain poncho	A B C D
Comfortable clothing worn in bed—and changed often—promotes feeling better. Heavy or wrinkly fabrics can be uncomfortable		E

Table 11 ■ TIPS FOR DAILY LIVING: FOOD PREPARATION

Technique	Special aids	Disability*
GENERAL PREPARATIONS		
Use a damp sponge cloth or suction cups to stabilize bowls and boards	Suction cups	A B C D
A tap turner increases leverage for turning sink faucets on or off	Tap turner	A B C D

Disability key:

A One-handed	C With ambulation aids	E Bed-bound
B Limited reach	D Using wheelchair	

Table 11 (continued)

Technique	Special aids	Disability*
A knob turner increases leverage for turning dials on a stove	Knob turner	A B C D
A "contour" turning handle helps in operating any rotating knob or handle, increasing leverage for the user	Contour turning handle	A B C D
Organize and store dishes and pots and pans to minimize lifting or moving other items to reach the most frequently used items. Carefully store often-used appliances and other heavy items so they are within safe and easy reach		A B C D
Use a "reacher" (similar to old-fashioned grocery store tongs) to reach for and grasp items stored beyond the range of reach or motion	Reacher	A B C D
Use a lazy Susan to limit reaching for items stored on a deep shelf	Lazy Susan	A B C D
Organize food stored in the refrigerator to permit easy access with minimal need to lift and push items around		A B C D
If seated at the stove (on a chair, stool, or wheelchair) a well-placed mirror hung over the stove and angled properly will allow you to see the contents of pots and pans		B C D
If in a wheelchair and countertops are too high, use a lap board attachment to the wheelchair to put your work surface at the right height. The lap board can also be used to carry items around the kitchen	Wheelchair lap board attachment	D
If the sink and faucets are difficult to reach, keep a water container in an easy-to-reach location		B C D

Table 11 (continued)

Technique	Special aids	Disability*
If feasible, the kitchen can be modified to provide open-space leg room under the counters so the person can work while seated or in a wheelchair		BCD

OPENING CANS

Technique	Special aids	Disability*
Use a hand-held electric can opener or a table top opener to permit easy opening of cans	Electric can opener	ABCD

OPENING JARS AND BOTTLES

Technique	Special aids	Disability*
Use a screw cap opener to increase leverage when opening jars and bottles. The opener is made of flexible rubber and is tapered inside to fit most bottle caps	Screw cap opener	ABCD
Mount a Zim jar opener on the wall near the work area. This opener has a deep V-shaped wedge lined with steel teeth that grasp the cover as you turn the jar. Wall-mounted jar and bottle openers of various types are available in stores and by mail order	Zim jar opener	ABCD
Portable lightweight Zyliss jar openers can open tubes of tooth-paste and instant coffee jars	Zyliss jar opener	AB
Use an "Un-Skru" jar opener to increase leverage and permit opening jars with one hand	"Un-Skru" jar opener	AB
Use a hip-high drawer to help open a jar. Place the jar upright inside the drawer with the jar top protruding above the top of the drawer. Close the drawer against the jar and hold the drawer shut with your hip. This		AB

Table 11 (continued)

Technique	Special aids	Disability*
will steady the jar while you use your good hand to unscrew the top		

OPENING CONTAINERS

Technique	Special aids	Disability*
Use your knees to hold firmly boxes or bags to be opened		A B C

CARRYING AND MOVING FOOD AND EQUIPMENT

Technique	Special aids	Disability*
Use a cart on wheels to move several items at one time	Wheeled cart	A B C D
Use a wheelchair lap board to carry items	Wheelchair lap board	D
Canvas and plastic pouches and carrying aids can be fastened to a wheelchair or walker	Pouches and carrying aids	C D

FOOD AND UTENSIL STORAGE

Technique	Special aids	Disability*
Group items in the kitchen by use, and store items where they will be used. Create a baking area, a food slicing and cutting area, a cooking area, etc.		A B C D
Add storage aids that are easy to reach and use—pegboards, open shelves, pull-out trays—to permit easy access to frequently used utensils, foods, bowls, and spices	Pegboards, shelves, pullout trays	A B C D
When storing leftovers, ladle soups out of a large pot on the stove before lifting the pot. Store leftovers in cook-and-serve containers	Cook-and-serve containers	A B C D

Disability key:

A	One-handed	**C**	With ambulation aids	**E**	Bed-bound
B	Limited reach	**D**	Using wheelchair		

Table 11 (continued)

Technique	Special aids	Disability*
POURING LIQUIDS FROM LARGE CONTAINERS		
Use a half-gallon carton grip to hold a milk carton while pouring the milk into a pitcher	Half-gallon carton grip	A B C D
CLEANING VEGETABLES		
Use a suction-mounted vegetable brush and clean vegetables by rubbing against brush. (A suction-mounted nail brush will work as well.)	Suction-mounted brush	A B
PEELING OR PARING VEGETABLES		
Use a cutting board equipped with upright stainless steel or aluminum nails. Secure food on nails; lift and rotate to peel or pare underside. A U-shaped peeler will help person with a weak grasp	Cutting board with nails, U-shaped peeler	A B
CUTTING MEATS, FRUITS, AND VEGETABLES		
Stabilize food on cutting board. Use a rocker knife; the curved blade gives a back-and-forth rocking motion that allows easy cutting with one hand	Rocker knife and cutting board	A B
If shoulder or elbow movement is restricted, use a food scissors to cut meats and vegetables rather than a knife	Food scissors	A B
CHOPPING AND BLENDING		
A food processor or electric blender is a helpful aid for chopping, mixing, and blending	Food processor; electric blender	A B C D

Table 11 (continued)

Technique	Special aids	Disability*
LIFTING AND TURNING MEATS AND POULTRY		
An auto fork will help turn and lift meats and poultry. Food is pushed off the tines when the handle of the fork is squeezed, allowing one-handed operation	Auto fork	A B
Use small kitchen tongs for lighter lifting tasks	Kitchen tongs	A B
COOKING VEGETABLES		
Use a wire frying basket, or a pasta cooker basket, to cook vegetables in water. Once the cooking is completed, the food can easily be lifted and removed from the boiling water. Use pot holder mitts to avoid injury	Frying basket or pasta cooker basket	A B C D
SETTING AND CLEARING THE TABLE		
Assemble items on a serving cart with wheels to allow minimum trips back and forth	Wheeled serving cart	A B C
Use wheelchair lap board to assemble items to be moved	Wheelchair lap board	D
CONSERVE ENERGY		
Use a sturdy folding chair in the kitchen, or sit on a rolling chair on wheels	Folding or rolling chair	A B C
While working at the counter, slide bowls or other items along the counter rather than lifting or carrying items		A B C D

*__Disability key:__

A	One-handed	**C**	With ambulation aids	**E**	Bed-bound
B	Limited reach	**D**	Using wheelchair		

Table 11 (continued)

Technique	Special aids	Disability*
Sit to work whenever possible. Use a high stool for working at high counters	High stool	A B C
Use a wheeled cart that can be pushed by hand or with your body to carry things back and forth	Wheeled cart	A B C
When filling pots with water or other liquids to be cooked on the stove, place and empty pot on the stove first and then fill it		A B C D

Table 12 ■ TIPS FOR DAILY LIVING: EATING AND DRINKING

Technique	Special aids	Disability*
USING UTENSILS AND FORKS, KNIVES, AND SPOONS		
If there is limited arm motion, utensils and forks, knives, and spoons with extension handles will permit easier use. Handle shafts usually can be adjusted to a variety of angles	Utensils and forks, knives, and spoons with extension handles and adjustable shafts	A B D E
If there is a spilling problem with spoons or forks, a swivel spoon or fork can overcome the problem. The swivel motion keeps the inner curve of the fork or the bowl of the spoon level no matter how the handle slips or turns in the person's grasp	Swivel spoon or fork	A B D E
Cut food with a small rocker knife, allowing one-handed operation	Rocker knife	A B E
Use tape or foam rollers around the handles of forks, knives, and spoons to provide an easier grip. Utensils with built-up grips can be purchased	Adhesive tape, foam rollers, and built-up utensils	A B E

Table 12 (continued)

Technique	Special aids	Disability*
If the grasp is very weak, there are special utensils available that can be inserted in a cuff designed to slip over the hand, eliminating the need to grasp the utensil by its handle	Cuff-mounted utensils	A B E

DRINKING FROM GLASS AND CUP		
Adhesive strips around a glass provide a more secure grip	Adhesive tape	A B E
Use a glass holder or a mug-shaped cup with handle for easy grasp	Glass holder	A B E
Special cups are available that enable safe, no-spill drinking from a reclining position. A flexible straw may also do the trick	FLO-Trol invalid feeding cup	E
Drinking glasses with handles help if it is difficult to grasp or hold a glass	Glasses with handles	A B E
A plastic glass with a cut-out portion to accommodate the nose will allow a person to drink without tilting or bending the head	Special cut-out glass	A B E
Extra long glass straws, usually with a bend, allow drinking without bending the head. Glass can be stabilized on a rubber pad or with rubber suction cups	Bent glass straws; rubber pads; rubber suction cups	A B E
Use a glass and straw set in a tilting glass holder. The holder will keep the glass steady and will tip to allow the person to reach the straw without bending the head	Tilting glass holder	A B E

Disability key:

A One-handed	**C** With ambulation aids	**E** Bed-bound
B Limited reach	**D** Using wheelchair	

Table 12 (continued)

Technique	Special aids	Disability*
SPECIAL DEVICES AND TECHNIQUES		
Use a sandwich holder to raise a sandwich to the mouth when there is limited arm motion	Sandwich holder	A B E
Box holders and milk carton holders can be used if the person's grasp is weak	Box holders and milk carton holders	A B
Plates and glasses can be kept in place on a serving tray by using a nonslip placemat or tacky material (Dycem™) under plates	Dycem and nonslip placemat	A B E
A piece of bread held in place by a nonfunctioning hand can work as a food pusher		A B E
Use dishes with a raised bumper guard ridge to keep food from spilling off the plate and to allow food to be pushed onto a fork or spoon	Special bumper guard dishes	A B E
Healthful snacks and a beverage (if not medically contraindicated) can be made available and accessible to the bed-bound person to enable the person to snack without assistance when hungry		E

Table 13 ■ TIPS FOR DAILY LIVING: HOUSEHOLD CHORES

Technique	Special aids	Disability*
LAUNDERING AND IRONING		
Use a laundry cart or basket on wheels to transport clothing	Laundry cart or basket on wheels	A B C D
Do small, manageable loads of laundry		A B C D

Disability key:

A	One-handed	C	With ambulation aids	E	Bed-bound
B	Limited reach	D	Using wheelchair		

Table 13 (continued)

Technique	Special aids	Disability*
Place hand washables in a net bag	Net bag	A B C D
Tongs may help to remove clothing from washer	Tongs	A B C D
Presoak laundry in sink if hand washing is preferred. Press clothing into a towel to wring dry		A B C D
Place blouses, slips, and shirts on a hanger while still wet, then hang up to dry		A B C D
Drape hand washables over drying rack or travel clothesline to dry	Drying rack or travel clothesline	A B C D
Spread shirts, towels, and large sheets on table to fold		A B C D
Conserve energy by sitting down to fold laundry. Take frequent rest periods. Use both hands, if possible, to reduce stress on one-handed activity		B C D
Conserve energy by sitting down to iron and using a lightweight iron with a "cord minder"	Lightweight iron with a "cord minder"	A B C D

| VACUUMING, SWEEPING, AND MOPPING |||

Technique	Special aids	Disability*
Use an electric broom on floors and carpeting. Use a sponge mop with a lever for wringing out sponge on floors	Electric broom and sponge mop	A B C D
Use a long-handled dust pan to pick up dirt and debris without bending	Long-handled dust pan	A B C D

| WASHING DISHES |||

Technique	Special aids	Disability*
Use a rubber mat in the sink to reduce risk of breakage	Rubber sink mat	A B C D
Use a suction-mounted brush to wash glasses, bottles, and flatware	Suction-mounted brush	A B C D

Table 13 (continued)

Technique	Special aids	Disability*
If one hand is impaired, have rinse water and drying rack near the functional hand		A B
Dishes can be air-dried rather than wiped dry with a dish towel		A B C D

MAKING THE BED

Technique	Special aids	Disability*
Use a flat sheet for the bottom sheet. Lay the sheet on the center of the bed, using tongs or a reacher if necessary, to open up and spread out the sheet. Use a wooden spatula (similar to a baker's oven paddle with a short handle) to tuck in the sheet all around. If using a fitted sheet, try replacing one corner with extra fabric and a Velcro closure	Tongs, reacher, wooden spatula, Velcro closure	A B C D
Pin top sheet to blanket (or fasten with Velcro) to facilitate bed making		A B C D
Use oversize pillow cases to make slipping on easier		A B C D
Completely make up one side of the bed before going to the other side		A B C D

GENERAL HOUSEKEEPING

Technique	Special aids	Disability*
Store cleaning supplies in various locations in the house where they will be used, for example, extra cleanser in the bathroom, dust cloths in the bedroom		A B C D
Wear an apron with pockets to carry small items		
Plan cleaning activities to assure frequent rest periods		A B C D

Table 13 (continued)

Technique	Special aids	Disability*
Use carts with wheels wherever possible to carry necessary items	Wheeled carts	A B C
A pouch or a caddy can be attached to a walker to provide hands-free carrying. Be careful not to overload the bag, as extra weight may affect the balance of the walker	Walker pouch or caddy	C
Use a waist-tied pouch or a knap-sack to leave your hands free when moving about or working	Waist pouch or knap-sack	A B C
For the bed-bound patient, remove soiled articles and empty wastebaskets as required to keep the room fresh and clean. Arrange items on the bedside table so they are within easy reach of the person		E
Provide a bell or buzzer or cord-less phone for the bed-bound patient and place it within easy reach	Bell, buzzer, or cord-less phone	E
Provide a rope ladder or knotted rope attached to the foot of the bed of the bedbound patient. Let the ladder or rope extend along the top of the bedcovers so the person can use it to pull himself upright. A trapeze bar arrange-ment suspended from the ceil-ing or overhead bed frame can also serve the same purpose	Rope ladder or knotted rope or trapeze bar	E

Disability key:

A One-handed	**C** With ambulation aids	**E** Bed-bound
B Limited reach	**D** Using wheelchair	

Table 14 ■ TIPS FOR DAILY LIVING: SPORTS AND RECREATION

Technique	Special aids	Disability*
PLAYING CARDS		
Extra large cards are easy to see and easier to hold	Oversize cards	A B E
A grooved block of wood can serve as a card holder or use a firm cardboard box turned upside down, placing cards between top and bottom of box	Grooved block of wood	A B E
GARDENING		
A small, sturdy bench will work well in the garden. Sit on it to plant or weed	Small bench	B C
HOBBIES		
A universal support arm attachment can be fastened to a wheelchair or a sturdy folding chair to hold and mount cameras, binoculars, soldering irons, radios, instruction books, etc.	Universal support arm	A B C D
CONCERTS, THEATERS, SPORT EVENTS, ETC.		
The key to attendance at these events is accessibility. Check ahead to learn accessible routes and entrances		B C D
ATHLETIC ACTIVITIES		
There are wheelchair athletic teams and sports events, also a special Olympics for the handicapped. Unless a person is fully		A B C D

Disability key:

A One-handed   **C** With ambulation aids   **E** Bed-bound
B Limited reach   **D** Using wheelchair

Table 14 (continued)

Technique	Special aids	Disability*
homebound or bedbound, athletics are possible. (See the Appendix under "Physical Disability.")		

KNITTING

Technique	Special aids	Disability*
A knitting needle holder allows one-handed work	Knitting needle holder	A B

EMBROIDERY

Technique	Special aids	Disability*
An embroidery hoop with a clamp will stabilize the fabric and permit one-handed operation	Clamp-on embroidery hoop	A B E

Table 15 ▪ TIPS FOR DAILY LIVING: GENERAL ACTIVITIES

Technique	Special aids	Disability*
USING THE TELEPHONE		
A push-button phone with large buttons may be easier to use	Push-button phone with large buttons	B E
Use a pen to dial a rotary phone		A B E
Use a shoulder support for phone to leave hands free	Phone shoulder support	A B C D E
Mount the phone receiver on a gooseneck and place ear to phone, leaving hands free, or rent an operator head set from your local telephone company	Gooseneck mount	A B E
Use a speaker phone attachment for hands-free phone use	Speaker phone attachment	A B C D E
An automatic dialer will allow easy calling of frequently called numbers	Automatic dialer	A B C D E
A lightweight cordless phone can be carried and used anywhere in the house as both a convenience and a safety measure	Cordless phone	A B C D E

Table 15 (continued)

Technique	Special aids	Disability*
WRITING		
Use a clipboard to hold paper steady, or hold the paper on a desk or table with paperweights	Clipboard and paper-weights	A B E
Use an electric typewriter or word processor for ease in writing	Electric typewriter or word processor	A B C D
Dictate notes into a cassette tape recorder	Cassette recorder	A B C D E
A ball-shaped pen or pencil holder permits easier writing for people with limited finger grasping action. The ball is held in the hand, with the pen or pencil protruding through the ball, and writing is accomplished through arm and hand motion	Ball-shaped holder ("Arthwriter")	B
Use a foam rubber roller to build up the grip on a conventional pen. Commercially manufactured built-up pens are also available	Built-up pens	B
Use a tilting tray table for writing in bed, or if in a chair, use a desk pillow for lap writing	Tilting tray table and desk pillow	E
For those who have to remain flat on their backs, the Fabrian Reading/Writing Aid is a versatile device that permits reading and writing with hands free while lying flat in bed. This device can also secure and hold magnetic games. Be sure to use a felt-tip pen when writing "against gravity"	Fabrian Reading/ Writing Aid	E
READING		
A simple book holder will allow tilting the book for easier viewing without needing to hold the book	Book holder	A B E

Table 15 (continued)

Technique	Special aids	Disability*
Use the tilting tray table or the Fabrian Reading/Writing Aid (see above). Or use the Bedspecs Prism glasses (see below)	Tilting table tray, Fabrian Reading/ Writing Aid, Bed- specs Prism glasses	E
Talking books from the public library are free and are not lim- ited to people with low vision		

WATCHING TV		
The prisms in Bedspecs Prism glasses change the angle of vision, helping the person to view TV or to read without lift- ing his head	Bedspecs Prism glasses	E
A TV remote control permits changing channels and adjust- ing sound without leaving chair or bed	TV remote control	A B C D E

TRAVEL		
A cushion that swivels helps to guide the person in and out of a car seat	Swivel cushion	C D
Depending on the style of car, a "rain gutter hook" and handle can provide additional leverage as the person gets in and out of a car	Rain gutter hook	A B C D
Airlines and airports do accommo- date people who need help when sufficient notice is given		C D
Cars can be modified to provide hand controls	Modified car controls	C D

__Disability key:__

A	One-handed	**C**	With ambulation aids	**E**	Bed-bound
B	Limited reach	**D**	Using wheelchair		

Table 15 (continued)

Technique	Special aids	Disability*
Vans can be specially modified to lift wheelchairs inside	Modified vans	D
Sliding boards may permit safe and easier transfer from wheelchair to car	Transfer board	D
Ramps and special "Handicapped" parking spaces are provided at many buildings to allow easier entry		C D

SITTING DOWN, STANDING UP, AND RECLINING

Technique	Special aids	Disability*
Elevating furniture a bit (even 2 or 3 inches) can lessen the strain on legs and back. Furniture leg extenders can be attached to the legs of a chair or bed	Furniture leg extenders	B C D E
A spring-assisted Assisto-seat helps overcome the initial difficulty in getting up from a chair by pushing the person up and out. (Trained professional help will be needed—usually from a therapist—to select the right spring tension and demonstrate the device.)	Assisto-seat	B C
Special chairs with a built-in ejector are available	Ejector chairs	B C
Adding an extra cushion to a chair will raise the seat and shorten the distance required to sit down. Be sure the cushion has nonslip strips to prevent the cushion from slipping	Nonslip cushion	B C
Bed wedges of varying thicknesses and elevation can provide extra comfort for the back. Chairlike backrests often have adjustable backs	Bed wedges and back rests	C D E

Table 15 (continued)

Technique	Special aids	Disability*
EASY ACCESS TO AID		
Mount cane or walker clips on often used tables, chairs, or nearby shelves. This keeps the walking aid at hand and within easy reach	Cane and walker clips	C
Add a wrist strap to a cane to assure the cane remains within easy reach	Wrist strap	C
Folding walkers are available for transport in a car or bus	Folding walker	C

Disability key:

A One-handed	**C** With ambulation aids	**E** Bed-bound
B Limited reach	**D** Using wheelchair	

6

Nutrition, Plain and Special

What Is Good Nutrition?

OR SOMEONE receiving home health care, good nutrition is of vital importance. You're likely to find as many different ideas as to what constitutes good nutrition as there are foods available—including all the various food fads that crop up from year to year. However, certain basic facts about nutrition are generally agreed upon, and they should serve as useful guidelines.

To begin with, there is the familiar breakdown of nutrients into proteins, fats, and carbohydrates—the "macronutrients." Table 16 lists these essential nutrients, their functions in nutrition, and the food sources containing them.

Next we have the division of foods into five basic groups. Table 17 covers these food groups—meat, milk, fruits and vegetables, breads and cereals, fats and oils—and lists the nutrients to be found in each group. Since no one food contains all the nutrients necessary for good health, a balanced diet must be planned drawing from the five groups listed. In drawing up such a diet plan for the person on home health care, keep three key words in mind: variety, moderation, and individuality.

Variety can be the "spice of life" in eating as well as in any other activity. We have access to many kinds of foods, including a good ethnic variety, and these foods can be prepared in many different ways to please the palate. Eating a variety of foods makes good nutritional sense also. The more different kinds of foods a diet includes, the better the chances of providing all the nutrients the body needs for optimum health. If you ate mostly milk and cheese, for example, barely touching other

Table 16 ■ THE MACRONUTRIENTS

Macronutrient	Best sources	Function(s)
Proteins	Meat, eggs, poultry, fish, cheese, milk, yogurt, legumes (e.g. soybeans, peanuts, black-eyed peas, kidney beans, pinto beans, lima beans), nuts, seeds, grains (e.g. oats, rice, wheat, barley, corn)	Constituent of muscle, bone, cartilage, skin, blood, lymph, enzymes. Helps body form new tissues and replace old ones. Regulates balance of water and acids and bases. Transports nutrients and oxygen. Needed to make antibodies, clot blood, and form scar tissue
Fats	Butter, margarine, lard, oil, meat, cream, ice cream, milk, cheese, yogurt, eggs, poultry, fish, nuts	Protects vital organs, provides insulation. Concentrated source of energy. Prevents skin and hair from dryness. Provides construction material for hormone-like substance known as prostaglandins
Carbohydrates	Grains (e.g. oats, rice, wheat, barley, corn); fruits, vegetables, legumes (e.g. soybeans, peanuts, black-eyed peas, kidney beans, pinto beans, lima beans), seeds, milk	Provides energy (in the form of glucose), which enables the body to carry out all of its functions

foods, you wouldn't have any problem getting enough calories, protein, calcium, and riboflavin—but you would risk becoming anemic because your diet would lack iron.

Variety is important, but don't misinterpret a varied diet to mean "anything goes." Moderation in a diet is just as essential as variety. Some foods are not as nutritious as others and so should be limited in any diet. These are foods that contain "empty calories," a term used for foods that are high in energy-producing calories but low in nutrients. Most foods high in sugar are full of empty calories.

Table 17 ▪ THE FIVE BASIC FOOD GROUPS

Food group	Sources	Nutrients
Meat	Red meat, veal, poultry, fish, seafood, eggs, cheese, nuts, seeds, legumes (e.g. dried beans, dried peas)	Protein, fat, iron (meat eggs), vitamin A, ribo-flavin (liver), thiamine (pork)
Milk	Milk, cheese, yogurt, ice cream, ice milk (Includes all whole, low-fat, and nonfat products)	Protein, fat (whole milk products), calcium, vitamins A and D (milk, ice cream), riboflavin
Fruits and vegetables	All fruits and vegetables	Carbohydrate, vitamin A (yellow fruits and veg-etables), vitamin C (citrus, dark green vegetables), vitamin B and iron (green leafy vegetables)
Breads and cereals	(Includes all whole wheat and enriched products) bread, cereal, noodles, rice, all pasta	Carbohydrate, B vita-mins (thiamine, ribo-flavin, etc.), iron
Fats and oils	Butter, margarine, vetetable oil, lard	Fat, vitamin A (butter), vitamin E (vegetable oil, margarine)

Individuality should be a key factor when planning a diet or when making modifications in a present diet. In addition to consulting the U.S. Recommended Daily Allowances (USRDAs) established to provide guidelines for many nutrients, there are other factors to be considered: How much exercise does the person get? It there a need to lose or gain weight, or just maintain the present weight? Are there any special health problems that would influence the diet?

VITAMINS

Vitamins are organic substances that are necessary to good nutrition. They perform important functions, such as assisting enzymes in the digestive system to process the fats, carbohydrates, and proteins we eat. And a little bit of vitamin goes a long way. Only minute quantities of vitamins are needed to accomplish these vital functions, which is why they are called micronutrients. Carbohydrates, proteins, and fats, on the other hand, are required in larger quantities and are, logically, called macronutrients.

Of the thirteen known vitamins, four of them—A, D, E, and K—are what is called fat-soluble. The remaining nine—vitamin C and the various B vitamins—are water-soluble. Fat-soluble vitamins can be stored in body fat and so do not have to be replenished on a daily basis. The water-soluble vitamins, however, cannot be stored by the body, and any of these vitamins not used by the body are washed out in urine or in perspiration. Water-soluble vitamins, therefore, have to be replenished on a regular basis.

It's often not possible to eat all the right foods every day, nor can we be sure we are always getting the right amount of nutrients. In such cases, vitamin supplements are often effective in providing good nutrition. If you have any question as to whether a vitamin supplement is needed, check with your physician—but make sure he has a good working knowledge of nutrition. Some doctors have been known simply to hand out printed diets to patients. Discuss nutrition requirements in detail with your doctor.

MINERALS

Minerals, unlike vitamins, are inorganic substances. Like vitamins, however, they play an important role in nutrition, assisting enzymes and helping build bones and muscles, as well as functioning in the formation of red blood cells, among other benefits.

The minerals our bodies require come in the form of macrominerals of which large quantities are needed, and microminerals—or trace minerals—which the body uses in very small amounts.

The most common and well-known minerals used by our bodies are calcium, iron, potassium, and zinc: calcium for good bones and teeth; iron for the blood; potassium for proper muscle nourishment; and zinc for the effective healing of wounds. Of course, these are only a few of the many functions of minerals in our bodies, and we need other minerals as well, such as iodine, copper, and manganese, to name a few.

The proper use of mineral supplements is as important as the use of vitamin supplements, and the same precautions apply: Check with a knowledgeable physician if there is any doubt.

The best way to get necessary vitamins and minerals is, of course, through a balanced diet. Try to stick with fresh foods as much as possible. Processing foods, especially fruits and vegetables, destroys many of the nutrients present in the original food. Since many of the water-soluble vitamins are also susceptible to heat, make sure that vegetables and fruits are cooked in small amounts of water for a minimum length of time.

In addition to consulting a doctor, nutritional therapist, or other health professional, you can learn much about the benefits of good nutrition by checking the many magazine articles and other publications available at the local library. One of the best sources of nutritional guidance is *Jane Brody's Nutrition Book* (New York: Norton, 1981), a recognized authority in the field. This book, as well as many good cookbooks, can also help in planning some of the special meals sometimes required as part of home health care—bland diets, salt-free diets, special mineral needs, liquid diets, adding taste without using salt, and so on. Individuals vary and so do their health and nutritional needs. The goal to be kept in mind is simple: Eating well means being well.

When Eating Is Not Possible

Unfortunately, there are some health problems—cancer or abdominal surgery, for example—that prevent an individual from the physical act of eating and swallowing food or, in some cases, of digesting it. Nutrition is, nevertheless, still required, both for survival and for good health, and other means have been devised for making sure the individual gets the proper nourishment.

Everyday, Ellen R. feeds herself highly nutritious meals—although not a morsel of food passes her lips.

Every night, as Kevin G. gets ready for bed, he prepares an all-night "meal" for himself—to be consumed while he sleeps.

These two individuals are typical of the many people who, for various reasons, cannot obtain nutrition by eating regular meals. They bypass chewing and swallowing and nourish themselves by depositing liquid nutrition directly to the digestive system (enteral nutrition, as in Ellen's case) or by supplying nutritional elements directly to the bloodstream (parenteral nutrition, as in Kevin's method).

Enteral nutrition means nutrition obtained through or by means of the gastrointestinal tract. Parenteral nutrition refers to nourishment derived without—or outside of—the gastrointestinal tract.

In enteral nutrition, often known as tube feeding, the individual is fed through a tube rather than through the mouth. The tube can be inserted through the nose and into the stomach (nasogastric tube), or the tube can be surgically inserted into the stomach with an opening outside the abdominal wall (gastrostomy tube), or the tube can be located in the small intestine (jejunostomy tube).

In parenteral nutrition, the individual is fed nutrient solutions intravenously through a catheter (a small tube) inserted surgically into a large vein near the shoulder blade.

Effective, safe, and proper use of either of these two methods in home health care will require a learning period for both the caregiver and the patient, but once the requirements and techniques are mastered, the results can be extremely beneficial.

In essence, there will no longer be the danger—as there was not too long ago—of a patient literally starving to death because of an inability to obtain proper nourishment.

Enteral Nutrition

This is the preferred method of nourishing those individuals who, although unable to maintain an adequate intake of food orally, still remain sufficient functioning of the gastrointestinal tract to allow digestion.

This type of condition can be brought about by cancer of the esophagus, which can prevent the passage of food from the mouth to the stomach, or cancer of the mouth or jaw, which does not allow chewing of food. Also, any disorder that affects the ability to swallow—such as a stroke or ALS (amyotrophic lateral sclerosis)—can necessitate the use of enteral feeding. Additionally, any illness or procedure that compromises the person's nutritional status—chemotherapy, radiation therapy, or inflammatory bowel disease, for example—can lead to the decision to supplement regular meals with enteral formula.

Frequently, enteral nutrition is initiated when the patient is in the hospital, usually after surgery. Physicians, nurses, and nutritionists monitor the patient's progress and adjust the enteral feeding and formulas used to suit the needs of the individual. Also, while the patient is healing after surgery, the health care team has time to instruct the patient and the caregiver in the procedures, techniques, and precautions involved in enteral nutrition so that it can be continued successfully at home. In other circumstances, the doctor may suggest adding special formulas to the daily diet of someone cared for at home during chemotherapy or radiation therapy.

If the enteral formula is used as a complete food replacement, many adjustments, both physical and psychological, have to be made by the patient, by family members, and by the caregiver. It's a difficult period for all concerned, and the members of the health care team, especially the social worker, can provide the support and encouragement needed to help the patient adjust and start on the way to recovery and acceptance of his condition.

If a feeding tube is used, the type of feeding tube and its location will be determined by the physician, who will take into consideration the nature of the patient's illness or injury and whether or not the enteral nutrition will be required on a short-term, long-term, or permanent basis.

Modern enteral feeding tubes are made of polyurethane or silicone. They are softer and generally more flexible than the older tube types, which were made of rubber or polyvinyl chloride (PVC). Although the newer tubes are smaller in diameter than the older types, which could accommodate heavier and more viscous food formulas, the smaller diameter and softer material of the newer tubes make them much less irritating to mucous membranes and easier for the patient to tolerate. A disadvantage of the small diameter tube, however, is that it can clog when thicker food formulas are used, which means that certain formula restrictions have to be observed.

The type of food formula provided for patients on enteral nutrition depends on the amount of digestive capability remaining. If almost the entire gastrointestinal tract is functional, the formula fed into the tube may consist of blended natural foods such as meat, fruit, and vegetables. If digestive capability is restricted, the formula may consist of special chemical mixtures of proteins, carbohydrates, fats, vitamins, and minerals.

The formula is poured into a bag or pouch and, with the assistance of gravity or a feeding pump, is dripped into the system. Commercially prepared formulas are available and offer the safest and most reliable way of obtaining proper enteral nutrition.

Home enteral nutrition requires much careful advance planning in addition to thorough training of the patient and the caregiver. Teaching can take place in the hospital or at home, by specially trained health professionals.

Over a period of time, the patient's nutritional needs may change. A careful check has to be kept on the progress of the patient on the formulas being used. This means regular weight checks and keeping accurate records on intake and output. Everything fed to the patient may need to be recorded, and urine testing to check for the presence of sugar and acetone is often done. The physician will explain what is required, and the other members of the health care team will show how to accomplish it.

Assistance will be required for the initial period at home, and this assistance will not only be provided by the health care team but may also come from the local pharmacist who provides the supplies and equipment needed, or from a home alimentation service that the patient can employ.

Regardless of where the help comes from, the patient and the caregiver will learn all about formulas and how to mix and store them safely, how to maintain cleanliness, how to use all the equipment, and what to do in case of emergencies (a tube that comes loose, for example).

Generally, a commercial food formula can be kept unopened until used, since it is in a sterile container. Many formulas can be stored in a dry place at room temperature until used. However, once opened, it must be used immediately, and if there is an unused portion, it should be refrigerated in a clean, air-tight container. The manufacturer's label or printed instructions will state just how long (usually twenty-four hours) and under what conditions the opened formula can be kept before it has to be discarded.

Since formulas should be at room temperature when used, any refrigerated portions should be taken out about half an hour before use in order to warm to room temperature.

FEEDING METHODS

Enteral feedings can be administered by gravity (continuous or intermittent drip) or by an infusion pump, which feeds the formula at a steady rate.

Delivery systems for enteral feeding usually consist of a container for the formula (plastic or glass), a hanger (usually a pole), a drip chamber (transparent so the drip rate can be monitored), tubing and connectors, and flow regulators (clamps for the tubing), or specially developed pumps.

The continuous drip method is usually the preferred method because it will produce less abdominal discomfort or diarrhea. However the method to be used should be determined by the physician with the needs and medical condition of the patient in mind. Regular evaluations will allow room for flexibility in both the formulas used and the method of administering them.

SPECIAL TECHNIQUES

Experience and practice will generate confidence in home enteral feeding, and that confidence can be more quickly achieved by using certain helpful techniques.

When receiving an enteral feeding, the patient should be sitting up. This will prevent vomiting or aspirating (breathing in) the formula.

If you're using a nasogastric tube, tape it in place to keep it from slipping. A piece of tape can be placed on the tube to mark its position in relation to the nostril to make it easier to determine whether it has moved. The tube usually remains in place between meals and is changed every two to three weeks. Some patients on long-term enteral feeding are trained to remove and reinsert their nasogastric tubes as required.

Feeding rates should be varied according to the fomula being used, the main consideration: do not feed it to the patient at too fast a rate or in large quantities. This can lead to stomach distention, nausea, cramps, diarrhea, and other discomforts. If any problems of this nature should arise, the patient and the caregiver should first check to make sure that all equipment is being properly used and that the feeding is being administered as directed. If the problem cannot be resolved by these checks, then the feeding should be stopped and a health care professional consulted (by phone if necessary) to determine what to do next.

In time, enteral feeding will become a part of the daily routine, allowing a near-normal life style for the individual.

Parenteral Nutrition

This type of nutrition has to be used when the gastrointestinal tract must be bypassed, a condition that can have a number of causes, for example, the surgical removal of sections of the intestines (as occurs in Crohn's disease, an inflammation of the gastrointestinal tract). There are others who cannot eat enough—burn victims who need extraordinary amounts of nutrients. Still other individuals refuse to eat for various reasons, and there are some who should not eat because of recent gastrointestinal surgery that should be given time to heal.

In some cases (all those cited above except for Crohn's disease), parenteral nutrition will be a temporary measure until artificial feeding is no longer needed. In other cases, such as major chronic gastrointestinal disorders, for example, when portions of the intestines have been removed, or other instances when permanent intestinal damage has been caused by radiation therapy for cancer, parenteral nutrition can be required permanently.

Usually parenteral feeding is the only means of providing nourishment, regardless of whether it is temporary or permanent, and in such cases, it's referred to as total parenteral nutrition (TPN).

Since the gastrointestinal tract is being completely bypassed in TPN, some other means has to be employed to get the proper nutrients into the patient's system. For many years, there was no really effective way of doing this, and many patients died as a result of malnutrition and accompanying diseases that the patient was too weak to resist.

Attempts were made to meet the body's nutritional requirements by introducing nutrient solutions into a small vein in the hand or foot or into the scalp. However, to provide the needed nourishment, large fluid volumes of the nutrient solution were required, and the body couldn't tolerate them. If the fluid volume was reduced, then the proportion of nutrients in the solution had to be increased. This high concentration caused destruction of the small veins being used.

It wasn't until the late 1960s that Dr. Stanley Dudrick, of St. Luke's Episcopal Hospital in Houston, devised a method for infusing the nutrient solution into the superior vena cava, the large vein near the heart, where the solution was diluted by the large quantity of blood being pumped through the heart. The technique worked, and this is the method now used in TPN.

The nutrient solution is introduced into the superior vena cava through a permanent catheter in the vein inserted surgically in the hospital. The catheter is made of silicone, and the most recent version of it is known as the Hickman catheter.

Since silicone is a rather slippery material, there is a possibility that the catheter might slip out of place in the vein. This problem is resolved by creating a subcutaneous (under-the-skin) tunnel along the chest wall. The catheter is drawn up through this tunnel to an exit near the top of the chest on the right side. Another incision is made in the hollow beneath the collarbone, and the catheter is threaded into the large vein and sutured into place. A dacron cuff is placed around the catheter under the skin. In time, tissues under the skin form and grow around the cuff, anchoring the catheter into place. The catheter is capped when not being used to infuse nutrient solutions into the vein.

The nutrient solutions are specially prescribed for each individual to supply the needed nutrition. The solutions can be purchased commercially or the patient can mix the ingredients at home. Usually, these solutions are mixtures of dextrose, vitamins, minerals, and other nutrients. They must be kept sterile and administered on a sterile basis. Because of the high potential for infection, strict procedures must be followed to avoid the possibility of bacterial infection.

The catheter has to be cleaned regularly, and the site where it enters the body must also be cleaned. In the hospital, the patient and the caregiver will be given full instructions on the cleaning procedures to be followed by the health care team. Also, as with enteral feeding, assistance will be needed during the initial period of home health care until the routines and procedure are learned and can be used effectively and safely.

For many patients, parenteral feeding is done at night while they sleep. A controller or an infusion pump can be used to administer the feeding. The controller is a gravity device whereby drops of the solution fall into a drip chamber and then into the tubing leading to the catheter. A sensor monitors the drip rate and sounds an alarm if the rate falls below or exceeds what has been set into the controller. If the tube or the catheter become clogged, the drip rate decreases, and if the tubing somehow disconnects, the drip rate increases. In either case, the sensor sets off the alarm, awakening and alerting the patient of the problem.

If an infusion pump is used, the solution is delivered at a set rate, forcing the fluid into the tubing and the catheter at a certain number of drops per minute. Pressure is involved here, and if a partial clogging occurs, the pressure may increase to the point of rupturing the tubing. Precautions must be taken to keep the catheter and the tubing open and to prevent blood clots in the catheter. Usually a sodium heparin solution is used for this purpose. The physician and the health care team will explain its function and how to use it.

Infusion of the nutrient solution overnight (a total of ten to twelve hours, including sleeping time) is the preferred method. However, some individuals may require continuous infusion on a twenty-four-hour basis. To avoid the necessity of being confined to home because of this, a portable infusion vest has been developed. The vest is worn under the outside clothing. Two pockets in the vest hold the nutrient solutions, and a small pump operated by a rechargeable battery pack infuses the solution into the vein through the permanently installed catheter.

In such a case, the patient is, of course, always aware of being nourished parenterally. There is no respite—and this can lead to depression. In fact, depression is always a potential problem when total nutritional needs are obtained without eating food.

Depression can come about because the individual concerned feels that the loss of bowel function or the ability to chew and swallow food or to function as a "normal" person in these most vital aspects of living is too much of a burden to bear. A negative self-image builds up. The individual sees himself or herself as an abnormal, deformed, sick person. If depression is allowed to take too strong a hold, it can completely devastate his or her life. The caregiver, the family, and the members of the health care team have to work hard to prevent this. Support, encouragement, compassion, and understanding are needed.

Additionally, the individual usually has many fears and anxieties. The presence of a surgically inserted tube or catheter is a constant reminder that something might go wrong, something might malfunction, a catheter might rip loose, an enteral feeding tube might slip out—

the list of fears is large and can be terrifying. Once again, the caregiver and the others involved will have to give support and understanding. When necessary—if the depression or the fears or anxieties cannot be controlled even with help—professional assistance should be sought. A psychiatrist or social worker has the expertise and the training to provide the necessary help.

Still another factor the patient and the caregiver have to contend with is the tremendous financial burden enteral or parenteral nutrition entails. Although enteral nutrition is considerably less expensive, the costs are nevertheless high. Home health care involving TPN can cost anywhere from $40,000 to $70,000 per year—and more. Medicare and private medical insurance policies can help, but even with third-party reimbursement the costs can be staggering. Organizations, especially the Lifeline Foundation (see Appendix) are working to get more financial aid for enteral and TPN patients. Also, companies that offer home enteral nutrition and TPN will work with you and your doctor to prequalify the level of third-party reimbursement to which you are entitled.

Despite all these burdens, fears, and problems the individual being nourished enterally or parenterally can build and maintain a good quality of life. It isn't easy, but it can be done. As in so many other situations involving health problems, the prime requirement is a strong, positive mental attitude.

With this as a basis, all the rest is possible.

7

Drugs and Medication

BECAUSE MEDICATION AND DRUGS are such an integral part of health care, it's important that both the patient and the caregiver become knowledgeable not only about medicine and drugs in general but also about the specific medication being taken. The major source of information on the matter of prescribed medication is, of course, the physician who originally makes out the prescription—and the time to get this information is when the prescription is being written.

Be prepared to ask questions. Get the facts. Don't just blindly accept the prescription from the doctor. Too many of us hesitate to "impose" on the doctor by asking him questions, or even asking him to repeat his instructions about when to take the medication, the assumption being that it will all be written on the label by the pharmacist, so why annoy the doctor with silly questions.

Even though this may go against the way you've been conditioned by doctors, it's important to remember that the medications and drugs they prescribe are potent chemicals. This certainly gives you the right— indeed, the obligation—to find out all you can about what's being prescribed. There's no reason for a doctor to refuse to answer legitimate questions about the medication he is prescribing for a patient. If your doctor does refuse, or shows unreasonable irritation, it might be a good time to start thinking about finding another doctor. At the very least, you must persist until all your questions are answered and you understand why this particular medication has been prescribed.

Make sure the doctor tells you the exact name of the medication (write it down!) and whether he's prescribing a brand name medication or has indicated that the pharmacist can substitute a generic drug, which will be less expensive. In writing the prescription, the doctor will indicate to the pharmacist whether the medication should be in the form of tablets, capsules, or liquid and will also state how much of the medication he wants the pharmacist to supply for the patient and how many times it can be refilled. He will also specify the strength of the medication, how frequently you should take it, and whether it should be on an empty stomach, before or after meals, or at bedtime.

Make sure you understand all there is to know about the medication. Ask the doctor. Write down what he tells you for future reference. Don't trust your memory in such an important matter. Ask the doctor how to spell the name of the medication if you're not sure. Never mind that the pharmacist will type the name on the label. You want to know it beforehand. You might want to look it up on your own. (I'll tell you how to do this a little further on.)

Equally as important as finding out what this medication is supposed to accomplish is knowing how the desired effect will be achieved (what part of the body or brain it will act on) and what the side effects can be. Frequently, these can range from mild reactions—a slight headache or rash or feeling sleepy or a little bit nauseated—to more severe adverse reactions, such as increased blood pressure, impaired vision, heavy and persistent vomiting, or severe abdominal pain. Don't get alarmed at the list of possible side effects, and above all, do not let this deter the patient from taking the medication as prescribed by the doctor.

However, do not neglect to discuss this matter with the doctor. Statistics have shown that the elderly, who are the ones most likely to be on home health care, take about 25 percent of all the drugs dispensed in this country—and the risk of adverse reactions to drugs increases with age. Individuals between seventy and ninety years of age take three times as many drugs and have three times as many adverse reactions as those under age fifty.

The doctor can advise you and discuss possible side effects of medications with you. Remember, though, that he isn't a mind reader. He won't know what you're concerned about unless you tell him, and if you don't ask questions, he may well assume that there's no need to give you additional information. Don't leave the doctor's office (or don't let him leave the hospital bedside) until you find out everything you want to know.

By the same token, don't let the doctor's visit end until he has been told everything he has to know. The doctor should be informed of any reactions the patient may have had to previously prescribed medications and should also be told of any physical or medical problems the patient may have had recently. If he has been the patient's regular doctor for some time, his own records will tell him much that he has to know. If, he's a new doctor, however, he should be informed of any medications the patient is now taking, any allergies, and any problems or adverse reactions to medicines or drugs in the past. Do not neglect to tell him what nonprescription drugs the patient is now taking on his or her own (aspirin, antihistamines, antacids, etc.) as over-the-counter (OTC) drugs can also affect the system, especially when taken in conjunction with prescribed medication.

One other necessary precaution is to take the medication exactly as prescribed by the doctor: at the times indicated, in the manner specified, and in the quantities prescribed. If the doctor has said to take all of a certain medication, he means just that. If the prescription, for example, calls for thirty capsules and the doctor wants the patient to take all of them at the rate of three a day, his instructions should be followed to the letter. Even if the patient starts feeling much better after a few days, the medication should continue to be taken as prescribed. The thirty capsules represent the total dose the doctor wants the patient to take, and the patient who cuts down on this total dosage will not get the full benefits of the medication the doctor has prescribed.

Also, make sure you follow the doctor's instructions as to when and how to take the medication. For example, certain drugs lose their effectiveness if mixed with food, so they should be taken on an empty stomach or at a set time before meals. Equally important are the doctor's instructions about taking the medication with food or with water. One elderly woman, who was occasionally incontinent, had a serious adverse reaction because she did not drink water with the medication, as prescribed by her doctor. She was afraid of having an "accident" if she drank too much water. The doctor's instructions have to be followed carefully and conscientiously. If you or the patient have any doubts, ask the doctor.

When the doctor prescribes a certain medication, he will be taking into consideration many factors of which neither the caregiver nor the patient may be aware. For instance, as we get older, there is a decrease in gastric juice activity. This may result in slower absorption of drugs in the digestive system. The doctor has to take this into consideration when prescribing drugs. The excretion of drugs by the kidneys decreases with age—another factor for the doctor to consider. Metabolism also changes with age, and so the rate of drug metabolism changes, too. Since metabolism occurs primarily in the liver and it's in the liver that drugs are metabolized into a water-soluble form for excretion, the doctor has still another factor to contend with.

As a group, older people have different physiological responses to drugs than younger individuals, and there are also differing psychological or emotional responses. Moreover, elderly people have decreased visual acuity, which can present problems in reading labels on medications. There is also a change in color perception, which affects the ability to distinguish pills or capsules of different colors. Hearing difficulties, quite prevalent in older people, can cause confusion in hearing the doctor's instructions and interpreting them properly. Additionally, there can be problems in opening some of the child-safety caps on medication bottles (the pharmacist can change these on request) and in keeping track of the many drugs the elderly often have to take each day (medication scheduling charts and other devices are available at your pharmacist's to make this task easier).

If both the caregiver and the patient are elderly and if the caregiver is also somewhat infirm—as can happen with an older couple when one spouse is taking care of the other at home—the doctor will have to review carefully the medications he has prescribed and make sure the couple can manage the required home health care program. For example, if the caregiver's hearing is weak, the doctor may have to write out all his instructions in full and make sure the caregiver understands them. Also, the doctor may have to spend a bit more time taking the caregiver and the patient through a "dry run" to make sure the medication is being properly administered.

Whether you are an older caregiver or comparatively young, there are methods and techniques you can use in managing the medication schedule for the patient. Here are some guidelines:

1) If the patient is a diabetic and requires a daily insulin injection, the doctor or the health care nurse will show you how to accomplish it (see Chapter 16.)

2) If the patient has difficulty swallowing pills, ask the doctor if it is all right to mix the medication with food.

3) Some patients, especially the elderly, will sometimes suddenly balk at taking medication. If this happens, do not force the patient. Wait it out calmly; do not sit or stand in front of the seated patient with a spoonful of medication held to the patient's lips. It won't work. Wait it out calmly, and the patient will soon come around. If not, consult the doctor.

4) Do not try to imitate the brisk efficiency of the hospital setting in administering the medication. Remember, this is *home* health care. Let the patient take the medication himself, if possible, while you are nearby.

5) Do not feel guilty if your performance as a caregiver is not up to par on some days. Nobody is perfect, and if you forget and bring the medication to the patient a little off schedule, or if you accidentally spill it, or if anything else of a minor nature goes wrong, take it in stride. You and the patient will be the better off for it.

In dealing with medications as a part of home health care, it would be a good idea to have on hand (either purchased for your own use or available at the local library) one or more of the following books, or similar ones:

- *The Physicians' and Pharmacists' Guide to Your Medicines,* prepared by the United States Pharmacopeial Convention (New York: Ballantine Books, 1981)
- James W. Long, M.D., *The Essential Guide to Prescription Drugs* (New York: Harper & Row, 1982)
- Harold L. Silverman and Gilbert I. Simon, *The Pill Book,* (New York: Bantam Books, 1982)
- H. Winter Griffith, M.D., *Complete Guide to Prescription and Non-Prescription Drugs* (Tuscon: HP Books, 1983)

Each of these books lists a great variety of prescription and nonprescription drugs, giving you details on the type of drug, generic name, brand name, precautions, side effects, how the drug works, interactions with other drugs and substances (alcohol, for example), interactions with different foods, and other important information.

You can use these books to supplement what you've learned from the doctor, or to refresh your memory, or to gain additional knowledge about medication and drugs. Obviously, you will not have the background, the training, or the expertise of a physician or pharmacist. However, the knowledge you gain from questioning your doctor and consulting these books will, if used wisely, enrich your understanding of the treatment and medication recommended by the doctor and will allow you to deal effectively with this important aspect of home health care.

Drug–Drug Interactions

Medications or drugs (the terms are generally interchangeable in common usage) can be dangerous, despite having been prescribed by a doctor. Although originally intended for beneficial reasons—to bring about better health or to combat an illness—medications can, if care is not exercised, have an unwanted and adverse effect.

There are many drugs on the market today, giving the physician a full range of resources from which to choose. However, this multiplicity of beneficial drugs carries with it the seeds for potential misuse. This is especially true when an individual is taking more than one drug, as is often the case with elderly patients. If you are the caregiver for someone who is taking several prescription drugs, be aware that the interactions of drugs within the patient's body can sometimes result, at best, in less effective drug action and, at worst, in real harm to the individual.

New drugs must, by law, be tested before being approved by the Food and Drug Administration (FDA). Most people know this and feel reassured that no drug will be permitted on the market until exhaustive laboratory and clinical tests have been conducted to prove both the effectiveness and safety of the drug. However, at present, the law does not require drug manufacturers to conduct tests on possible interactions of all drugs with each other. Tests such as these are not feasible because of the vast number of drugs available by doctor's prescription. Morever, the subject of drug interactions is exceedingly complex and is still being actively researched.

At present, the most reliable source of information about the interaction of drugs with each other is the pool of knowledge acquired through the continued reporting of drug reactions and interaction by physicians and pharmacists. Once such information becomes known, the FDA requires that it be made available to all physicians and pharmacists. If the information applies to nonprescription, over-the-counter (OTC) drugs, that must appear on the label. Additionally, the FDA publishes and distributes a monthly bulletin with details of drug side effects and interactions.

What is a drug interaction? Essentially, it is the action one drug has upon another drug's effectiveness or toxicity when the two of them are taken together, either simultaneously or within a short interval of time. It's a complex matter, involving chemistry, body metabolism, and a host of other factors.

A drug interaction can involve one drug either reducing or enhancing the effectiveness of another drug. A particular drug may act upon another drug in such a way that the action of the second drug is speeded up, which can result in harm to the patient. Conversely, one drug can slow down the action of a second drug to the point where the patient does not derive the benefit from it intended by the doctor when he wrote the prescription.

Physicians keep themselves up to date about drug interactions, and a doctor is not likely to prescribe two or more drugs that will interact in the wrong way in a patient's body. However, if a patient changes doctors and continues to take an old medication and does not tell the new doctor about this, the doctor may unknowingly prescribe a drug that will interact adversely with the old medication. It's for this reason that a doctor treating a new patient will take a complete medical history and ask what medications the patient is now taking. Too often, though, people do not give the doctor all the required information. This is not necessarily deliberate. An elderly person whose health has not been good for a number of years and who has been taking all sorts of medications may just not remember all of them. To avoid this situation, it's an excellent idea for the caregiver to keep a written record of all the medications presently being taken by the patient and give a copy of this to the new doctor for his records. Along with this, it would also be a good idea to keep a record of any reactions the patient has had to particular drugs.

Bear in mind, too, that nonprescription medications, the kind you can buy over the counter, are also considered drugs. This holds true for aspirin, antihistamines, digestive aids, laxatives, and so on. The doctor should be made aware of all the OTC medications being taken by the patient on a more or less regular basis. For example, if the patient has been taking aspirin regularly for any number of reasons and the doctor decides an anticoagulant is needed to keep blood clots from forming in the patient's system, the aspirin can enhance the effect of the anticoagulant to the point where the patient can be in danger of excessive bleeding. If the doctor knows the patient is taking aspirin in quantity, he can avoid this problem.

Alcohol, which is also considered a drug, represents a great danger in many cases when people will inadvertently mix it with a prescribed medication. For example, if the doctor has prescribed Valium, a common tranquilizer, he probably will caution you against allowing the patient to mix the medication with alcohol. Combining Valium with alcohol can cause death—and the alcohol doesn't necessarily have to be ingested in the form of a drink. Some cough or cold medicines that can be purchased without a prescription and that are often found in home medicine cabinets do contain alcohol. Make it a habit to check the label on all preparations to determine the percentage of alcohol.

The indiscriminate combining of Valium and alcohol provides an excellent example of the phenomenon of "potentiation." Potentiation occurs when two drugs are mixed and instead of producing an additive effect (the effects of one drug being added to the other) a multiplying action takes place. The results of the mixture go beyond the mere sum of the effects of the two drugs. What you have then is a dangerously increased and accelerated combined drug action. The alcohol has increased the sedative effect of the Valium, and the Valium has done the same for the intoxicating effect of the alcohol.

An extra word of caution here. Alcohol does not mix well with many medications. A person does not necessarily have to be a heavy drinker to observe this precaution. Many doctors are now displaying in their offices a poster warning of the risks of consuming alcohol while taking medication. Be guided by this and by what the doctor tells you when he writes out the prescription. If he doesn't mention alcohol and you know that the patient in your care likes to have an occasional drink or a glass of wine with meals, ask the doctor about this. Don't feel foolish. It's better to be reassured by the doctor that it's all right than to continue a practice that may be harmful to the patient. Potentiation is nothing to fool around with.

On the other hand, physicians sometimes deliberately employ potentiation to increase the effect of a beneficial drug, such as an antibiotic. In this case, the physician will prescribe a second drug known to potentiate the action of the antibiotic, thus increasing and speeding up the activity of the desired drug and getting the patient well faster.

If you have occasion to consult any of the books on drugs I mentioned previously, you'll note that they pay particular attention to the effects of drug interactions. These drug guides caution the reader not to take a particular drug if he is presently taking other specified medications. When in doubt, the safest course is to consult your doctor.

Consulting the doctor is always a good idea. He will have compiled a very thorough medical history on the patient, determining, among other things, what medications the patient is now taking and the kinds of reactions to certain drugs the patient may have had in the past. This type of medical history allows the doctor to prescribe medication he knows will not produce adverse reactions or drug interactions.

All of this will have been to no avail, however, if you go into a store and purchase for the patient an OTC cough medicine, antihistamine, or laxative that should not be taken with his present medication. A phone call to the doctor will not take long or take up much of his time, and you will have aided the doctor's efforts to safeguard the patient's health.

Often the pharmacist can provide the same information. Although the pharmacist is not licensed to practice medicine and cannot prescribe medications or drugs, he is licensed and qualified through training and experience to warn you of the dangers of drug interactions. He has the resources and the publications on hand to help you in this respect.

Many pharmacists are now starting to keep computerized records on their patients, listing such important items as allergies, medications taken in the past, presently prescribed medications, and any adverse reactions previously reported by the patient. (A pharmacist, like a physician, will think of a customer as a patient because the pharmacist is part of the health care team and is assisting the doctor in treating the patient.) With the computer there to help him, the pharmacist can quickly determine any potential danger, either in a newly prescribed medication from a new doctor or in an OTC preparation you have picked from the shelf. When something like this happens—and there are cases on record—a phone call from the pharmacist to the doctor quickly sets everything right.

Both the doctor and the pharmacist will depend on you, the caregiver, to keep them informed of any adverse reactions or drug interactions you have observed in the patient. Even though the reaction may seem mild to you, note it down and report it. Leave nothing to chance. Check out everything that gives you cause to think the patient in your care might be having a drug reaction or interaction. Every little twitch or ache or pain doesn't have to be investigated, of course, but don't gloss over any symptom that might be important.

For example, if the patient develops a rash some time after taking a new medication, this may well be an indication of possible problems with the medication. If the rash goes away, it doesn't necessarily mean that the problem has also gone away. The human skin has been called the body's early warning system. Any rash, outbreak of hives, skin eruptions, discolorations, or similar reactions should be brought to the attention of the doctor—and later to the pharmacist if the doctor confirms that there has indeed been a reaction.

The books on drugs I have previously mentioned will aid you in becoming more knowledgeable about drug–drug interactions. Remember, medications prescribed by a doctor are meant to be taken into the patient's body. Make sure you know all you can about these medications, and be alert and aware of all possible reactions and interactions. Play it safe!

Food–Drug and Drug–Nutrient Interactions

Check the labels on medications prescribed by the patient's doctor, and you'll find that each one will have specific instructions about when to take it, usually in relation to mealtimes. Why is it so important to take the medication either before, during, or after meals? Some might say it's to prevent an upset stomach, and this would be true in certain cases. But there's another reason for the doctor to be so specific about this. He is taking into consideration the possibility of food–drug or drug–nutrient interactions.

Food contains natural or added chemicals and substances, which can interact with medications the patient may be taking. One form of interaction results in either slowing down or speeding up the time it takes for the drug to be processed by the digestive system and get to the part of your body where it's needed. This is a matter of the drug's "bioavailability," which refers to how quickly the drug enters the bloodstream and how long it stays there. If the bioavailability of a drug is changed because of an interaction, the medication may not be as effective as originally anticipated.

Also, interaction with food can either enhance or impede the absorption of the drug. Impeding the absorption of a drug can mean that not enough of the drug gets to act as intended by the doctor.

For example, tetracycline is a well-known antibiotic that has been on the market for over thirty years and is dispensed under many brand names by several pharmaceutical firms. Physicians and pharmacists are familiar with this drug, and it is frequently prescribed. To do its work well, however, tetracycline should not be taken in conjunction with milk or other dairy products. The calcium in milk, cheese, yogurt, and various other dairy foods will bind up the tetracycline and impair absorption of the drug. For this reason patients are advised to avoid milk for at least one hour before and after taking tetracycline and to take the tetracycline one hour before or two hours after meals.

Although no serious long-term health damage is likely to result from slowing down the absorption of tetracycline, there are other food–drug interactions that can be very dangerous. One of the most serious interactions of this type can take place when a mono amine oxidase (MAO) inhibitor is prescribed for treating severe depression. If the patient is taking one of the MAO inhibitors (some brand names are Marplan, Nardil, Parnate, and Eutonyl), the doctor will undoubtedly caution the patient against eating any foods containing a high content of a substance called tyramine. The interaction could have fatal results. Blood pressure can suddenly rise to dangerous levels, causing severe headaches and, if unchecked, the bursting of small blood vessels and death due to brain hemorrhaging.

Some of the foods rich in tyramine are aged cheeses, yogurt, pickled herring, bananas, chicken livers, Chianti wine, canned figs, sour cream, avocados, and broad bean pods. The doctor or the pharmacist can give you more details on which foods to avoid. Generally, no aged or fermented foods should be consumed, and there has even been some question as to the advisability of drinking large quantities of coffee, tea, or cola beverages while taking an MAO inhibitor.

Individuals with Parkinson's disease are often treated with levodopa, which helps reduce the tremors, rigidity, and other symptoms of the disease. Pyridoxine (vitamin B_6) has been found to reduce seriously the beneficial effects of levodopa. If the patient is taking a vitamin supplement containing pyridoxine at the same time that levodopa has been prescribed, it's a simple matter to eliminate the vitamin supplement. However, pyridoxine is also present in many foods, and foods high in pyridoxine content should be avoided. Some of these foods are bacon, beef liver, oatmeal, beans, pork, sweet potatoes, and vitamin-enriched cereals. Check with the doctor as to food limitations to observe in this instance.

The interaction of pyridoxine and levodopa is essentially one between a drug and a vitamin—a drug–nutrient interaction. There are many other interactions that take place between drugs and vitamins and minerals (referred to as micronutrients because they are required in such small quantities) and between drugs and carbohydrates, fats, proteins, and other minerals (the common nutrients). Since nutrients and micronutrients are in the foods we eat, any drug interaction that impairs the absorption of these necessary substances into the patient's system will reduce the nutritional benefits that can be derived from a well-balanced diet. A vitamin or mineral deficiency can result.

One of the micronutrients, vitamin B-12, is directly affected by the use of colchicine, a drug prescribed in treating gout. Contrary to the old myth, gout is not exclusively a disease of the wealthy, who can afford to indulge in rich foods. An excess of uric acid usually brings on an attack of gout, and individuals are susceptible to this regardless of economic circumstances. Colchicine, through its effect on the bowel wall, inhibits absorption of vitamine B-12, and for this reason the doctor is likely to prescribe a vitamin supplement along with the colchicine needed to ward off gout attacks.

Mineral oil, an important ingredient of some laxatives, impairs the absorption of the fat-soluble vitamins, A, D, E, and K. Since most laxatives can be bought over the counter, the doctor will not be aware that the patient is taking a laxative on a regular basis unless he is so informed. The patient may well be offsetting the nutritional value of his food by use of a common laxative.

The absorption of vitamins A, D, E, and K is also impaired by Questran, a brand-name medication prescribed for reducing high levels of cholesterol in the blood. In this case, since Questran can be obtained only through a doctor's prescription, the doctor or the pharmacist will caution about the possible loss of the nutritional benefits of these vitamins, especially if the medication is to be taken on a long-term basis.

Taking any medication on a regular basis for long periods of time increases the risk of adverse interactions. One of the means for controlling high blood pressure, for example, is through the use of diuretics—medications designed to reduce the volume of water retained by the body. Regular and prolonged use of a diuretic can lead to a serious loss of potassium from the body. This can be counteracted by a diet that includes foods providing a good source of potassium, such as bananas, tomatoes, oranges, figs, raisins, prunes, and potatoes.

It's always a good idea to adapt your diet to provide foods that will replace any of the nutrients or micro-nutrients that have been depleted through drug interactions. Physicians usually prefer this method instead of prescribing vitamin or mineral supplements, either in capsule form or through injections.

Sometimes a diet has to be modified not to replace a vitamin but to restrict its presence in the system. Warfarin is a drug prescribed as an anticoagulant (Coumadin and Panwarfin are brand names). An anticoagulant will reduce the clotting ability of the blood, a very necessary effect for treating blood clots that, if not dissolved, might travel from a vein to the lungs, causing a pulmonary embolism. Vitamin K provides the natural clotting factors in our blood. The presence of too much vitamin K will decrease the effectiveness of the medication and impair its anticoagulant action. Therefore, it's advisable not to eat large quantities of leafy vegetables, such as cabbage, cauliflower, and spinach, which are rich in vitamin K. Consumption of potatoes, fish, and liver should also be restricted.

Not all interactions of drugs with foods and nutrients are adverse and undesirable. In some cases, physicians take advantage of a known interaction to increase the effectiveness of a medication. For example, when the doctor prescribes an iron supplement he will probably tell the patient to eat plenty of citrus fruits and juices. These contain absorbic acid, which enhances the absorption of iron into the system.

In another case, in fighting a fungus infection of the skin, hair, or nails, an antifungal agent known as Griseofulvin (brand names: Grifulvin, Grisactin) is often prescribed by physicians. Eating foods high in fat content, such as pork and bacon, with lots of butter or margarine (not usually recommended), will increase the absorption of the drug and thus increase the effectiveness of the medication.

There are many other interactions, both adverse and desirable, that are important and should be considered when taking medication. The books on drugs previously mentioned will give you guidelines to drug interactions with foods and nutrients. However, as I've cautioned before, the doctor, aided by the pharmacist, has to be the primary source of information and guidance in this matter.

Self-Medication

Don't be misled by the above heading. I'm not advocating that as part of commendably taking responsibility for his own health the patient prescribe and dispense medication for himself. Only a physician can order prescription drugs, and only a pharmacist or a nurse (usually in the hospital) can dispense these drugs.

Self-medication refers to the use of various over-the-counter (OTC) preparations available in any pharmacy and in many supermarkets or discount chain stores. In other words, we're talking about such items as aspirin, antacid tablets, laxatives, cough medicines, antidiarrhea preparations, and so on. The list is a long one, as you'll note just from looking at the shelves in your local store.

All of these preparations are available without a physician's prescription and, of course, without question by the salesclerk selling any of them to the caregiver for use by the patient. All of them are safe to use as directed. However, there is some risk involved, especially if the patient is presently taking medications prescribed by the doctor, or on a special diet, or under some kind of medical or therapeutic care or supervision.

What are the risks? Take aspirin, for an example. Aspirin, either by itself or as the major part of other OTC drugs, is used by a vast number of people to ease the pain and tension of headaches and toothaches, to help reduce fever, and to alleviate the discomfort of colds and sore throats. It is one of the largest-selling OTC preparations in the country, running a close second to cough and cold remedies. Cautions and warnings concerning the use of aspirin are included with every package, yet not too many people read them.

One of the mildest reactions to the use of aspirin can be stomach irritation, which is not always avoided by using buffered aspirin. However, in addition to stomach irritation, aspirin can cause internal bleeding in the stomach, sometimes in such small amounts that no noticeable symptoms appear until the condition has existed for an extended period of time and the individual develops anemia.

Other problems that can develop from the extended or excessive use of aspirin are stomach ulcers, kidney damage, and failure of the blood to clot properly. If aspirin is taken in conjunction with oral anti-diabetic drugs, the effects of these drugs can be increased, resulting in hypoglycemia (low blood sugar). If the patient has high blood pressure or congestive heart failure and the doctor has prescribed Lasix, a strong diuretic used to rid the body of excess fluid, taking aspirin at the same time can cause aspirin toxicity.

There are many other reactions and interactions that can occur from the use of aspirin, but don't be frightened off from the necessary use of this drug. Remember, though, that *aspirin is a drug,* so when the doctor starts to write out a prescription and asks what medications the patient is now taking, the doctor has to be informed if the patient is taking aspirin on a regular basis.

Many elderly people suffer from what they usually refer to as the "aches and pains" of getting older. To ease the pain and discomfort, an

OTC ointment or liniment is often massaged into the affected body area. This is a very common practice and is usually quite safe. However, such preparations should not be used indiscriminately, and proper caution should be taken. These preparations are known as topical analgesics, which means they are locally applied pain relievers. Actually, they produce their "soothing" effect through use of a counter-irritant or an anesthetic action, or both combined. A counter-irritant stimulates the nerve endings in the skin and produces the well-known sensation of warmth. The anesthetic action of the preparation blocks the nerve impulses in the area being massaged and produces a sensation of numbness. The total sensory stimulation of the preparation acts to distract the user's mind from the aching muscle or joint, producing a true feeling of temporary relief.

Many drugs and chemicals are combined to provide the effective action of the ointment, which is intended for external use only. However, although care is exercised, some of these substances are absorbed into the body in small quantities through the skin. Normally, this presents no danger, although people tend to have thinner skins as they get older and this adds to the introduction of the substances into the system.

The risk of possible adverse effects increases unless certain precautions are taken when using this form of self-medication. The ointment should not be applied to broken or bruised skin. Avoid spreading it over large areas of the body. Do not apply heat to any portion of the body where the ointment has just been used. Do not wrap tight bandages or other airtight coverings over the affected area. Use the preparation sparingly on any areas of the body where skin folds will provide warmth and moisture that will increase the absorption of the drugs into the system.

These two very common examples—the use of aspirin and ointments—point up some of the risks inherent in using any OTC products in self-medication. However, since self-medication is being practiced much more these days and has been estimated to represent 65 to 85 percent of all medical care today, it's important for the caregiver to know the pertinent facts. It is often the caregiver who, by purchasing OTC drugs for the patient, effectively allows the patient to practice self-medication.

Being on home health care is far different from being cared for in a hospital or other institution. When the patient is living at home and being cared for in that environment, he is not being watched and supervised every minute of the day. He is independent within the limitations of his illness or disability, and this means he will be thinking in terms of taking care of himself as much as possible—with, if necessary, the assistance of the caregiver. This is where self-care and self-medication comes in.

As with self-medication, self-care does not mean that the patient or the caregiver acts as the doctor. It does mean that minor discomforts, illnesses, and injuries are handled without calling in the doctor. If you have a slight cold, you take OTC products for it—aspirin, perhaps, and maybe some cough syrup—all of which can be purchased locally in many different kinds of stores. If your stomach is slightly upset, you take any of the various OTC products designed to combat stomach acidity. If you cut or burn your finger, you treat it with a first aid cream. This is normal, everyday behavior, and there's no reason at all to change it even though the patient is now on home health care.

The patient has a right to self-medicate if he so wishes. Physicians generally recognize this. The physician asks only that the patient keep him informed of what the patient is doing, either in person or, more likely, through the reports the doctor receives from the nurse supervising the home health care. If the doctor knows what OTC products the patient is taking, either for a specific problem or on a regular basis, he can advise the patient accordingly of any possible risks or problems.

But the doctor should not be counted on as an all-seeing, all-knowing entity. He's a human being, and so is the nurse supervising the home health care. Even though they do their jobs well and conscientiously, they cannot be expected to be on top of everything every moment of the day and to monitor the patient's every activity. Therefore, a lot of the health care is up to both the patient and the caregiver, and they have to take responsibility themselves.

The government aids in the tasks of self-medication and self-care. The Food and Drug Administration (FDA), which has to approve all OTC medicines, has established strict regulations concerning which products can be sold over the counter and which can be obtained only through a physician's prescription. Also, professional associations, such as the Proprietary Association, have also established standards. Thus, when a person goes to the store to purchase as OTC medicine, he can be sure that it will be safe if used as directed—and if a preliminary check has been made with the pharmacist or the physician concerning possible interactions with other medication the patient may be taking.

You'll also find an additional safeguard in the labeling of the product. Information presented on an OTC label will give you just about everything you need to know to make an informed choice—product name; type of medication; active ingredients; name and address of manufacturer, distributor, or packager; dosage instructions; warnings and cautionary statements; and expiration date. Take the time to read each label thoroughly. After all, this is something the patient will be taking into his system, and you, as the caregiver, have an obligation to the patient's health to know what you're doing. Pay particular attention to the warnings and cautionary statements, and don't hesitate to ask your pharmacist about any point on which you are unsure.

The OTC field is growing rapidly. A recent survey indicated that, in the United States, at least 40 million people a day take an OTC drug. More and more OTC products are coming on the market. You can't possibly know about all of them, but your pharmacist can help you find the product that will best serve your purposes.

Along with your pharmacist, you'll find that good old Madison Avenue—the advertising industry—can also be used as a guide. Most OTC products, old and new, are advertised in the media. The advertising campaign for each product will serve to alert you to what's available when you are seeking particular OTC medications for the patient. Once you know you have several products to choose from, you can start reading labels and conduct your own inquiry into which will be the best OTC product for the patient to use.

8

Personal Health Care

LTHOUGH THE PATIENT may have a team of health care professionals looking after him, it's important he maintains his own sense of self—his independence—to the greatest extent possible. To this end, the patient should care for *himself* as much as possible within the limits of his illness and disability. Accomplishing this personal care involves knowing not only what to do but why certain care procedures are necessary.

In this chapter, we'll be covering the most important aspects of personal care encountered during home health care. Obviously, each individual will have different needs, but the guidelines presented here should give a good general picture of what the patient can and should accomplish on his own.

Eye Care

One of the most precious abilities we have is the ability to see. Even with poor or blurred vision, we can somehow manage to orient ourselves in the world around us. If vision goes—if blindness sets in—the results can be devastating.

Although home health care involves no unusual risks to the eyes and special care is usually required only if eye problems are already present (see Chapter 15), it's important that the patient and the caregiver be aware of proper eye care to prevent future problems.

First and most obvious, the patient should visit an ophthalmologist (a physician specializing in treatment of the eyes and eye diseases) on a regular basis. He will check visual acuity, test for glaucoma (a leading cause of blindness), discuss any vision problems with the patient, and take any preventive action required to help maintain good vision.

As we get older, our eyes do not function as well as they did in our youth. This is a normal and expected development of the aging process.

We find that we need glasses for reading as well as for distant vision, and quite often bifocals are prescribed.

In addition to regular checkups from the ophthalmologist (he will decide how often these are needed, depending on the condition of the patient's eyes), the patient can take certain precautions between checkups, such as the following:

Avoid eyestrain by taking occasional breaks and looking off in the distance, or even closing your eyes, when reading for any length of time or when watching television.

Keep at least one light on in the room where you are watching TV so as to cut down on the glare from the screen.

Make sure you have enough light in a room to enable you to perform regular tasks without squinting or straining. If necessary, add lamps or increase the wattage of the bulbs you're using.

If you have to be out at night, especially for an extended period of time, be sure to wear your glasses. Night vision diminishes with age, and accidents are always a possibility unless you exercise extreme care.

Both the patient and the caregiver can help the doctor by being aware of the signs of possible eye problems. The National Society to Prevent Blindness lists the following signs you should look for as indicating the need for a professional eye examination:

Difficulty in focusing on near objects
Faces or objects look blurred or foggy
Spots, ghostlike images
Impression of a "skin" over eyes
Frequent changes in glasses, none of which is satisfactory
Trouble adjusting to darkened rooms, as at movies
Halos (rainbow-colored rings around lights)
A dark spot in the center of viewing
A curtainlike blotting out of vision
Vertical lines look distorted, wavy
Difficulty in seeing clearly at long distances (as in driving) or for close work (reading, sewing)
Excess tearing or "watery eyes"
Dry eyes with itching or burning

None of these signs are reasons to panic. However, a visit to the ophthalmologist should be arranged as soon as possible as some of these signs could indicate possible eye problems.

One of the major causes of blindness in the United States (it heads the list for new cases of blindness) is an eye disorder called macular degeneration. The macula is the central portion of the retina at the back of the eye, and it controls our close reading vision. If the macula is damaged, serious vision problems result, leading to blindness.

A simple test, called the Amsler grid test, can be performed at home to detect the presence of macular degeneration. The test consists of observing a grid of sharply delineated lines in a manner specified in the test instructions. If the results of the home test indicate possible eye problems, you are advised to see an ophthalmologist right away. Macular degeneration can be treated with laser surgery in the doctor's office or as an outpatient at a hospital—but it has to be done without delay. The National Society to Prevent Blindness (79 Madison Avenue, New York, New York 10016) will send you a home eye test for adults, which includes the Amsler grid test, for a one-dollar handling charge.

Keep an eye on your eyesight—it's much too precious to lose.

Keeping Fit: Your Own Program

Whether you're seven or seventy, frail or hearty, ailing or well, one of the most effective ways to safeguard your health is through the full and frequent exercise of your physical abilities. Our bodies work best when they are used often and well.

Basically, exercise involves anything that moves you—walking to the corner, reaching for your hat, dancing the foxtrot, or doing the laundry. Whether you are moving gently or vigorously, physical activity brings benefits that can be yours no matter what your age or current state of health. Moreover, these benefits cannot be derived by any other means. There is no diet, no medication, no substitute for the simple, natural act of moving around.

It's an accepted fact that we can deteriorate physically if we don't keep our bodies moving. The first signs of this deterioration are usually general fatigue or vague aches and pains. We begin to tire easily; we feel stiff, sluggish, and out of sorts; we get short of breath from minimum exertion; we suffer indigestion and sleep poorly.

If we continue our sedentary habits over the years, we allow the natural defenses of our bodies to weaken and, in effect, invite any number of diseases or disorders to move right in and take over.

Obviously, all illness is not caused by lack of exercise, and conversely, regular exercise will not guarantee complete freedom from degenerative disease. There are many other factors that interact to influence our health—genetic makeup, diet, environment, emotional well-being. Nevertheless, becoming physically active is an excellent way to assure ourselves greater strength to resist illness or to recover from surgery, especially in our later years.

Even if you've been inactive most of your life, or if your strength and your abilities have been diminished by illness or injury, all is not lost. Our bodies have remarkable recuperative powers that can be brought into play by physical activitiy. In fact, movement of some sort is a fundamental part of treatment programs for nearly all injuries and illnesses—even progressively degenerative diseases such as Parkinson's and Alzheimer's. So whether you spend most of your time in a rocking chair, in a wheelchair, or in bed, you can start now to claim the health benefits that are yours when you keep moving.

Exercise works on your body in different ways, depending on the types of movements you perform. Some activities are very effective in increasing joint flexibility and keeping muscles relaxed. Others work primarily to strengthen specific muscles or to develop balance and coordination.

Even if you are now coping with one of the chronic illness, such as arthritis or diabetes, regular movement and exercise offer definite advantages (see "Special Considerations for Special Conditions" later on in this section).

The best fitness program is the one you feel works for you. With the help of a good physical therapist or doctor, plus a little trial and error, you should be able to find activities that are not only effective but enjoyable as well.

Let's take a closer look at the types of movements recommended for therapeutic purposes as well as for your general health and well-being. We'll start with the most gentle movements and build up to the more strenuous.

RANGE-OF-MOTION EXERCISES

Range of motion exercises are simply the motions we ordinarily make as part of everyday activities. In physical therapy, however, these motions have been broken down into smaller movements, each of which is repeated several times.

For example, one range of motion exercise may involve moving your head from side to side, then up and down. Another exercise will consist of slowly lifting your right arm in front of you until it is pointing straight at the ceiling, then lowering it slowly to your side. Still another exercise will have you simply opening and closing your hands.

Sometimes, if you cannot move by yourself, the therapist will help you do the exercises—by holding your arm, for example, while you move it around—or she will actually do all the moving for you while you remain completely passive. This procedure is often useful during pain-

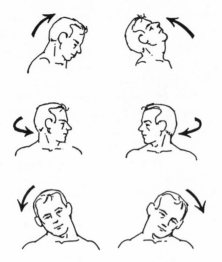

NECK MOVEMENTS

Nod your head as far forward and backward as you can without discomfort or pain.

Turn your head to the left and to the right as far as you can.

Move your head to each side—again, as far as you can.

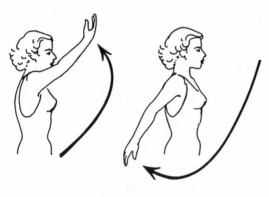

SHOULDER MOVEMENTS

Slowly raise your arm as high and straight as it will go, then bring it straight down and as far back as possible.

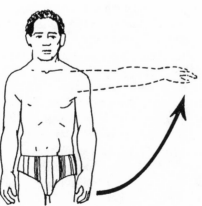

Lift each arm to the side to shoulder height.

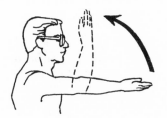

ELBOW MOVEMENTS

   Start with the arm straight out, then bend at the elbow, palms up.

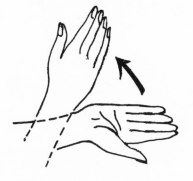

   With arms bent at the elbow, rotate palms up and palms down.

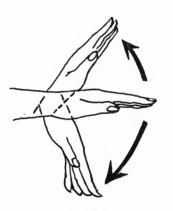

WRIST MOVEMENTS

   Keeping your hand relaxed and straight, lift and lower each hand, using your wrist as the "hinge."

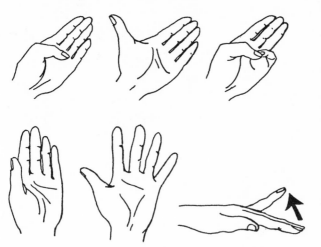

THUMB AND
FINGER
MOVEMENTS

Bend thumb to
palm, then extend
thumb, then bend
thumb to pinkie.

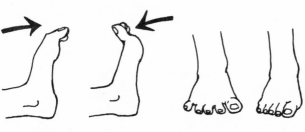

Place fingers
together; spread
fingers apart; lift
and lower the fin-
gers, using your
knuckle as a hinge.

ANKLE, TOE, AND
FOOT
MOVEMENTS

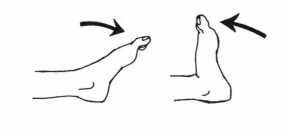

For the ankle:
Point the toe and
flex the foot.

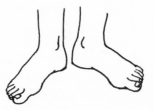

For the toes:
Bend the toes for-
ward and back as far
as you can; spread
the toes; squeeze the
toes together.

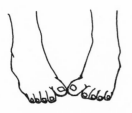

For the foot:
Touch big toe to big
toe; touch heel to
heel.

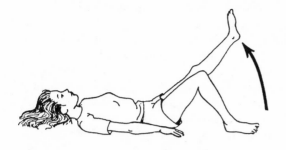

KNEE AND HIP
MOVEMENTS

For the knee: In a chair
or on your bed, bend the
knee and straighten the
leg.

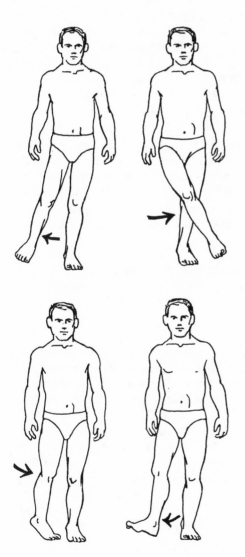

For the hip: Move your
leg to the side; move one leg
across the other; rotate
your leg to the inside; rotate your leg to the outside.

ful attacks of arthritis, when your joints are so inflamed that even carrying the weight of your arm is too stressful.

Range-of-motion exercises have been designed by physical therapists to increase your body's natural ability to flex, bend, stretch, and twist. These exercises are commonly used to help stroke patients regain mobility and coordinaton and also to counter the debilitating effects of arthritis or neurological diseases such as Parkinson's, ALS, and multiple sclerosis. Range-of-motion exercises are also a basic part of the rehabilitation of muscles traumatized by surgery, such as after a mastectomy or a hip replacement.

Exercises such as these are essential for anyone confined to bed for any length of time. Without continued. movement—even very gentle motion—joints and muscles soon get stiff and painful to move. Range-of-motion exercises will help maintain function, prevent deterioration of movement, and even increase the motion of a joint.

For the more active exerciser, range-of-motion movements give your body a chance to start circulating more blood to the muscles and to "oil" the joints with synovial fluid. Always begin any strenuous activity with warmups to help loosen the muscles and joints. Range-of-motion exercises are the essential base to any planned program of exercise.

Ideally, you should move each joint through its range of motion three times each day. Do it smoothly and slowly. Avoid pushing a joint beyond its free range of motion—do not force it. If there is inflammation or pain, consult with your physical therapist for specific guidance and assistance.

No matter what the extent or limitation of your range of motion, you'll find that these exercises will help promote flexibility, and they are especially valuable if there are few other opportunities for movement available to you.

ISOMETRIC EXERCISES

Isometric exercises are the kind used by bodybuilders to develop their physiques—and also by individuals to strengthen muscles that have been weakened by illness or injury. With isometrics, the muscles gradually get stronger through repeated pushing or pulling against a resisting object or force. Whenever you lift, carry, or press against something, you are performing isometric movement.

Isometric exercises can be done with equipment such as hand exercisers or weights, but they can also be done by working against the resistance supplied by another person. If your therapist or doctor prescribes certain equipment or machines, be sure they also tell you how to use these devices correctly and also how often you should repeat an exercise or how much weight you should be using. One of the most common mistakes patients make is to overtax themselves right at the start, thus aggravating their condition instead of helping it.

One more word of caution: Isometric exercises can strengthen all muscles except the heart. In fact, this kind of activity can put a strain on your heart and elevate your blood pressure—still another reason why it's important to work under the supervision of trained medical professionals.

ISOTONIC (DYNAMIC) EXERCISES

Isotonic, or dynamic, exercises consist of all movements that both contract (shorten) and extend (lengthen) the muscles. Unless you are pushing against a resisting force, you are performing dynamic movement. Common examples of dynamic movement are walking, twisting from side to side, bending down to touch your toes, gardening, and skiing.

If some of these seem like the range-of-motion exercises discussed earlier, you're right—but they are also dynamic movements. The effect of dynamic movement on your body varies according to the level of energy the activity demands. In general, however, dynamic movement both strengthens muscle groups—including the heart—and increases flexibility and stamina.

AEROBIC EXERCISES

The word "aerobic" refers to the use of oxygen. Your muscles require oxygen to work and "burn" calories. As you demand more of your muscles, they demand more of your heart, which pumps the blood carrying oxygen from your lungs. The heart, in order to meet this greater demand, must either pump faster or pump more blood with each beat.

Aerobic exercise gradually strengthens the heart so that it supplies a maximum amount of oxygen-rich blood to your system with a minimum of effort. In other words, a strong heart delivers more but works less.

How fast do you have to move to be doing aerobic exercise? That depends on your present state of fitness. If you've been inactive or ill for quite some time, it won't take much to get your heart beating faster— maybe even as little as walking at the rate of one mile per hour. But another person walking at the same pace may not even be breathing hard. You can feel when movement becomes strenuous. The important thing to remember, no matter what kind of movement you do, is not to strain. Straining is not strengthening.

Any kind of movement provides you with tangible benefits whenever you do it regularly. The kind of movement you decide to do depends not only on your personal preference but also on your state of health and your doctor's advice. If it is possible to work in some kind of aerobic activity, by all means try to do so.

Special Considerations for Special Conditions

There are many diseases, ailments, and illnesses that can require home health care. No matter what the health problem, though, keeping fit is vital. Special conditions require special considerations in the matter of keeping physically active. We'll cover some of the major ones here.

ARTHRITIS

Gentle movement increases flexibility in the joints by stimulating the production and circulation of synovial fluid, the "oil" in the joints. Joint swelling and inflammation are reduced with gentle exercise—especially if it's done in the water, where the weight of the body on the joints is lessened by the buoyancy of the water. Warm water is especially soothing.

More vigorous exercise—from walking to swimming or dancing—is particularly helpful between attacks of rheumatoid arthritis. By keeping your entire body in good shape, you build up a reserve of strength to resist the debilitating effects of recurrent attacks. Remember, it's crucial to warm up the muscles and joints before starting any exercise program, then gently stretch them out afterward to avoid stiffness.

DEPRESSION/ANXIETY

Whatever the cause of depression or anxiety, exercise has truly therapeutic effects. Aerobic exercise, especially, has the physiological effect of a tranquilizer. By increasing the circulation of blood to the muscles, exercise helps them relax.

There are also psychological benefits to be derived from engaging in some activity that demands your attention, or puts you in a social situation. It can get your mind off your troubles. Sometimes simply doing things with other people can have a very soothing effect, especially if the activity is not competitive.

HEART DISEASE

A strong heart doesn't need to work hard. It pumps a maximum amount of blood with a minimum of effort. As with any other muscle, the heart needs to be used to be kept in optimum condition.

The important thing to remember here is that only *aerobic* exercise benefits the cardiovascular system. Do something that requires rhythmic movement strenuous enough to raise your heart rate—and sustain the effort until you become pleasantly tired, not exhausted. The more you exercise, the greater your endurance will become, and the stronger your heart.

Cardiac patients must exercise under the supervision of a doctor or physical therapist to make sure they don't overtax their capacities. The point is to strengthen the heart, not strain it.

HYPERTENSION

Even without certain dietary restrictions (low sodium, low fat), regular aerobic exercise can lower blood pressure. In combination with dietary changes, this form of exercise has enabled some patients to stop using their blood pressure medication entirely. Exercise will raise the level of high density lipoproteins (HDL) in the blood and lower the cholesterol—both desirable goals in combatting hypertension and the related risk factors that can lead to heart disease or stroke.

POSTSURGICAL RECOVERY

Physicians and surgeons want to get a patient out of bed and moving around as soon as possible after surgery. Even if all the patient can do at first is to sit on the edge of the bed and dangle his feet, he is urged to do so. Experience has shown that recovery proceeds much faster if the patient becomes physically active as soon as possible after surgery. Because each case is different and each patient is different, the surgeon is the one to decide when the patient should start exercise-type movement, how much to do, and how often.

OSTEOPOROSIS

Osteoporosis is a condition most common in women, especially those over forty, in which calcium is lost from the bones, making them porous, brittle, and prone to fractures. Any exercise that puts stress on the bone through muscle pull or body weight (isometrics, walking, easy movement) stimulates the body to build up calcium and other minerals in the bone that's being worked. If you play tennis, for example, the bone in your playing arm will be stronger (more dense) than in your other arm. In other words, the benefit of exercise to bones is specific to the bone being stressed (in the good sense of the word).

STROKE

Aerobic exercise and proper diet are the best preventive measures against cardiovascular illness, including stroke. However, once a person suffers a stroke, exercise is also the best rehabilitative tool to regain strength and coordination, or to maximize those capabilities that remain.

Simple, gentle, repetitive movements, under the guidance of a physical therapist, can retrain stricken nerves and muscles to function properly once again.

Exercise pays—especially with stroke.

The Skin—a True Miracle Fabric

It warms; it cools; it's waterproof; it's elastic; it can be washed thousands of times over many decades before it wrinkles and creases. It is two square yards of body stocking that encloses us and informs us on a continual basis of our environment. Heat, cold, itch, touch, and some pain messages all start here. Yet most of us take this, our largest sense organ, for granted—and have little real knowledge of its wonders.

BASIC FUNCTIONS

Skin is a multilayered membrane that forms the outer packaging of our body, helping us to retain body fluids and other vital substances. More sensitive than most thermostats, our skin controls our body temperature. It lowers the temperature by opening blood vessels at the surface of the skin, allowing heat to escape, and raises the temperature by closing these vessels. When our body temperature gets too high, sweating helps to reduce further and control our body heat.

We are protected, soothed, and comforted by the skin's sensory functions. The skin on a big toe often serves as a temperature tester so we can check out how hot a bathtub full of water is or how cold the surf is before we take the plunge (assuming the toe is healthy and there is no nerve damage or circulatory impairment). And when comforting is needed, our skin lovingly conveys the sensation of being hugged, stroked, and caressed.

Skin protects us from solar radiation. When the sun beams down on us, the top layer of skin thickens to protect us. Additionally, pigmentation of the skin increases and our skin darkens, thus adding further protection. Rabid sun worshippers abuse this protective system by overexposure—sometimes with very unpleasant results. Medical researchers have confirmed the relationship between certain kinds of skin cancer and excessive exposure to the sun. Excess sun damages "sensor cells" in the skin. These cells would ordinarily summon other cells to destroy early cancer cells, which are really foreign bodies. Thus, excessive exposure to the sun allows skin cancer to develop.

Our skin has an amazing "built-in computer" that works to identify any and all foreign substances that may come into contact with the skin. Skin cells, acting as sensors, help to determine whether the foreign substance is to be considered friendly and so to be tolerated. On the other hand, the sensor cells may not be "tuned in" to the substance and, in refusing to accept it, will trigger an allergic reaction.

Allergic reactions are highly specific reactions to specific substances in specific people. The reaction occurs because the "sensors" have not accepted the substance. This does not necessarily mean that the substance is a harmful one, just that the sensors have not "passed" it. An allergic response can also be beneficial. The allergic reaction to bacteria, viruses, and fungi can serve to confine these invaders as well as attempt a curative process.

PROPER CARE AND FEEDING

Sidney I. Rogers, a Downstate Medical Center (New York) dermatologist, when asked for the secrets of proper skin care, says: "Normal skin under normal conditions needs a minimum of care. Just simple washing to clean off external dirt, accumulated cells on the surface, and excess oils and sweat is all that is often necessary." Under other than normal conditions, special care should be taken. A cold environment may result in dry skin. Creams or creamy lotions will help keep the skin smoother and more supple. Under very warm and humid conditions, more washing and less creaming is in order.

Individuals with naturally dry skin, or with dryness due to aging or sun damage, would naturally require more lubrication. Although the effect of creams and moisturizers is only temporary, they do help to add and retain moisture in the top layer of skin. Most creams or lubricating lotions will do the trick; there is no known value to many fancy additives or expensive beauty creams.

The skin of the scalp should not be overlooked either. Shampooing, under normal conditions, is best done at least once a week.

Home health care does not preclude getting out in the sun. Sunscreen preparations can be used for protection, and men as well as women can benefit from the use of creams or lotions on their skin. Time as well as sun and weather take their toll of skin, and it must be properly cared for both for cosmetic and health reasons.

With the passage of time, our skin, our outer body stocking, seems to reflect the years of care as well as wear and tear. Changes that are visible—in our hair, skin, and nails—are the flags of growing older. Although some changes are inevitable—our skin does get thinner and loses some of its elasticity—other changes can be the result of a lifetime of overexposure to the sun and unrelieved dryness, both of which can be controlled or avoided.

Some exposed areas like the hands and forearms may become freckled, and dryness can give skin a leathery look and feel. Also, sun damage to areas of the skin may produce little reddish scaly or wartlike growths called actinic kerotoses. These growths can become malignant and should be examined by a doctor and treated early. Other sun damages that may be encountered are pigmentation changes and skin growths that can range from benign to highly malignant cancers (melanomas). While avoiding the sun will not reverse previous sun damage, it most certainly will prevent further damage.

ITCH—A COMMON COMPLAINT

Itch is probably the most common skin symptom, with a long list of possible causes. Dry skin seems to be the most common cause of skin itch. Prickly heat, fungus (athlete's foot or jock itch, for example), insect bites, and allergic reactions are also on the list and add their groups of itching sufferers.

The most common and most readily available "treatment" for itch seems to be scratching. Unfortunately, this can aggravate both the itch and the condition that caused it. There is even a name for this phenomenon—the itch–scratch cycle. The more our skin itches, the more we scratch it, and the more we scratch, the more we aggravate and inflame the area that itches. Should this cycle persist, it can result in thickened, leathery areas of skin and, sometimes, infected, oozing, and painful lesions that require the attention of a doctor, preferably a dermatologist.

Itch can be brought on by depression or anxiety—the body is reacting to the emotional turmoil. Poor hygiene can lead to itch and infection. Diabetics sometimes have a tendency to itch. People who are senile or depressed may ignore problems related to the skin. They may not wash, rinse, or dry themselves properly, leading to the appearance of a rash and frequently an infection. People with neurological disorders with lessened sensations may be unaware of trauma or injury to the nerve-damaged area, and this can lead to sores or ulcers.

Shingles is more common in older people and is very painful. Also, nonmalignant growths may develop and, because of their location on the body and the tendency of clothing to irritate the area, may cause annoyance and irritation.

Some rules to follow in attempting to prevent the symptoms of itch are to eat well, practice good hygiene, exercise regularly, and maintain a level of physical and mental activity that will result in good overall body tone. It's not a good idea to overbathe in the winter, and it's important to keep cool and dry in summer. After bathing or washing, the application of lubricating creams and lotions may help if dryness becomes a problem.

You will know it's time to call for help should any itch, sore, scab, or growth persist, increase in size, or change shape or color. If there is bleeding from a skin growth, it is important to see a dermatologist right away. A change in color of the skin or a propensity to bruise easily should be brought to the attention of a physician. At times, a rash may appear shortly after starting a medication. The physician who prescribed the medication should be informed of this development. Occasionally, medications can cause reactions after a long period of usage.

Special Skin Care Problems

DIABETES

People with diabetes are subject to yeast infections, especially in the finger webs, the groin area, under the arms, and under the breasts. Vascular (circulatory) changes can lead to thinning of the skin, hair loss (usually on the legs), and coolness of the toes. Due to circulatory impairment, infections may develop more easily. Wounds may not heal readily, and ulcers or even gangrene may develop. Itching of the genital and anal areas is common. Diabetics may have other itchy rashes or may react to diabetic medication with a rash or ultrasensitivity of the skin to the sun. Repeatedly injecting insulin into the same area of the skin may result in a "hollowing" depression in the skin at the injection site, a condition that will gradually improve once the practice is stopped.

ARTHRITIS

In rheumatoid arthritis, the skin may be thin and shiny over the affected joints of the fingers, hands, or toes. Blisters, ulcers, or skin hemorrhages may occur on the feet or ankles. During an acute attack of rheumatoid arthritis, the skin may become red and swollen. In gout, a form of arthritis, uric acid accumulates in excessive quantities in the blood and uric acid crystals eventually settle in the joints and sometimes the cartilage, forming white or yellowish lumps. Acute attacks of gout often involve the large toe, the ankle, or the foot, with the skin becoming hot, swollen, and tender.

STROKE

Those individuals who have had a stroke that has resulted in numbness of an arm or leg have to be extra careful to avoid injury to the area. Since the nerve pathways have been affected, injury to the skin may not be immediately noticed and serious harm may result.

INTERNAL CANCER

Occasionally, an internal cancer can manifest itself on the skin, especially cancers of the breast, stomach, lung, uterus, kidney, ovary, or large bowel. Skin lesions will appear, usually few in number, and range in color from pink to violet to brown. They are often what is known as nonsymptomatic—that is, they do not exhibit the symptoms of cancer—which is why any persistent or suspicious skin lesion should be examined by a doctor.

Certain cancers of the white blood cells can invade the skin, causing severe and persistent itch and rash. Several types of skin rash—some related to hives—can appear from an internal cancer. Sometimes there is a rather sudden thickening of the palms of the hands and the soles of the feet. A generalized scaling and redness of the skin may be related to cancer of the white blood cells, known as lymphomas.

Occasionally an internal cancer may "seed" itself into the skin. A sudden onset of velvety darkening and thickening of the skin in the groin area, under the arms, or under the breasts may be a sign of internal cancer, although this symptom may also be found in extreme obesity or in endocrine gland disorders.

If any skin problems appear, do not attempt to diagnose them yourself, and don't panic about the possible implications of the skin condition that has appeared. Consult a dermatologist, and he will determine what the skin problem is and how to treat it.

MEDICATION REACTIONS

Medications are a frequent source of skin problems, usually causing an itch because of an allergic reaction. Some medications may cause flushing, hot skin, or excessive perspiration; others may cause a reaction on exposure to the sun. As mentioned before, report any reactions or side effects from medication to your doctor.

ALLERGIES

By the time we are older, most of us know whether we are allergic to any particular foods (although not all reactions to foods are allergic reactions). For example, spiced foods or alcohol may produce flushing of the skin in some people, especially those with a tendency toward a ruddy complexion. Occasionally, however, a new allergy may develop, accompanied by hives or a rash. If you have started eating a new food, you can experiment by cutting out the food to see if the allergy goes away. In any event, do not ignore it. If it persists, check with your physician.

FUNGAL INFECTIONS

If the skin is excessively moist for long periods of time, for example, between the toes, this provides an excellent breeding ground for fungi and bacteria to grow and cause disease and infections. Proper skin hygiene can prevent this.

In general, over-the-counter medications may be helpful for alleviating itch or dryness or an acute self-limiting eruption such as sunburn, athlete's foot, or mild skin irritations. However, see a dermatologist for any persistent itch, rash, or skin sore, especially a growth or mole that changes shape or color.

A dermatologist is a doctor highly trained as a specialist in skin diseases. He can recognize many skin conditions that may or may not be related to internal disorders. Many of these problems are acute; some are chronic. Some are of small consequence; others are more serious. Whenever a skin problem is chronic and recurrent or does not respond to treatment in a short period of time, a dermatologist should be consulted.

Good skin care is mostly up to you. A home health aide or a home care nurse may be needed to apply medications or dress ulcers or wounds (as in the case of bedsores, discussed in the next section), but for the most part, you can take care of your skin yourself. Keep your skin clean and make sure it's neither too dry nor too moist. You'll *feel* as well as see the results.

Incontinence

A middle-aged married woman prepares for a very rare evening out with her husband—rare because she has steadily resisted attending social functions for the past two years, ever since her "problem" developed. Now, unable to refuse still another time, she has agreed to go to a dinner at which her husband will receive a business award.

She dresses carefully, choosing a black polyester outfit, not because it's fashionable or because she looks good in it (she doesn't!) but for one reason only—the color of the dress and the polyester material are least likely to show the embarrassing wet spot.

A man in his fifties hesitantly clears his throat in his doctor's office and stares at a spot above the doctor's head, refusing to look him in the eye. The physical examination has been concluded, the doctor has been encouraging. The problem isn't all that bad. Certain tests will have to be made, but the doctor assures the man that what has happened is not unusual or life-threatening, although it's not something to ignore. The man, his face suddenly reddening, interrupts the doctor and, after a stammering start, finally blurts out what is on his mind. How will this—this "thing" that has happened to him—how will it affect his virility?

An elderly woman sits on a chair in her darkened bedroom and listens to the voices drifting up from the family conference being held downstairs. She can hear the murmur of voices—her daughter and her son-in-law and their two grown children discussing what's to be done with Grandma. She cannot hear the words, but it doesn't matter. She's seen their attempts to hide the looks of revulsion at what has happened to her. It will be a hospital and then probably a nursing home for her. She's no longer the plump, cheerful Grandma, always smiling and sweet-smelling. Now she's become an old woman that her family finds unpleasant to have around.

These three are typical of individuals with urinary incontinence. It has been estimated that there are anywhere from 7 to 12 million people of all ages in the United States who have "bladder control" problems; after age sixty-five, one in eight are incontinent. Incontinence is the inability to control the excretion of bodily wastes. Urinary incontinence is by far the most common. Fecal incontinence, although not as prevalent, can be even more devastating in its effects.

Incontinence itself is not a disease. You can't "catch it" from someone else, nor is there a virus that can be held responsible for it. Incontinence is a symptom of other problems, some of them treatable, some of them temporary. An acute illness in an elderly person, for example, can bring on confusion, disorientation, and fatigue, all of which can lead to incontinence. The emotional impact of extreme anxiety, severe stress, or rising anger can produce a sudden urge to urinate, which, in an elderly person, may not be controllable at the moment.

Several types of urinary incontinence have been recognized by health professionals. One of the most common is "stress" incontinence. This can be brought on by any sudden physical strain, even a mild one, such as that involved in coughing, sneezing, lifting, jumping, or outbursts of laughter. When this occurs, small amounts of urine can be unexpectedly expelled.

Women are subject to stress incontinence more than men. It rarely occurs in men except after surgical removal of the prostate. In women, however, 43 percent of those who have had at least one child and 15 percent of those who have never borne children have had "significant" stress incontinence.

What is known as "urge" incontinence is also common. This is characterized by a sudden desire to urinate that is so strong that there isn't enough time to get to the bathroom, resulting in involuntary urination. This condition can be brought on by certain medications (diuretics, for example), by a bladder infection, by pregnancy in women, or by an enlarged prostate in men.

In "locomotor" incontinence, the urge to urinate may not be overpowering. However, especially in elderly people, some physical difficulty or impairment may prevent the person from moving fast enough to the bathroom.

"Overflow" incontinence is what the name implies—urine overflows from a full bladder. The bladder muscles have lost the ability to contract in a normal manner (sometimes due to nerve damage), and urine accumulates until it overflows. In this type of incontinence, the bladder is almost always full, and overflow (leakage or dribbling) occurs readily and unexpectedly, often just from a change in body position.

The causes of incontinence are many, including: disease, physical injury leading to paralysis, and neurological disorders such as stroke, Parkinson's, or multiple sclerosis. Whatever the cause, whether treatable or untreatable, temporary or permanent, incontinence unfortunately carries with it social stigma as well as physical and medical difficulties. It can start in childhood accompanied by cruel derision for a child who "wets his pants" and go on from there to adulthood, when elderly people are placed in hospitals or nursing homes because the families just don't know how to cope with the problem at home.

Incontinence *can* be coped with. To do so takes a combined effort on the part of the caregiver and the one being cared for, but it can be done. Here is what the *Encyclopedia and Dictionary of Medicine, Nursing, and Allied Health* (Benjamin F. Miller, M.D., and Claire Keane, R.N., B.S., M.Ed., W. B. Saunders Co., Philadelphia, 3rd Edition, 1983) has to say on the matter:

Finding a way to keep the incontinent patient clean and dry can be a very real challenge. It requires knowing the patient as a person and making no assumptions about his ability to cooperate and achieve control until an effort has been made to involve him in a plan for control. It demands ingenuity, perseverance, and patience and a very real desire to help the patient cope with his problem.

The key words here are "clean and dry." This has to be your ultimate goal as the caregiver. It's essential, also, that you do not decide to ease the "burden" on the incontinent person by mentioning it as little as possible. This would be a serious mistake. Incontinence is not a pleasant subject, and it's certainly not easy for many people to talk about it. However, the discussion and planning have to be right out in the open and *must* include the person being cared for because he or she is the one who has to cope most directly with incontinence and all its social, emotional, and physical ramifications.

A real attempt must be made to rid our minds of the association of incontinence with infant behavior or with memories of child bed-wetters. An adult—usually an elderly person—who has to struggle with incontinence has to be helped to maintain a sense of dignity, a realization of personal worth, a feeling of confidence in the ability to go on functioning despite what has happened.

Incontinence can't be ignored, or made light of, but it must be viewed in proper perspective. It's a problem that can strike at many of us— and there are methods of dealing with it. Techniques have been developed, equipment has been designed and tested, and many people have set their minds to the task of how to help others learn to live with this problem.

Some urinary difficulties can be resolved with a simple procedure. For example, there are many elderly people who, during the night, find that they awaken moments too late to do anything about the need to urinate. By the time they are fully awake and ready to move, the "accident" has already happened. If this is a frequent occurrence, try to time these episodes. If they occur at about the same time during the night, arrange to have the person awakened just before that time so there will be ample opportunity to get to the bathroom, use the bedside commode, or use the urinal, if these are necessary.

If these episodes occur duing the day, the same method can be used. If there is any regularity about when these incidents take place, then a schedule can be worked out that may resolve the whole matter.

Assuming, though, that the solution is not that simple, there's still much that can be done. A great variety of specially made underclothes are available, as well as several types of pads, creams, lotions, and other preparations for dealing with incontinence and staying "clean and dry."

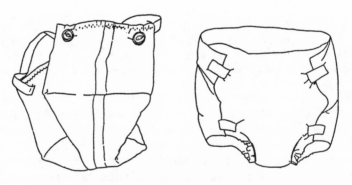

Disposable products: briefs (left), and diapers (right),
help patients with bladder control problems.

Illustrated are typical disposable products for those who are incontinent. These can be purchased at a pharmacy that deals in home health care products, or, if more privacy is desired, delivery can be arranged.

Literature giving facts about the incontinence product being sold, such as how to pick the right size brief, special features (zippered insert pads, for example), and how to select and use the product best suited to your needs can usually be found on a pharmacy rack. Also, of course, the patient's physician, therapist, health care nurse, or pharmacist can provide advice.

Most of these items are designed for dealing with urinary incontinence. Where fecal incontinence is concerned, there's not that much choice. In such cases, especially when the individual is bed-bound, an "adult diaper" is the most practical answer. A combination of a diaper and a bed underpad will aid greatly in dealing with the problem. With this type of incontinence, or with heavy voiding of urine, it's of utmost importance that the individual be cleaned right away. It's unpleasant—there's no getting around that—but it must be done. Special lotions, creams, and deodorant sprays are available that will facilitate the cleansing process and will ensure dryness afterward. Superabsorbents have been added to many incontinence pads to further aid in maintaining dryness. Thus, wetness and odor are kept to a minimum.

Disposable pads are used for both men and women. These are external devices that absorb urine. In some cases, though, it's necessary for a nurse or doctor to insert a catheter—a thin tube inserted through the urethra and into the bladder to drain the urine. The physician will be the best judge of the need for catheterization and how the catheter is to be used. Cleanliness is of paramount importance when dealing with catheters.

For men, there is an additional device that can be used for incontinence. It's called a sheath catheter or a condom catheter, and while not really a catheter since no tube is inserted into the bladder, it does act as an external collecting device. Urine drains into a sheath fastened on the penis and then flows through a flexible tube to a bag fastened on the leg of the person.

At present, external collecting devices have not proved practical for women, although companies are at work perfecting such devices, and there is one on the market that the manufacturer claims can be used by many women.

Women, though, do have the advantage of a special set of exercises that physicians and therapists sometimes recommend as helpful in controlling incontinence. These are called Kegel exercises and were originally devised to strengthen women's pelvic-vaginal muscles. By learning to exercise these muscles, women can contract them and shut off the flow of urine. The exercises require concentration and much practice, but by repeatedly stopping and starting the flow of urine, women can strengthen the muscles involved and, if successful, can achieve control, especially over stress incontinence.

Both men and women have to be extremely careful to maintain scrupulous cleanliness. This is of critical importance. Urine on the skin, if not cleansed off thoroughly, can bring about skin irritation and in some instances can lead to a decubitus ulcer (bedsore) in an individual who is confined to bed or who has to spend much time in bed and cannot move around and change position readily.

Our skin ages along with us, and older people do not have the natural protection a young and supple skin provides. Therefore, urine (and feces) can do much damage to an elderly person's skin in a comparatively short period of time. Infections and ulcers can be prevented if proper care is taken. Immediate disposal of urine-soaked pads, diapers, or clothing is imperative. After that, the person must be cleaned thoroughly and gently, using appropriate lotions, barrier creams, and whatever other preparations the physician or nurse or therapist recommends.

At present Medicare does not provide reimbursement for use of incontinence products, either disposable or reusable. However, these products are not usually exorbitantly expensive. With careful selection your funds will go a long way.

In any event, incontinence cannot be ignored. It must be dealt with on a daily basis with no letup. Persistence, patience, and understanding (above all, understanding) are the vital factors.

Remember, incontinence is not a disease, and there may be no way to stop it. But the individual on home health care can learn to live with incontinence and can learn, also, to function capably in daily living.

Oral Care

To many of us, brushing our teeth is something we all do regularly and almost automatically. Unfortunately, this is not always so, especially for someone distracted by other health problems. A chronic illness, an injury, or a disability often represents such a profound change in life style that normal activities, such as regular brushing of the teeth and other oral hygiene, are frequently neglected.

It's important, therefore, that you, as the caregiver, see to it that the person being cared for does not overlook the need for good oral hygiene. The teeth and their supporting tissues represent one of our most valuable health assets. Good oral health affects how we feel, how we look, how we eat, and how we sound—aspects of our lives that help determine the quality of life we enjoy.

There is no question that proper diet contributes to good oral health. A well-balanced diet will include all the basic foods and nutrients we need for proper nourishment. But a diet such as this does no good unless it can be eaten. A functioning set of teeth (natural or dentures) makes it possible to chew an adequate quantity of meat, fruits, vegetables, bread, and cereals. If chewing is difficult or painful, proper nutrition suffers. Too few calories may be eaten, or, even worse, there may be inadequate nutrition in the foods that are eaten. For example, a lack of fiber from breads, cereals, or vegetables could induce problems with regularity. It simply makes more sense to eat the right foods rather than to rely on laxatives and other preparations to make up for the lack of a proper diet.

Moreover, eating can be one of the more pleasurable activities of daily living. The smell, the taste, and the texture of good food is enjoyable, and there's no reason to deny ourselves this pleasure. Without good oral care, however, an individual can find eating so fraught with difficulties that a general lack of interest in food can develop. If this occurs, it can only serve to aggravate and perhaps deteriorate the general health of the person already being cared for at home because of a health problem. At the very least, it will directly affect the way that person feels about himself.

The ability to communicate can be limited by the absence of a full set of teeth. The clear consonant sounds we use in everyday speech can become slurred and mushy if we do not have good teeth or sufficient teeth to help form words and sentences. The result can be an inability to make oneself understood, and this, too, can affect the way an individual feels about himself and his relationships with others. If we can't communicate with other people, especially those close to us, we cannot adequately express our feelings—and it's harmful to keep emotions locked up inside ourselves.

If teeth are missing, broken, yellowed, or otherwise discolored, an individual will not be able to feel good about his appearance. We have all seen people who unconsciously cover their mouths while talking. This type of stress and restraint is not good for someone who is trying to maintain good health at home despite a disability or a chronic illness.

Poor oral hygiene can lead to the loss of teeth and sometimes to a bad bite (malocclusion). In severe cases, the joint that holds the lower jaw to the skull (the temporomandibular joint, usually referred to as the TMJ) can develop a painful dysfunction because of overclosure, or overbite, as it's more commonly called. The teeth click and grind together, and the TMJ becomes inflamed. There is often pain around the ears, sometimes very severe, and stiffness of the jaw. Dental treatment is needed to correct the malocclusion and to relieve the TMJ pain.

Obviously, many dental problems take years to develop and these problems may have been present or in the process of formation long before the individual was placed on home health care. However, there may be added discomfort and stress if dental problems are allowed to develop or to worsen while an individual is being cared for at home.

Brushing and flossing thoroughly at least once a day—preferably several times a day, especially after a meal or snack—helps prevent the collection of food debris in the mouth and the formation of plaque, that hard substance that the dentist has to scrape from the enamel of the teeth.

If the patient can leave home for brief periods, regular visits to a dentist and hygienist for professional cleaning and polishing of the teeth is important. A person cannot possibly do as thorough a job of cleaning as can be done in the dentist's office. Also, such visits will allow the dentist to check the condition of the patient's teeth and gums, especially for the presence of periodontal disease of the gums, which is the major cause of tooth loss in adults.

Mouthwashes help to rinse the teeth and sweeten the breath, but they do not replace the need for regular brushing and flossing. Inadequate dental hygiene can result in bad breath, stained teeth, and the development of heavy plaque deposits. In addition, bleeding gums, which may be an indication of the onset of periodontal disease, can be quite painful. These symptoms can be prevented through regular checkups by a dentist, regular cleaning by a dental hygienist, and proper dental care at home.

An example of how this three-pronged approach can effectively solve dental problems is the case reported by a dentist who had a patient troubled with bleeding gums. The patient constantly had a bad taste

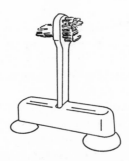

A suction-mounted toothbrush permits "one-handed"
brushing of removable dentures.

in her mouth. At first she thought she could eliminate the bad taste and stop the bleeding gums by taking large doses of vitamins. This method, of course, did not work. Vitamins will not get rid of impacted food and heavy plaque, which is what the dentist found on examining her. There were areas between her teeth that allowed food particles to collect and become impacted.

With a few new fillings and some crowns, the dentist was able to shape her teeth to provide less opportunity for food impaction. In addition, a thorough cleaning by a hygienist gave her mouth a fresh start. She was taught proper dental self-care and subsequently reported that her gums had stopped bleeding. The fresh taste in her mouth she now enjoyed was evidence of the return to health of her oral tissues.

In another case, Mrs. S. had a tumor removed from the floor of her mouth. She had received radiation therapy and was recovering well at home. Then she and her dentist noted a marked increase in the number of cavities she developed. Her dentist discussed the matter with the surgeon who had operated on her mouth, and the two of them agreed that the quantity and type of saliva now being formed in her mouth was a factor in the increasing incidence of tooth decay Mrs. S. was experiencing. Flouride treatment and the prescription of a flouride gel significantly reduced the tooth decay.

Oral Care for Special Situations

THE DIABETIC PATIENT

Gum problems for this group of patients can be severe. Proper care is critical because the diabetic's resistance to infection and his healing capacities often are impaired. The diabetic may need to visit the dentist more than the usual twice a year and certainly should be meticulous in his oral hygiene. If a dental infection develops in a diabetic, the dentist can use immediate application of antibiotics to control the infection.

THE POSTSURGICAL PATIENT

Following major surgery, many patients are not able to participate to any great extent in their own oral care. Dentists suggest that prior to surgery patients make sure that any dentures, bridgework, partial dentures, or other removable dental prostheses have been inscribed with the patient's name. The dentist can do this or else it can be done by a dental laboratory. It's unfortunately true that hospitals often lose dentures, and proper and permanent identification will help prevent such a loss.

It is also suggested that when the patient is able to sit up again it would be a loving gesture that the caregiver clean the patient's dentures for him or, if dentures are not used, to help the patient clean his teeth. Flossing the patient's teeth would be both thoughtful and helpful, but it would be best to seek the doctor's advice before attempting this as the patient's ailment or condition might preclude this.

THE CANCER PATIENT

If there has been a diagnosis of head, neck, or oral cancer, any questionable teeth (those with potential for decay) should be removed before radiation treatment is begun. After radiation of the mouth there is an extended healing process involved. Also, after radiation or oral surgery, the quantity and quality of the saliva can change. This may necessitate the use of artificial saliva for the patient who depends on saliva to keep dentures in place. Changes in saliva increase the susceptibility to tooth decay, especially cavities that develop at the root of the tooth. The daily application of flouride gel, prescribed by the dentist, may be helpful in this situation.

HEART PATIENTS AND OTHERS

There is a group of patients who must avoid any possible injection of bacteria into the bloodstream, which may result in an infection of the heart called endocarditis. When visiting their dentists, these patients almost always have been premedicated with an antibiotic to prevent bacteria from growing in the bloodstream. This group includes heart surgery patients, those with a history of rheumatic carditis, patients with artificial heart valves or with prolapsed mitral valves, and those who have had a joint replaced with an implanted artificial joint.

THE BEDRIDDEN PATIENT

The individual who is confined to bed at home should be encouraged to do as much for himself as possible. The tools for oral care are quite portable, and, if a patient is able, he should take care of his own oral hygiene. Proper lighting and the use of magnifying mirrors can be of assistance to the patient with poor or limited vision. When there are problems involving dexterity or grasping ability, the patient can more easily handle the toothbrush if the grip is made larger by inserting the handle through a rubber ball or tennis ball, or by customizing the grip in a similar way to help the patient hold the brush more securely. Special built-up toothbrushes can be purchased at a surgical supply house or a pharmacy that specializes in such products. Floss holders designed to allow the patient to floss his teeth with one hand are also available.

Customizing the handles of dental water irrigating devices may also prove helpful.

Improvement in the quality of life of a person on home health care is of significant importance. Dr. Richard S. Harold, a dentist in private practice in Malden, Massachusetts, specializes in contributing to an improved quality of life for people being cared for at home. Dr. Harold makes house calls, bringing with him completely portable dental equipment.

Not all communities are fortunate enough to have someone like Dr. Harold to provide the added touch of compassionate health care by making dental house calls. You can determine what services are available in your community by contacting your local dental society or the Academy of General Dentistry, 211 East Chicago Avenue, Chicago, IL 60611 ([312] 440-4300).

Your local Office on Aging or other community centers may be able to identify dentists who, while they do not make house calls, may have fully equipped vans that can park outside your home to bring dental services closer to those who can't travel too far. Also, transportation or van service to take you to your family dentist may be available. Be sure to check out all possibilities.

Oral Care Aids

There are many regularly available products that can help you in maintaining good oral health care at home. *The Dentist's Desk Reference* identifies the following aids to oral hygiene and oral health, some of which may prove helpful to you.

Powered Toothbrushes • Battery-powered electric toothbrushes are available. The brushing motion can be back and forth or up and down, a combination of both, or a rotating motion. The brushes are usually made of nylon filament bristles, set in different configurations by each manufacturer. Powered toothbrushes can be useful replacements for hand-held brushes for those on home health care who might have problems with hand dexterity.

Dental Floss, Dental Tape, and Floss and Tape Holders • Dental floss comes in waxed and unwaxed forms, and both types can be used in interdental (between the teeth) cleaning to loosen and remove plaque and food debris. Dental tape is sometimes referred to as "flat floss" and is wider than floss and covered with a soft wax coating. It is used for the same purpose and in the same way as dental floss.

Several devices are available to hold the floss or tape in a taut position for one-handed operation—a technique that may have to be used by an individual who does not have the full use of both hands.

In addition, although they do not fall into the category of floss or tapes, there are numerous products designed to do what floss and tape do—clean between the teeth. Among these products are round and triangular toothpicks of wood or plastic, small tapered brushes consisting of a wire core with bristles in various configurations, and small handles with rubber tips of different shapes. The effective use of any of these products depends on the spaces between the teeth and the size and flexibility of the mouth of the person using them.

Oral Irrigating Devices • The popular Water Pik is an example of this type of device. Whether attached to a faucet or to a motor-driven pump, these oral irrigating devices generate a stream of water, either pulsating or continuous, that can be used for removing debris between the teeth. While these devices are not recommended to replace brushing or flossing, they do seem to remove accumulated food particles that brushing or flossing may miss.

It's best to clean your teeth with a toothbrush and dental floss or tape before using the water device. You will then be able to see the additional debris it may dislodge. Use it at its lowest pressure setting and keep the tip moving continuously about one-half inch from the gums. Do not use this device if your gums are inflamed.

Denture Adherents • These are powders or pastes sprinkled or spread on dentures before they are inserted into the mouth. The product is designed to make the dentures adhere to the gums and remain in place. They do not "glue" the dentures in place and will not make ill-fitting dentures fit better. However, they can be used as an emergency measure to stabilize an ill-fitting denture until it can be adjusted by the dentist or a new denture is made.

In certain circumstances, such as for patients who have very flat ridges on their gums or who may have a postcancer prosthesis in the mouth, these powders and pastes may be helpful in keeping the dentures more firmly in place.

It is suggested that no more than a thin, even coating of powder or paste be used and that this material be cleaned twice daily from the denture-bearing tissues in the mouth, accompanied by thorough rinsing. Powder or paste should not be used on a continual basis unless prescribed by a dentist.

Dental Cleaning Agents • These products are used to remove soft debris and stains from dentures and to prevent the dentures from acquiring an unpleasant odor. There are many of these agents available, as you can see from a glance at the shelves in a pharmacy. Dentures should be rinsed thoroughly before applying the cleaning agent. The denture should be brushed thoroughly but carefully so as not to bend any clasps or abrade the denture. Rinse the denture several times before inserting into the mouth.

The denture should be professionally cleaned by your dentist at least once a year.

Mechanical Denture Cleaners • These are sonic or ultrasonic devices for cleaning dentures through high frequency sound waves. The sound waves break up debris and food particles, which can then be washed away. Leaving a denture in a mechanical cleaner for an extended period of time may damage the denture.

Sexuality

Sexual drive—as well as sexual ability—extends for many people into their sixties, seventies, and eighties. Society has recognized the sexuality of the young and their need to express it and is now beginning to extend the same consideration to the elderly—but not as fully.

There are still far too many hang-ups apparent in the way many individuals—including some health professionals—look upon the matter of sexuality, especially when older people are concerned. A fairly common reason for this attitude is that we do not like to think of older people making love since this conflicts with our image of our parents. Another reason is that we are at this moment a youth-oriented society (more people are getting older all the time, though!) and old age just cannot be equated in the minds of some people with the "youthful" activity of sex.

It was an accepted concept not so many years ago that one went to the family doctor for advice about sexual problems. (Books on sex were shelved in separate rooms at the local library, and only doctors or qualified social workers were allowed to use them.) Trouble was, physicians were not that well informed about sexuality and, on the whole, tended to express the more conservative views about sex and sexual activities.

Physicians are more knowledgeable about such matters today. However, there is still some reluctance on the part of some physicians and other health professionals—nurses, therapists, and social workers—to discuss sex with their patients.

This is not true of the majority of health professionals, of course, but this reluctance can be encountered sometimes when least expected—such as while filling out questionnaires and medical histories. Some health professionals may gloss over questions about sexual activity, either out of a misplaced desire not to embarrass their patients or on the assumption that sex just couldn't be an important factor in this sick or disabled or elderly person's life, and if by some chance it were, he or she would bring the matter up.

Assumptions such as these cannot be allowed to deter the person being cared for at home from expressing his or her sexuality. In a sense, it's a right all of us have, and it should not be denied—as it sometimes is in nursing homes where the owners and the staff segregate the patients by sex and do not allow even married couples to share any moments of sexual intimacy because this just isn't what the "old folks" are supposed to do.

We're all human—including physicians, nurses, and health professionals—and we are all subject to the same foibles, follies, and false concepts. Consequently, a health professional may be talking to an elderly patient—someone complete with a chronic illness or disability and the usual assortment of wrinkles and other marks of age—and will avoid bringing up the matter of sexuality, assuming that it is not one of the prime concerns of the patient.

Clearly, it *is* a prime concern for many individuals, regardless of age or disability, and the matter should be openly discussed by patients, caregivers, social workers, health professionals, and, above all, by the two individuals most directly involved—the husband and wife, couples living together, or just plain lovers.

A case in point is what happened to Dora, a married woman in her early sixties who had a colostomy—a procedure in which an artificial opening is made in the large intestine for the purpose of evacuating the bowels through the abdominal wall rather than through the anus, which in Dora's case had been surgically removed. When Dora returned home from the hospital she was very apprehensive about what life would now be like for her husband and herself. She had made a good start in adjusting to the new way her body now had to function, and her husband had attended sessions with her at the hospital and knew what a colostomy involved. This wasn't what troubled Dora. She was concerned about their sex life.

Dora and her husband, Everett, had had an active sex life for many years. Until Dora's operation, they had lived a full and vigorous existence in which lovemaking was an enjoyable and frequent activity. Things would be different now, Dora realized, but she had not been able to bring herself to discuss sex with her husband, and Everett, sensing her feelings and not too sure of his own emotions at the moment, also did not talk about it.

The situation remained at this uncertain level until an enterostomal therapist (a health professional trained in the care of people who have had colostomies or similar operations) came to the house as part of a home health care visit and sensed what was on Dora's mind from a few words that Dora let slip. The therapist talked to Dora and her husband briefly that day and then set things in motion to ensure that Dora and Everett would be able to get the kind of counseling they needed.

It took time, but the two of them came to realize that there was no reason to give up sex. For one thing, sex for them had always involved more than just the act of intercourse. They had enjoyed touching and cuddling and caressing and sometimes just sharing in the warmth of each other's closeness. There was no reason why they could not continue to do this now. True, Dora had to wear a collection pouch on her stomach to cover the stoma (the hole through which her bowels could be emptied), but she and Everett learned how to deal with this. In time, it did not interfere with their closeness.

They also found that they could consummate the sex act without much difficulty, and while they couldn't be as lusty and physically vigorous as they had been in the past, they could still enjoy a satisfactory sexual relationship.

While Dora and Everett's situation may not be typical of the sexual problems faced by people being cared for at home, it does reveal the fact that sexuality cannot be ignored.

There are many avenues for sexual expression and for the enjoyment of sex. It's a highly personal matter, to be sure, but it cannot be pushed to one side. There has to be communication. First, there must be communication between the patient and whoever is counseling him, be it a nurse, a physician, a social worker, or a therapist. The discussion has to be open and honest and cover all the questions the patient may have. Not everything can be covered at one session, of course. Other questions are bound to arise later. However, the fact that an avenue of communication has been opened is what is important.

Next, there must also be communication between the patient and his sexual partner. Assuming for the moment that this partner is a wife and it's the husband who has become disabled and must be cared for at home, the two of them have to talk freely and frankly. Talking it over will be much easier if they have had this kind of open relationship in the past. If not, they must make a start at developing that kind of relationship now—that is, if they want to keep sexuality alive in their marriage.

Finally—and this may not be necessary if things work out well between husband and wife—there can be communication among the husband, the wife, and the counselor. Quite often a third party, someone who is trusted and will have a more objective viewpoint, can be a great help in guiding the partners to a new understanding of how to express their sexuality.

Once the lines of communication are established, the couple can work things out further in the privacy of their bedroom. If, for example, the nature of the disability or illness precludes much physical mobility for the husband, different sexual positions and techniques can be tried out until both feel at ease and can concentrate on giving each other pleasure. Sexual experimentation can be fun, and if a sense of humor is maintained, even the inevitable awkwardness and difficulties that will arise can be overcome with a minimum of stress.

Sex is not defined by the number of different positions that can be attained. Nor must it necessarily involve an orgasmic conclusion. Sex is closeness, touching, sharing. Expressions of sexuality can vary infinitely with the couples involved.

There's room for many varieties of sexual expression. An older couple—especially if one of them has a chronic illness—can still enjoy a high degree of sexuality by just ordinary caressing that doesn't even involve the genital areas or other erogenous zones. For some people, a gentle back rub from a caring partner is a beautiful expression of sexuality. For others, a little kissing and cuddling on a relaxed level may be all that's needed. For still others, gentle smiles and whispered conversation while holding each other close can be both stimulating and rewarding.

The one common element in almost all expressions of sexuality is physical closeness—touching. The number of ways this closeness and touching can be accomplished will depend only on the imaginations, desires, and life styles of the people involved.

There is no "right" or "proper" way to express sexuality. Whatever feels right to the two people involved is what's right and proper for the two of them.

SPECIAL CONSIDERATIONS

The Heart Patient • Because sexual intercourse involves bodily activity, a common fear of men (and women) who have had heart attacks is that from now on sex will be dangerous for them. This fear, although understandable, is unfounded. After a suitable period of rest in which the heart has had time to heal (the physician can tell the patient how long this should be in his particular case), sexual relations can be resumed. Usually, the physician will first want to test the patient's exercise tolerance level to assess how strong the recovery has been. A rough rule of thumb is that if the patient can take brisk walks without tiring and can climb two flights of stairs without becoming breathless, then sexual relations can be resumed. No patient should attempt to make this assessment on his own. The physician (usually a cardiologist) will be the one to make the final determination. If the patient lacks stamina, limited sexual activity (perhaps just cuddling, touching, and kissing) can be enjoyed.

The resumption of sexual activity need not necessarily be vigorous. Also, former heart attack patients should avoid sex after a heavy meal, when tired or after drinking alcohol.

The Arthritis Patient • Arthritis sufferers have problems with mobility and flexibility of joints. Pain—especially arthritic pain—can often put a damper on sexual activity. Nevertheless, sexuality does not have to be banished forever from the life of the arthritic patient. Sexual activity can be timed to coordinate with the period when medication taken by the person will have its strongest effect and pain will be diminished. Positions and techniques can be worked out by the couple so that sexuality can be freely expressed—and enjoyed.

Masturbation • Up to now, we've been discussing sexuality as it relates to two partners. Obviously, the single person has to express his or her sexuality also—and the term "single" can also apply to a married man or woman whose spouse has lost interest in sex because of illness or other reasons related to being a home health care patient. (Lack of privacy, for example, if a bed has had to be set up in the living room or the family room instead of the bedroom.)

How does a single person express sexuality? At its core, sexuality is not necessarily expressed by sexual activity. Sexuality reflects how a person feels about himself or herself. Masculinity and femininity can be demonstrated by what the person says or does. Words and actions delineate the self-image which the individual creates for himself or herself and projects to others.

Sometimes this is enough; other times, it isn't. This brings us right up against a once taboo word: masturbation.

The word itself may no longer be taboo, but attitudes still linger and are difficult to erase. No matter how many research studies show the prevalence of masturbation, and no matter how many medical experts, psychiatrists, therapists, and sex counselors emphasize that masturbation is a healthy and normal expression of individual sexuality, it is still too frequently spoken of in hushed tones or written about in circumlocutions.

Perhaps this is because there is something guilt-inducing about giving yourself sexual gratification. Or it may be that since masturbation is almost always a secret activity, the person is afraid of being found out.

A young man, crippled and confined to a wheelchair, spending most of his time at home, expressed this fear in confidence to a therapist. He told the therapist that he was constantly dreading what his mother might say to him when she changed his bedding and realized that he had been masturbating. It was his sole outlet for his sexuality, and yet he could not enjoy it fully.

Fears and guilt feelings about masturbation are not confined to the young alone. The isolation that sometimes accompanies being cared for at home—or caring for someone's health at home—can cause the person to repress his or her sexuality until secret masturbation brings a quickly lost moment of release.

Then again, masturbation can be used by a couple or by one member of a couple as a means of sexual expression and to bring sexual pleasure to a partner when full sexual activity by both partners may not be possible. In such an instance, there can be no guilt or hidden fears—sexuality will have been expressed openly and fully.

Impotence • One of the more disturbing aspects of sex for those in a home health care setting is impotence on the part of the man. Impotence—the inability to bring about and maintain an erection—is a subject so fraught with fears, misinformation, and hidden shame that it is extremely difficult for many people to discuss it, especially the man involved. Far too often, it's never mentioned at all—not between the man and woman or to a doctor or professional counselor.

As recently as five years ago, it was thought that 90 to 95 percent of all cases of male impotence were caused by emotional or psychological stress on the part of the man. The usual advice was: "It's all in your head. Relax, and everything will be all right." Research has shown that this diagnosis was not correct for many cases of impotence. It is now known that there can be many organic causes of male impotence, among them spinal cord injury, diabetes, radical prostate surgery, heart and blood vessel disease, thyroid problems, kidney disease, and the use of certain medications for hypertension.

The latest estimate is that about half of all cases of male impotence are caused by physical problems rather than psychological ones and that about 10 million American men have chronic impotence.

To determine whether impotence is physical or psychological in origin, doctors can conduct a test while the patient sleeps. Electronic monitors record whether the individual has any erections during periods of REM (rapid eye movements), which indicate normal sleep. If three to five erections are achieved while asleep, the impotence is psychological in origin. If there have been no erections, the impotence is, in all probability, caused by organic problems and is physical in origin.

If it has been definitely established through testing that a patient's impotence is not psychological, the urologist (a doctor specializing in the male genito-urinary system) may suggest a penile implant. This is an operation in which a device is implanted in the male penis to allow the patient to achieve and maintain an erection. It's not a natural erection, of course, but it does serve the purpose, and many men have testified to a new lease on life because of their penile implant.

At present, two types of implants are used. In the first, a semirigid silicon rod is implanted in the penis, and the man can adjust it's position when an erection is desired during sexual activity. The second type of implant produces a more natural effect but is a bit more complex. In this procedure, twin inflatable cylinders are implanted in the penis, a silicon reservoir containing a special fluid is placed in the body cavity near the bladder, and a pump with a release valve is implanted in the scrotum. All of these items are small in size and are placed inside the body. The length of the penis remains the same, although the width may be slightly altered.

Once the operation has been completed and recovery has progressed, the patient is taught how to manipulate the internal pump by squeezing the scrotum gently with his fingers. The pump takes fluid from the implanted reservoir and sends it to the two tubes implanted in the penis, which inflate and produce an erection. Pressing the release valve returns the fluid to the reservoir, deflating the erection. Ejaculation is not simulated by this device.

The inflatable implant was developed in 1973 and since then has been inserted in about 12,000 men. The success rate has been good, with about 92 percent of the men giving it a favorable report. The operation costs about $6,000, with a hospital stay of three days. Counseling is required afterward for both the man and his partner in order to learn how to use the prosthesis and to adjust to it physically and psychologically.

A recently formed support group, Impotents Anonymous, has started organizing chapters in several states, indicating a definite need for information about impotence, as well as a broader understanding of its physical and emotional impact (see the Appendix).

Aging • In addition to coping with expressing their sexuality under other than usual conditions, people at home with a chronic illness or other health problems also are subject to the normal sexual changes that come about with the aging process. These are physical as well as psychological changes. Men may find it takes longer to attain an erection, which will diminish rapidly after ejaculation, and that the ability to recover and be ready for another sexual encounter takes longer than it used to. Women may have difficulties with vaginal dryness and discomfort, along with needing more time spent in foreplay and stimulation than before. Both men and women may tire easily and will not be able to be as sexually athletic as in the past.

All this is the normal "slowing down" that comes with getting older. Sexual partners can learn to adjust to these changes as well as to the changes brought about by the health problems that have to be dealt with. As mentioned before, communication is very important. Not only should the partners talk things over, but their conversation should be open, honest, and unashamed. One should not hesitate to experiment or to seek out professional help when it is needed. The stress of daily living on home health care can be alleviated through doing things we enjoy, and sex is one of those enjoyments.

Sexuality is part of all of us, and to deny it or repress it because of age or because of an unrelated health condition is to diminish the quality of life.

Sleep

The words are just about the same every time it happens.

The elderly grandparent sitting with the rest of the family watching TV or reading the Sunday papers will nod and start to doze off, and one of the children will call out, "Look at Grandma (or Grandpa). Fast asleep!" And then Grandma (or Grandpa) will snap upright and claim, "I was just resting my eyes."

It's an inside joke, common to many families—the "just resting my eyes" response. Everybody chuckles about it, and the older person goes along with it because everybody knows that the older you get, the easier it is to doze off during the day.

There's some truth in this, of course, since an increase in involuntary dozing is often part of getting older. However, sometimes this can also be an indication of sleep difficulty the older person is having at night. Since many grandparents who live at home with their children and grandchildren don't like to complain, preferring to keep a low profile, it's possible that an uncomfortable bed is causing a poor sleep pattern during the night—or it might be something a lot more serious. But nothing is being said about it because the older person doesn't want to "make waves."

This same situation can prevail for an elderly person who is being cared for at home rather than in a hospital or other institution. He will refrain from saying anything about his sleep difficulties either for fear of drawing attention to his problem and perhaps having to return to the hospital or because he thinks sleeping difficulties are to be expected due to the combination of advancing age and health problems.

CHECK THE BED

Let's consider the simple, nonthreatening, and fairly common matter of a bad bed causing the sleep problem. Unless a hospital bed has been installed in the home, the condition of the older person's bed is sometimes neglected, especially if it's a bed that the individual has been using for many years. It's important, therefore, to check the mattress, box spring, and bed frame whenever an older person begins a period of home health care. It's even more important if the reason for being cared for at home is a chronic illness or a permanent disability, for this means that the bed is likely to see a lot more than normal use.

Take the bed completely apart. Examine the frame or the side rails and slats, depending on the type of bed. Is any part of the frame bent or out of alignment? Are the wheels all in place, none of them buckled in? Are the frame clamps secure? Is there a center crossbar if this is a queen-size or larger bed? If side rails are used, are they firm and not warped? Are the slats straight and not bowed?

After this, examine the box spring. Are there any holes in it? Have any of the springs popped through the cover? Does it sag? Are the edges still firm?

Look at the mattress next—and ask the same questions. Be especially thorough in checking for a sagging middle and for a too-soft structure. A mattress should neither be too hard nor too soft—unless, of course, a very hard mattress is required because of an individual's back problems. In such cases, a board is often put between the mattress and the box spring.

A well-designed and engineered bed is constructed so that the mattress and foundation complement each other, the two units working together to provide the desired body support. If the bed is of good quality, much more has gone into it than just manufacturing and merchandising skills. Orthopedic surgeons have helped design beds for major manufacturers to make sure that the mattress distributes the body weight evenly, one of the most important factors in preventing so-called morning backache.

All of this applies directly to the elderly person being cared for at home. A mattress or a mattress-and-foundation combination that is either too soft or too hard does not distribute body weight evenly. When this happens, the person's muscles have no real chance to relax. They are fighting the distorted position the person's body has been forced into by the softness or hardness of the bed.

If muscles have had to be active during the night, fatigue will develop during the day, which along with the effects of medication can account for the tendency of some older people to doze off repeatedly during daylight hours. Moreover, the muscles of older people are not as resilient as they used to be, and this can add further to the nighttime strain and perhaps increase the daytime fatigue.

A good bed—proper mattress and comfortable pillows—is far more important in providing health care for the elderly than most people would suppose. It cannot be taken for granted.

INSOMNIA

A certain amount of bed rest is important to the maintenance of good health. However, it's often difficult for the person at home to get this kind of rest. Some of the time this is due to insomnia. Many jokes have been made about insomniacs, but it's no joking matter to those who suffer from it. It's especially debilitating and emotionally disruptive for someone who has to be concerned on a daily basis about the state of his health.

There are several approaches to dealing with insomnia. First the person should have a complete physical examination by a physician to make sure there's nothing organically wrong that might be causing the insomnia. If the doctor concludes that there is nothing organically wrong, the next thing to do is to examine the person's daily routine to see if the cause of the insomnia might be something as simple as too many daytime naps. A short nap of about ten or twenty minutes does no harm. It's when too many of these naps are taken during the day that trouble with nighttime sleeping can occur.

Another cause of insomnia might be overstimulation at night before going to bed. If the person is in the habit of doing some mild calisthenics before going to bed, as some people do, he should try scheduling his exercise period for earlier in the day. If he has been drinking coffee or tea at night, he should cut it out. If he sips some cognac to help him sleep, he should try skipping this for a few nights. Some people are helped to sleep by a drink before bedtime, but alcohol can also be a stimulant. Warm milk often does the trick.

Another method is to try experimenting with different sleep times. We all have a regular sleep-wake cycle in every twenty-four-hour period. As we get older, especially after sixty or sixty-five, the natural rhythm of this cycle can change. It may become less stable, and older people may find themselves waking frequently during the night. Insomnia may result from forcing a sleeping time that isn't synchronized with the changed sleep-wake cycle. It has been found that sleep patterns in the elderly vary more than in other age groups. Some experimentation may help determine an individual's proper sleep time and sleep pattern.

Insomnia sometimes exists only in the mind of the individual. He is sure he has insomnia and that he cannot sleep at night, yet this is not the case. All-night studies of his sleep pattern and his cycles of sleep show that he is sleeping far more than he knows and that he has no insomnia. In fact, he has what is called pseudoinsomnia. This cannot be shrugged off. Although the individual may be getting sufficient sleep most nights, the fact that he feels he isn't sleeping is very serious to him and can be emotionally and mentally upsetting.

There is no medication that can be given for pseudoinsomnia. The only treatment is for the physician to talk to the person, show him the results of the sleep tests and all-night sleep recordings (if a visit to a sleep disorder clinic has been arranged), and reassure the patient that he has no problems with insomnia.

It often helps to affirm that the old saying that the older you get the less sleep you need is generally true. Infants and growing children need a lot of sleep. Young men and women usually require about eight hours sleep in order to maintain health and function properly in the everyday world. Elderly people over sixty-five can and do get along with much less sleep—four to six hours is usually sufficient. Once the older person realizes this, the problem of pseudoinsomnia can be resolved.

Do not attempt to diagnose pseudoinsomnia yourself. A competent physician must do this. The doctor may or may not recommend going to a sleep disorder clinic or sleep laboratory after taking into consideration the patient's general health, the results of any tests that were ordered, and the doctor's general knowledge of the patient's mental attitude. In any event, he can determine whether there is any other reason for the problem, by eliminating all other possibilities, before considering pseudoinsomnia as the diagnosis.

SLEEP APNEA

Sleeping difficulties are not always benign in nature. Older people may develop a sleep disturbance known as sleep apnea. They experience breathing difficulty during the night, sometimes awakening with a choking feeling. They may have episodes of gasping and snorting and will stop breathing for a few seconds.

Cessation of breathing is the danger. The individual snores and thrashes about and will sometimes awaken and not even realize that he has had a sleep apnea episode. Nevertheless, there has been an interruption in breathing. The experts consider any breathing stoppage during sleep in excess of ten seconds and occurring more than thirty times in seven hours as constituting sleep apnea.

If the sleep apnea episodes are repeated night after night, they can lead to a chronic oxygen shortage, hypertension (high blood pressure), and abnormal heart rhythms, which can cause heart failure. Additionally, there is much daytime fatigue, an excessive amount of daytime sleepiness, with periods of dozing off, and in some cases, mental lapses and other intellectual deficiencies.

It has been estimated that about 30 percent of elderly people have some form of sleep apnea, and 90 percent of those with sleep apnea are male—and mostly obese. Drastic weight loss will often help control or eliminate the apnea. In other more extreme cases, surgery may be needed. A hole is created in the trachea (windpipe) to allow uninterrupted breathing, eliminating the risks associated with apnea.

Sleep apnea is dangerous and potentially life-threatening. If this disorder is suspected because some of the symptoms appear, check with a physician. It may not be sleep apnea (perhaps only a heavy snoring problem). If it is apnea, however, proper steps can be taken to correct the problem.

MEDICATIONS AND SLEEP

Sometimes medications will cause sleeping difficulties. Diuretics, antiparkinson drugs, and antidepressants can cause sleep disturbances. The physician can check into this and perhaps change medications he has prescribed.

There is always the temptation to self-medicate when experiencing sleep disturbances. There are many over-the-counter (OTC) preparations available. And many people use them on an almost nightly basis. We Americans spend about $25 million a year on OTC sleep aids. Although some of these may actually help bring on sleep, excessive use of these preparations is not advisable. To be on the safe side, check with a doctor. If something is really needed to induce sleep at night, he may prescribe a sleeping pill.

Medications to help bring on sleep, whether OTC or prescription, cannot take the place of natural sleep. Although it's a truism that we require less sleep as we get older, the quality of the sleep is important. Poets have for many years become rhapsodic when attempting to describe the wonders of sleep. Older people, who have spent a lifetime of nights in sleep, or attempting to sleep, know what the poets mean.

A good night's sleep is a wonderful restorative. It's well worth striving for.

III

Special Care

THIS PART contains information on four health situations that require special home health care techniques: the control of pain; dealing with pressure sores; high tech home care; and caring for the dying patient. Because of the special nature of these health matters, the caregiver will need assistance from health professionals in setting up and maintaining a home health care program. The information is presented here for your guidance. Check with your doctor and other members of the health care team before undertaking any of the procedures described.

9

Pain and Pain Control

To those who deal with it on a professional basis—doctors, nurses, therapists, psychologists, pharmacists—the statistic is well known: About one out of every three persons in the United States suffers from some form of persistent or recurring pain. In terms of money, it costs $60 to $70 billion dollars a year. In terms of human agony, the cost is incalculable.

Countless attempts have been made to understand pain. Researchers have delved into its causes; scientists have categorized its types; others have experimented with animals in the name of easing human pain. Believers in home remedies have put their faith in formulas handed down over the generations; charlatans have offered instant cures. Philosophers have meditated on it; hypnotists have tried to drive it from the mind; pain sufferers have experimented on themselves.

Our knowledge of pain and how to cope with it and sometimes control it is expanding steadily. However, pain is still with us—and it should be. Without pain, we would have no internal alarm network, no way of knowing that something was going wrong in our bodies. There's no reason, though, why we should have to suffer excessively as the price for this natural warning system. Pain researchers are continually seeking ways to reap the benefits of the pain signal that alerts us to trouble and, at the same time, to control the pain to avoid the suffering it imposes.

What Is Pain?

That question is not as simple as it seems. In order to understand pain and to learn how to manage it, we first have to know what it is.

It's difficult to define pain. Not too long ago, researchers weren't even sure that they could place pain in a separate sensory category, complete with its own nerve cells and pain center in the brain. It was reasoned that perhaps pain was nothing more than excess pressure on nerve endings sensitive to touch. Later research showed that pain was much more than this and that the subject of pain encompassed many facets that had not been realized before.

As a very basic definition, we can say that the presence of pain is a warning signal that body tissues are being damaged. There's more to it than this, of course, but this definition will serve as a starting point for an exploration of pain: what it is, what it does, and what measures have been discovered for coping with it.

Two main types of pain have been recognized—acute and chronic. Acute pain ceases in time; chronic pain lasts.

Acute pain can be brought on by a thumb inadvertently placed in the path of a hammer blow, by a match that isn't blown out fast enough, by a child's knee scraping the sidewalk, and by other such accidents. Pain can also be considered acute during childbirth, or when tooth decay reaches the nerve, or when an appendix has been removed. No matter what the cause or how sharp its impact, acute pain can be dealt with and will eventually go away. This knowledge helps us to bear the pain. Also, it's a known fact that once the pain has passed, it's difficult to remember the severity of its sensation.

Chronic pain, on the other hand, stays with us, giving us no real chance to forget what it felt like. Even during respites from chronic pain, we know it's going to return. This is the pain of migraine, arthritis, gout, cancer, and many other diseases and neurological disorders.

Chronic pain wears away at the defenses of the body and mind. It debilitates and incapacitates us. It can bring on severe depression, cause sleepless nights, ravage the sensibilities—in a very real sense, it can destroy our lives.

The Perception of Pain

Pain, whether acute or chronic, is actually perceived in the brain, no matter where the original tissue damage originates. Pain receptors in the form of free nerve endings are located in vast numbers throughout the body, especially near the surface of the skin. Extremely fine nerve fibers connect these nerve endings with transfer locations in the spinal cord, where the pain signals ascend up the spinal cord to the brain.

The pain nerve cells are called nociceptors by researchers. The term derives from the word "noxious" and indicates that the nerve cells are responding to noxious, or harmful, stimuli. Certain nociceptors are sensitive to a particular type of pain stimulation—the pain caused by the familiar hammer blow to the thumb, for example—whereas other nociceptors will react to the pain of touching a hot stove or sticking your finger with a pin or spilling battery acid on your hand, and so on.

Nociceptors are especially sensitive to certain chemical substances (acetylcholine and prostaglandins, among others) that are released by cells that are destroyed when tissue is damaged. As has been mentioned, the pain signal is a warning that tissue damage is taking place. The nociceptor senses the presence of the chemical substance released during tissue damage, and the pain signal starts on its way.

Wherever and however the original pain stimulus originates, the brain is the eventual destination of the pain signal from the nociceptors. In certain cases, however, the pain signal takes a detour on the way to the brain. This occurs when the pain stimulus is sudden and unexpected and requires immediate action to withdraw from the origin of the pain, such as when touching a hot stove, to use the example given above.

In this situation, a reflex action takes place. The pain signal is sent to the spinal cord, but instead of being sent up the spinal cord to the brain, the signal is transferred to an interneuron (a nerve cell also called an association neuron) that takes the signal directly to a another nerve cell, a motor neuron, in the spinal cord. The motor neuron sends a signal down to the appropriate hand and arm muscles, instructing them to pull the hand back from the hot stove. Thus, the reflex process has functioned to provide the immediate action required.

The brain, however, will still get the message that a hot stove has been touched, and the perception of pain will take place. The reflex action has provided only a momentary branching side trip for the pain signal.

Under more "normal" circumstances, when a reflex action is not called for, the pain signal will be sent to the spinal cord and then, through what is known as a second order neuron, will be sent up the spinal cord to the brain.

There has been some slight disagreement among scientists and medical researchers as to just where in the brain the pain *signal* actually becomes the pain *sensation*. Some state that this happens in that portion of the brain known as the thalamus; others feel it takes place in a lower portion of the brain called the midbrain. Wherever the perception of pain takes place, the interpretation of the quality of the pain probably occurs in the cerebral cortex of the brain.

This is not nit-picking by scientists, by any means. Determining the exact locations in the brain where certain events occur is important to gaining a fuller understanding of pain and how to control it. And since pain is often an unpleasant aspect of home health care, the more knowledge that is gathered about pain the easier will be the task of managing pain at home.

The brain does more than just perceive pain. When a pain signal has been received, the autonomic nervous system—that division of the nervous system that acts as the caretaker of the body—goes into action. Depending on the type of pain stimulus and the perception in the brain of the nature of the pain and its extent and location, changes may be made in pulse rate, blood pressure, respiration, and digestive action. Adrenaline will be released to quicken body responses, and sugar stored in the liver will also be released to provide energy where needed.

Pain Relief Through Drugs

Not too long ago, all that was available for pain were the narcotic drugs—laudanum, opium, and morphine. Today, however, physicians have at their disposal many drugs that can be used for pain relief, from mild analgesics to narcotics (see Tables 18 and 19).

A common pain medication is aspirin, one of the many analgesics available as an OTC (over-the-counter) drug. Aspirin is very effective in reducing low intensity pain, such as that experienced in headaches, or the discomforts associated with colds or the flu. When heavy doses of aspirin are needed—to cope with arthritis pain, for example—stomach upset or, more seriously, internal bleeding may occur. A physician should be consulted if these side effects of aspirin use appear. Acetaminophen (Tylenol) can be used in place of aspirin, and Ibuprofen has recently been made available over the counter. Analgesics are also available as prescription medication.

Although physicians no longer use laudanum or opium, morphine is still in active use. On the whole, physicians are careful about prescribing narcotics for pain relief. Narcotics can bring on depression or addiction, and surveys have shown that up to 20 percent of those treated with narcotics did not obtain relief from pain, and 80 percent of those who did get relief found it was only temporary.

Nevertheless, morphine can be prescribed for the relief of pain caused by cancer. Often, increasing doses of morphine have to be given as the pain grows worse. In such cases, especially if the patient is terminal, the possibility of addiction is not considered relevant.

Presently, some controversy exists over the question of allowing doctors to prescribe heroin for terminal cancer patients in great pain. Some medical experts claim that it is no more effective than morphine, whereas others say the euphoria produced by heroin will ease the way for a dying patient. In any event, because of the overpowering and desperate need for heroin by addicts, as well as the many criminal activities associated with this narcotic, legislators are reluctant to make it medically legal, even in limited quantities.

When cardiac pain is experienced, especially pain brought on by angina (spasms of the coronary artery), the physician will probably prescribe nitroglycerin in any one of several forms. Tablets are placed under the tongue, capsules are swallowed, transdermal patches are placed on the skin. In whatever form prescribed the drug should bring very fast relief from angina pain.

The pain of arthritis in its various forms (gout, rheumatoid arthritis, osteoarthritis) can be quite severe. Medications for pain relief from this disease are listed in the discussion on arthritis in Chapter 20.

Pain Relief Without Drugs

Other methods, not involving drugs, are on hand for the physician to use. One of the most effective is based on what is known as the gate control theory of pain. When something painful occurs (a stubbed toe, for example), the pain signal, an electrochemical impulse, starts at the point of contact and travels along the nerve pathways to the spinal cord and then to the brain, where it is perceived as pain.

The gate control theory holds that the nervous system in our bodies can handle just so many sensory impulses. If too many signals are crowded into the spinal cord, then some of them will be shut off and blocked from the normal pathways to the brain.

Pain signals travel along very fine nerve fibers to the spinal cord. It has been determined that the finer the nerve fiber, the slower the nerve impulses travel. Tactile sensations are carried to the spinal cord along large diameter nerve fibers, and these signals travel much faster than those in the finer nerve fibers. Consequently, tactile signals will arrive at the spinal cord faster than will pain signals.

Applying the gate control theory to these conditions, it's reasoned that, if a preponderance of tactile signals are sent to the spinal cord, they will overwhelm and block out the slower arriving pain signals. The "gate" will be closed, and the pain signals will not be able to get through and ascend the spinal cord to the brain. Some indication of the validity of this theory can be seen from the fact that, if the stubbed toe is rubbed vigorously (as is usually the case) the pain seems to lessen. However, rubbing a sore spot doesn't seem to supply enough tactile stimulation to block out sufficient pain.

Table 18 ■ NONNARCOTIC ANALGESICS, FOR MILD TO MODERATE PAIN

Generic names	Brand names[a]	Usage information / precautions[b]	Possible side effects[c]
Acetaminophen	Arthralgen Campain Datril Liquiprin Phenaphen Robigesic Tylenol	Drug starts working 15 to 30 minutes after taken • Discontinue use in 2 days if symptoms do not improve • Be sure to consult your doctor before using if you have bronchial asthma, kidney or liver disease • Avoid driving if you feel drowsy • Take no more often than every 3 hours • Don't exceed recommended dose if you are over 60 years old *Overdose symptoms:* stomach upset, irritability, convulsions, coma	*Rare:* extreme fatigue, rash, itch, hives, unexplained bleeding or bruising, blood in urine, painful urination, frequent urge to urinate, less urine, jaundice, anemia
Mixture of Acetaminophen and Chlorzo-xazone (muscle relaxant)	Parafon Forte	Drug starts working 60 minutes after taken • Don't drive until you learn how drug affects you • Don't work with dangerous machinery • Periodic liver function tests recommended if used for a long time *Overdose symptoms:* nausea, vomiting, diarrhea, headache, severe weakness, breathing difficulty, sensation of paralysis	*Common:* drowsiness, dizziness, orange or red-purple urine *Infrequent:* agitation, constipation, diarrhea, nausea, cramps, vomiting *Rare:* rash, itch, sore throat, fever, jaundice, tiredness, weakness, bloody or black stool

	Brand names[a]	Directions and precautions[b]	Side effects[c]
Aspirin	Bayer Bufferin Empirin St. Joseph	Drug starts working 30 minutes after taken • Take no more often than every 4 hours • Do not take with tetracyclines • Space the two drugs at least 1 hour apart • Before taking, consult your doctor if you have ulcers, gout, asthma, or nasal polyps • Urine tests for blood sugar may be inaccurate	*Common:* Ringing in ears, nausea, vomiting, abdominal pain, heart burn, indigestion *Rare:* Drowsiness, rash/hives, black stools, black or bloody vomit, shortness of breath, wheezing, blood in urine, jaundice, allergic reaction[d]
Ibuprofen (anti-inflammatory)	Advil Motrin Nuprin Rufen	Take with liquid or food to lessen stomach irritation • Do not take if you are allergic to aspirin • Not recommended for anyone younger than 15 • Don't drive until you learn how drug affects you *Overdose symptoms:* confusion, agitation, incoherence, convulsions, possible bleeding from stomach or intestine, coma	*Common:* dizziness, headache, nausea, stomach pain *Infrequent:* depression, drowsiness, ringing in ears, constipation, diarrhea, vomiting, swollen feet and legs *Rare:* convulsions, confusion, rash, hives, itch, bloody stools, breathing difficulty, bloody urine, jaundice, fatigue, weakness

[a]These brand names are only a sampling. Several generics reviewed are available under additional names not listed here.

[b]Check with your doctor for specific directions and precautions when taking these and any other medications.

[c]This does not list all of the possible side effects. Check with your doctor regarding the safety and possible side effects when taking these and or any other medications.

[d]Severe allergic reaction (analphylaxis) symptoms: itching, rash, hives, runny nose, wheezing, paleness, cold sweats, low blood pressure, coma, cardiac arrest.

Source: H. Winter Griffith, M.D., *Complete Guide to Prescription and Non-Prescription Drugs* (Tucson: HP Books, 1983).

Table 19 ■ Narcotic Analgesics for Moderate to Severe Pain

Generic names	Brand names[a]	Usage information / precautions[b]	Possible side effects[c]
Codeine	Anaphen	Prescription required • Habit forming • Starts working 30 minutes after taken • Take no more often than every 4 hours • Prolonged use causes psychological and physical dependence • Don't drive until you learn how drug affects you • Don't work with dangerous machinery • Avoid alcohol • People over 60 are more likely to be drowsy, dizzy, unsteady, or constipated	*Common:* dizziness, flushed face, difficult urination, unusual tiredness
Mixtures of codeine with other generics	Ascriptin with Codeine, Empirin with Codeine, Darvocet-N100, Percocet, Tylenol with Codeine, Wygesic		*Rare:* depression, skin rash / itch, blurred vision, slow heartbeat, irregular breathing
		Overdose symptoms: deep sleep, slow breathing, slow pulse, flushed, warm skin, constricted pupils	*Common:* Flushed face, difficult urination, less urine, unusual tiredness, difficulty in swallowing (Talwin only)
Hydromorphone	Dilaudid		*Infrequent:* depression, confusion, hallucinations, severe constipation, abdominal pain, vomiting
Meperidine	Demerol		
Morphine			*Rare:* skin rash / itch, blurred vision slow heartbeat, irregular breathing
Nalbuphine	Nubain		
Opium	Pantopon		
Oxycodone	Percodan		
Oxymorphone	Numorphan		
Pentazocine	Talwin		
Propoxyphene	Darvon		

[a] These brand names are only a sampling. Several generics reviewed are available under additional names not listed here.
[b] Check with your doctor for specific directions and precautions when taking these and any other medications.
[c] This does not list all of the possible side effects. Check with your doctor regarding the safety and possible side effects when taking these and or any other medications.

Source: H. Winter Griffith, M.D., *Complete Guide to Prescription and Non-Prescription Drugs* (Tucson: HP Books, 1983).

The additional tactile signals needed to block out the pain signals are created through electrical stimulation of the nerves where the pain is located. Electrodes are attached to the surface of the skin, one electrode preferably being placed over the pain location and another further along the nerve path. Low voltage impulses of electricity are sent to the electrodes. Hundreds of impulses per second are poured into the nerves, creating a heavy flow of tactile signals to the spinal cord, effectively blocking the pain impulses from getting through.

This is a highly simplified explanation of a very complex theory, of course, but the main thing for us to consider here is that it works. The procedure is known as transcutaneous electrical nerve stimulation (TENS), and although a fairly recent development, it has progressed to the stage where TENS equipment is completely portable and can be worn on the person.

TENS is an important aspect of pain management in home health care. It doesn't have the frightening list of side effects that some medications have; it's noninvasive (the electrodes are placed on the skin, not under it); and it is not complicated to use.

Heat and cold also play their parts in controlling pain. Heat pads and heat packs are used to provide moist heat that penetrates deep into muscles. Warm baths, hot tubs, and whirlpool baths are familiar to most people, and they do bring pain relief, although sometimes only temporary.

An ice massage is a very effective use of cold therapy to relieve pain. A small block of ice wrapped in a towel is rubbed slowly over the

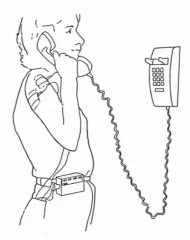

TENS devices are easy to wear, and offer many patients relief from chronic pain.

painful area for no more than about ten minutes, but in that time blood circulation can be slowed, and the pain can disappear and not return for several hours. This is *not* a technique you should practice at home without instructions in how to perform it and what precautions to take. The ice massage, for example, should not be used when poor circulation is the cause of the pain, since the cold will only add to the pain. Also, the ice should never be applied to the throat, since circulation of blood to the brain might be reduced.

Ice massage can be taught to individuals on home health care. For most applications, someone else—the caregiver, for example—will have to perform the massage because the painful areas may be out of reach for the individual. However, when the area can be reached without difficulty, the patient himself can do the massage after suitable instruction. One innovative method for self-massage involves placing an ice cream stick, wooden coffee stirrer, or even a tongue depressor into water and letting the water freeze around it. Then the individual can use the ice-on-a-stick to massage painful areas.

Health care professionals have found that distraction often helps mask pain. It doesn't remove the pain, but it does allow the patient to think of something other than his pain. Singing, talking, listening to music—anything that will distract the patient sufficiently to take his mind off the pain can be tried. As has been mentioned, Norman Cousins successfully used a form of this technique, as described in his book, *Anatomy of an Illness,* by watching old movie comedies. The laughter that was evoked by the movies helped him fight the effects of his painful disease. The distraction technique is one that can easily be employed as a part of home health care.

Massage has always been used to tone up muscles and help in relaxation. A form of massage called myotherapy, which concentrates on what are known as trigger points, can also be of great benefit in relieving pain.

Trigger points are tender spots on a muscle that normally do not cause trouble. However, under stress or sudden pain-producing trauma, they can become activated, and they cause the muscle to spasm. When this happens, the nervous system, in an attempt to protect the area, causes nearby muscles to spasm also. This action increases the tightening of the original muscle that went into spasm, causing more pain and bringing forth another protective muscle spasm from the nervous system. One spasm leads to another, and the pain can become much more severe than the original pain that started the whole process.

A gentle massage of the painful area by the caregiver, using only the fingertips, will usually disclose the trigger points. The patient will react to the sudden pain brought on by the contact with the trigger point. However, by touching the trigger point and holding slight pressure on it with your fingers or even your elbow for a few seconds, you will release it. You can then move on to the next trigger point on the muscle, probing gently until you find it and you release it also.

By releasing all the trigger points you can locate, you'll greatly reduce the pain for the patient. One word of caution, though: If you are the caregiver, make sure you receive sufficient instruction in the myotherapy technique from the physical therapist before you attempt to use it on the patient. If you find you cannot manage the light probing and application of slight pressure required on the trigger points, better leave this technique to the professionals.

Biofeedback is one more method that can be used at home to help relieve pain. It requires electronic equipment and a health professional who knows how to use it. The patient's active participation is crucial to the success of the biofeedback method, which has been found to be effective in relieving the pain of muscular spasm. (It is not recommended for all types of pain.)

Once the patient is hooked up to the equipment, the physical therapist can measure the patient's muscle activity and show him how to control this activity and reduce it until the pain is removed. In effect, the patient is taught how to relax the muscles involved, and the biofeedback equipment shows him when he is succeeding. It's a matter of practice and experimentation, assisted by the results indicated by the equipment. If you work at it, it works.

10

Pressure Sores

MOST PEOPLE call them bedsores; health professionals refer to them as decubitus ulcers; a more descriptive term for them is pressure sores. No matter what you call them, though, they are one of the most unpleasant, painful, and dangerous skin problems that can afflict a person receiving health care at home.

A pressure sore is just what the name implies—a skin sore caused by pressure. This pressure can be exerted in a number of ways: lying in one spot in bed without moving; sitting in a wheelchair in one position for too long; sliding down against the sheets in bed and creating repeated friction against the skin of the buttocks or shoulder blades; letting an arm or leg (usually paralyzed or otherwise immobilized) rest motionless against the bedclothes or a wheelchair support, with unrelieved pressure on an elbow or heel or ankle.

Usually, the point of pressure is located at the bony prominences of the body—hips, shoulders, elbows, ankles, heels, knees, base of the spine—any spot where a bone is close to the surface and skin can be compressed between the underlying bone and a resistant surface such as a mattress or chair cushion. Pressure can also be exerted against the skin by braces, plaster casts, or wheelchair parts.

If the pressure is not relieved, blood flow is cut off to the capillaries, the tiny blood vessels in the skin. The capillaries cannot carry blood and nutrients to the tissue cells in the skin, and eventually the cells die. A sore, or ulcer, then develops in the area of the dead cells, and unless treated, the ulcer grows in size and depth and can extend all the way down to the bone. The area of dead skin spreads, creating a festering sore that can take many months to heal and that can, in extreme cases, bring on conditions that will cause death.

Pressure sores can develop in as little as one to six hours of unrelieved pressure on the skin. Generally, the heavier the pressure, the less time it takes for the ulcer to form.

Other factors contributing to the development of pressure sores are incontinence (skin that stays wet is subject to deterioration), poor nutrition (vitamin and nutrient deficiencies will affect the skin), poor physical condition (adding to the general lack of mobility), impaired mental ability (disorientation and lethargy can lead to poor body hygiene), and lack of sensation (paraplegics and quadraplegics will not be aware of pressure on the skin or even of skin injury).

It has been estimated that there are about one million cases of pressure sores or "skin destruction" each year among individuals receiving health care at home because of disease or disability or injury. These cases will be either first-time occurrences or a continuation of already existing decubitus ulcers that have not yet healed.

Stages of Ulcer Development

Attempts have been made to standarize the classification of pressure sores according to the stage of ulcer development and size. There is at present no universal standard; however, there is general agreement that the ulcer progresses through four distinct stages:

Stage 1. At this stage, there is general reddening of the skin in the affected area. The skin is unbroken, but the redness will not whiten when pressed with a finger. If the pressure that caused the redness is relieved and the area returns to normal skin color in about seventy-two hours, the danger of an ulcer has passed.

Stage 2. A blister or superficial ulcer will have formed at this stage and the skin will be broken. There may be some pain, and drainage of the ulcer.

Stage 3. The wound is much deeper, penetrating both the outer skin layers and the subcutaneous tissue. Pain will be evident, and drainage is more likely. Dead tissue and a hard, black scab (eschar) may appear on top of the wound.

Stage 4. Extensive skin destruction is apparent. The wound is deep, the ulcer going into the muscle and clear to the bone in many cases. Eschar, dead tissue, and drainage are visible.

The size of the ulcer generally will increase as it progresses through the different stages, especially if treatment is delayed. Size is sometimes compared to various common objects—a coin such as a nickel or quarter, a golf ball, a baseball, an orange, and so on. This is not a very accurate way of recording data, and the more accepted method is to describe the shape of the ulcer (round, narrow, oblong, triangular, etc.)

and give its dimensions either in inches or centimeters.

This type of recordkeeping is essential in a hospital, but it should also be used for noting down information about any ulcers that may develop during home health care of the individual. The physician or visiting nurse will then be able to compare the original notation with the size and condition of the ulcer at the time of a medical examination.

Assessment of Risk

Another form of recordkeeping practiced in a hospital that can be adapted to the home environment is to make a periodic assessment of the potential of developing a pressure sore. In making this assessment, various factors are evaluated in order to arrive at a total picture of the individual's condition and the possible risk of a skin ulcer. Hospitals and other institutions usually devise a scoring method for making this evaluation, assigning numerical values to each factor, with a total score above or below a certain point indicating the degree of risk. It won't be necessary to do this as part of home health care; checking off the appropriate item, as indicated below, will be sufficient to show the physician or nurse when they visit the patient.

The factors to be evaluated are:

GENERAL PHYSICAL CONDITION

[   ] Very good
[   ] Good
[   ] Fair
[   ] Poor
[   ] Very poor

MENTAL CONDITION

[   ] Alert; well oriented
[   ] Apathetic; lethargic
[   ] Disoriented; confused
[   ] Not fully conscious most of the time

MOBILITY

[   ] Fully ambulant and mobile
[   ] Slightly limited; can walk with assistance
[   ] Limited; cannot walk far, even with assistance
[   ] Confined to wheelchair, but quite mobile
[   ] Confined to wheelchair; low mobility
[   ] Immobile; bedbound

INCONTINENCE

[   ] None
[   ] Occasional; nocturnal
[   ] Bladder only
[   ] Bowel and bladder

NUTRITION

[   ] Good; eats well; gets full nutrition
[   ] Diminished appetite
[   ] Poor; doesn't eat or drink much
[   ] Doesn't eat; I.V. feeding only

Skin Sensation   [   ] Poor
[   ] Normal   [   ] Partial; paraplegic
[   ] Diminished   [   ] None; quadraplegic

Using the above checklist, supplemented by their own observations, the physician or nurse can evaluate the home care patient's risk potential for development of a skin ulcer and can advise the patient and the caregiver accordingly.

Treatment

Although treatment of pressure sores is a task for a skilled health professional and, in severe cases, may require hospitalization of the patient, it will be valuable for you, as the caregiver or as the person receiving home health care, to have a basic idea of what is involved in the very serious matter of treating pressure sores.

Do *not,* however, attempt to perform any of the medical treatment described on your own. A decubitus ulcer is nothing to fool around with, and the information given here is strictly for general background information. A doctor or nurse should be the only ones to evaluate an ulcer and start a course of treatment.

Once a skin ulcer has developed, it must be cleaned and allowed to heal. If the ulcer is not large and is being treated early enough, cleaning can usually be accomplished with saline solutions and other preparations. The wound must be protected, and this can be done with a variety of dressings, vegetable gum, special antibacterial cream, powders, and other preparations. Observing sterile working conditions is of the utmost importance, and sterile gloves and applicators are part of the equipment the nurse or doctor will use.

For deeper ulcers, the treatment is even more exacting and can involve use of special dextranome "beads," which are placed in the cleaned and open wound. These beads are sterile, porous chemical spheres that are highly hydrophilic—that is, they absorb and retain fluids and exudates that could inhibit healing of the wound.

Other methods used involve surgical debridement (cutting away) of the eschar scab and dead tissue, irrigation of the wound, packing the wound with special gauze, and using plastic wrap and special foam dressing to protect the treated wound. Dressings have to be changed at scheduled intervals, and the nurse will usually check for drainage, pus, and odor when inspecting the ulcer and the dressing.

None of this is pleasant, and it can be quite painful for the patient.

What has been described here is, of course, not the full picture of all the treatment methods used. It should be enough, however, to give you some idea of the serious nature of pressure sores and ulcers.

Prevention

The one sure way to prevent pressure sores is to make certain pressure is never exerted on immobile skin for prolonged periods of time.

This is the ideal situation, of course, but the unfortunate fact is that it's almost impossible to achieve. Decubitus ulcers do develop in hospitals—an environment where health care professionals are in constant attendance—despite the best efforts of all involved. As has been mentioned, it can take as little as one hour of pressure to start forming a pressure sore. Obviously, neither at a hospital nor at home would it be reasonable to expect that an individual could be watched and tended to on an hourly basis.

However, many actions can be taken and aids used to help prevent skin ulcers from developing.

First and foremost must be the awareness on the part of the individual receiving the health care at home that pressure sores present a very real danger and that the potential risk should not be ignored. If at all possible, the individual must not remain immobile in one position for an excessive length of time. This requires alertness. Even though strain, effort, and perhaps even some pain may be involved, the individual if able has to turn and move himself on a regular basis.

If this isn't possible—either because of paralysis, mental impairment, semi-consciousnes, or any other reason—then the caregiver will have to make sure that the person is turned and moved regularly and that no portion of his body receives undue prolonged pressure against the skin.

Another means for preventing pressure sores is to distribute the weight of the individual over as wide an area as possible. This will keep pressure from building up in one spot. Weight distribution can be accomplished in some instances by using specially constructed chair cushions—especially those used in wheelchairs—that are anatomically shaped to support the individual as equally as possible over the entire body area in contact with the cushion.

Strategically placed pillows and foam cushions can be used for good weight distribution for the individual in bed. "Egg crate" pads (the rows of soft projections resemble egg crates) can also be used to help distribute weight under a person's body. Air mattresses are still another means of achieving effective weight distribution.

Avoidance of friction against the skin will help prevent pressure sores. Bedding has to be carefully arranged to minimize any sliding or slipping the individual might be subjected to. Sheepskin bed pads also help. The sheepskin helps spread pressure evenly with little friction and also provides good air circulation.

Heel and elbow protectors are also available. Usually, these are large foam pads or rolls that are placed around the ankle or elbow area to keep the limb elevated and the affected area away from sheets or other friction-causing surfaces.

Scrupulous cleanliness is vital. The individual and the caregiver have to work together to make sure all conditions that might bring on pressure sores are eliminated. The person's skin should be kept clean and not too dry or moist. Reddened areas must never be rubbed "to increase circulation" as this can abrade the skin, especially in an older person. Good personal hygiene is a must.

Remember, pressure sores are best treated by a skilled health professional. The use of any of the special aids described here should be approved by your physician or nurse before purchase. The risk of infection or making the ulcer worse is always present.

Much can be done during home health care to *prevent* pressure sores—and that should be the goal of both the caregiver and the person receiving the care.

11

High-Tech Home Care

THE PATIENT was surprised. Her doctor had just told her that she would be discharged from the hospital in a few days, but that her IV (intravenous) antibiotic treatment would have to continue for some time—at home. She looked at the plastic bag suspended from the rack next to her bed, and her eyes followed the tubing down to the needle taped in place in her forearm. Her surprised look began to change to a shocked and somewhat fearful expression.

It was all right, she was quickly told by the clinical nurse specialist who had come in with the doctor. Going home with an IV still in place was not that unusual. The nurse put it succinctly: "You're taking part of the hospital home with you. Many procedures that we used to do only in the hospital are now being done at home—by people just like you."

What the nurse was talking about is what I refer to as high-tech home care. Using equipment that was once found only in hospitals, patients are now learning how to manage hospital-type care for themselves at home. A family caregiver usually helps, and because of the complexity of some of the equipment and the techniques involved, a health care agency specializing in high-tech home care supervises and instructs the patient and the caregiver in all aspects of the medical procedure.

Table 20 lists therapies for which high-tech home care has proven useful for the patient being cared for at home.

The instruction of the patient and the caregiver in how to manage high-tech home care ideally starts in the hospital before the patient is discharged. The hospital discharge planner, together with the patient's physician, arranges for a health care agency to send in a clinical nurse specialist, who will work with the physician in setting up a treatment

Table 20 ▪ HIGH-TECH HOME CARE

Therapy	Equipment possibilities	Technical knowledge / skills required
Respiratory	Respirator, oxygen concentrator, nebulizer	Operation, care, maintenance of oxygen equipment
Diabetes	Insulin pump, glucometer	Interpretation of readings
Intravenous Chemotherapy Parenteral nutrition Antibiotic therapy	Needles / tubing, pumps, IV solutions	Strict sterile procedure care in handling solutions • Proper operation / maintenance of pumps (if used) • Storage
Kidney	Dialysis unit, peritoneal dialysis	
Tube feeding	Tubes, formula, flow-meter pumps	Proper tube position, irrigation, formula preparation or selection / storage

plan. The initial meeting can include many health professionals—the patient's physician, the clinical nurse specialist, the hospital discharge planner, a pharmacist, a medical social worker, a community health agency home care nurse—the reason being that high-tech home care requires much closer supervision and patient and family education than the more common situation in which a patient is sent home with a list of medications to take, a special diet to follow, and a planned exercise program. When complex high-tech equipment is involved, the initial setting up of the treatment plan has to allow for many additional factors.

One of the chief factors to be considered is whether the patient can benefit from this type of home health care. A careful screening program is necessary to make sure the patient—and the caregiver—can handle the complexities of advanced, high-tech home care. For one thing, the patient must be "clinically stable." This means the patient should be free from the effects of fever, for example, and should not be in such a weakened condition that serious complications could arise. Additionally, the patient and the caregiver should have already received some instruction and training in the hospital in the procedures involved and should be at least basically familiar with the equipment. Finally, the patient should be physically and emotionally ready and capable of managing his own health care program.

This last point is very important. The emotional stability of the patient is often the deciding factor. Regardless of how favorable the patient's physical condition and clinical status may be, health professionals could not approve the patient for high-tech home care if he did not exhibit a degree of inner strength and a clear determination and ability to manage his own health care at home—with, of course, the help of the caregiver. The caregiver, too, has to be someone who will not panic in an emergency and who has demonstrated an aptitude for working with the technically advanced equipment that will be supplied.

The reason for all this concern on the part of the health professionals meeting to evaluate the patient and work out a treatment plan is that high-tech home care involves a certain amount of risk as well as some obvious benefits.

Risk is, of course, present in just about any medical or health procedure. Even taking aspirin involves an element of risk. No surgical or medical procedure is completely free of possible trouble, even though the potential risk may be remote and unlikely. No medication or drug is completely free of some side effects, even though they may be minor in nature.

Thus, the patient who is managing a home health care program with high-tech equipment must be knowledgeable about the medical and technical procedure and any potential problems and must know what to do and whom to contact in an emergency. Although the health care agency supervising the high-tech home care may provide twenty-four-hour service and personnel who can respond in an emergency, it's not the same as being in a hospital room, where the nurse can be at hand in moments should a crisis develop.

The patient and the caregiver must weigh the problems and potential difficulties involved in dealing with sophisticated and complex home care equipment against the benefits to be derived—and the benefits can be many. First and foremost, is the fact that the patient is at home in familiar surroundings, away from the hospital regimentation and routine. At home, even though not in perfect health, the patient will feel more like a person again.

Another benefit is that the person can usually continue to lead a normal life in many respects. A high-tech home health care program can free the person for work and other activities instead of confining him to a hospital simply because that's where the equipment and the personnel to operate it are located.

Still another benefit is the cost. It has been shown that the savings per patient per treatment can amount to thousands of dollars when high-tech health care is practiced at home. Whether the funding comes from government programs, private insurance, or personal funds, the result is the same: it costs less to do it at home.

There's no doubt that being at home can be of prime importance to any individual whose health has been compromised and who needs long-term care and medical treatment. Despite the fact that this type of home care uses hospital type equipment with all its somewhat awesome dials, tubes, and controls, patients and families are more than willing to learn how to use this equipment. They put up with stringent requirements—as long as it can be done at home.

In one study, patients requiring IV antibiotic therapy at home were surveyed. Some of the patients had to be given antibiotics every twelve hours, which did not cause too much inconvenience or disruption of the regular household activities and normal sleep patterns. Other patients in the study were on six-hour schedules, and this did disturb both the patient and the families at night. Nevertheless, those on the six-hour schedule indicated that the inconveniences were not at all important when the advantages of the patient being at home rather than in the hospital were considered.

High-tech home care is the method of choice in many illnesses and disorders. Advances in technology have produced new methods of preparing and preserving medications so they can be administered in the home, usually requiring only refrigeration before use in many instances. Manufacturers of medical products and supplies are now dealing directly with the public, setting up special health care facilities as part of their operation, and providing service and instruction for the patient.

Medications and equipment are delivered directly to the patient's home on orders from the physician and the clinical nurse specialist. Company representatives are available for instruction and servicing of the equipment and are on call in case of emergencies. Thus, the home health care patient who is using high-tech equipment and procedures has both medical health professionals and the manufacturer's professional staff at his service.

The field is growing, and once patients learn about its advantages, they are no longer intimidated by the equipment.

Let's look at some examples of where this type of health care is now being used.

Diabetes

Diabetes, as explained in Chapter 16, is a chronic metabolic disease that affects millions of people. It is also a disease that, except for more advanced cases, has been successfully treated at home for many years. Home care for diabetes has usually consisted of the patient giving himself an insulin injection every day, watching his diet, and getting the proper amount of exercise. In order to check on the level of sugar in his system, the patient tested his urine with chemically treated strips of paper, recording the sugar level according to a color chart.

This method is still used, but recent advances have now added equipment and devices that help the diabetic manage his disease much more efficiently and effectively. A blood glucose monitor allows the patient to sample his blood glucose level several times a day, if necessary. This is a more accurate indication of the sugar in his system than urine testing and allows the patient to fine-tune his insulin requirements.

For those patients who need a more constant infusion of insulin, the portable insulin pump, worn on a belt at the patient's waist, allows the precise metering of insulin throughout the day. Measured doses of insulin are infused directly into the patient's body through the portable pump and a needle placed under the patient's skin, eliminating the need for self-administered injections.

Nutrition

In the matter of nutrition, technology has made it possible for individuals to obtain required nutrients at home despite conditions such as Crohn's disease, for example, where sections of the intestines sometimes have to be surgically removed (see Chapter 18). TPN (total parenteral nutrition, see Chapter 6) allows the person to hook up to a machine that sends a nutrient solution into a major vein in his body, providing his complete nutrition—and all of this can be done at home.

The equipment for TPN is sophisticated and requires that the patient learn how to use it effectively. Many patients have done so, with excellent results. Most important, they have been able to remain at home while they cared for their health.

In less severe cases of nutritional requirements, when there is still some digestive ability left, the individual can use enteral feeding, which makes use of tubes and pumps to introduce nutrients into the digestive system, bypassing the mouth. As with TPN, there is a learning period involved, but once this is completed, the person can live at home and obtain the required nutrition through this method.

Respiratory Disease

Emphysema and chronic bronchitis are major respiratory diseases, collectively known as chronic obstructive pulmonary disease (COPD), and as discussed in Chapter 22, are treated by the administration of oxygen to push more oxygen into the lungs and into the bloodstream to nourish the body cells.

COPD and other pulmonary problems require the use of oxygen equipment, nebulizers, and aerosol medications. These involve technical devices that have proved their worth in making home care possible for victims of respiratory ailments.

Renal Disease

An individual with end-stage renal disease, when the kidneys are failing and there is no cure, can be helped either by a kidney transplant or dialysis. There are dialysis centers where the machines are located that will cleanse the blood of the afflicted person, but this means being hooked up to a machine for several hours three or four times a week. High-tech home care now allows this person to make use of a home dialysis program (see Chapter 21).

During dialysis, the blood flows from the patient to the artificial kidney, where it is cleansed and returned to the patient. Inside the artificial kidney, the blood flows across one side of the membranous sheet or inside specially constructed tubes. On the other side of the membrane is a dialysate, a cleaning bath solution. Impurities in the blood flow through pores in the membrane, which are not large enough to pass the blood cells. With home dialysis the patient is able to lead an active life while regularly cleansing his blood at home.

Chemotherapy

Chemotherapy is used in the battle against cancer, and for many patients, the procedure was performed in a hospital room or doctor's office—until technical breakthroughs made it possible to perform this delicate and rather involved medical procedure at home.

Great care is taken when chemotherapy is to be administered at home. In addition to the careful screening of patients and caregivers, the physician and other health care professionals have many preparations to make to ensure that the home chemotherapy treatment will be effective.

Before the patient leaves the hospital, a nurse specialist visits the home to evaluate it as a site for the chemotherapy treatment. The nurse will check that proper refrigeration is available for the storage of the drugs to be used and will also inspect the electrical capacity of the house, specifically the availability of sufficient functioning electrical outlets needed for use of the equipment.

Additionally, the nurse will look into the family situation, attempting to get a clear picture of how much support the patient will get from the family. Understanding and encouragement from the family is an important factor in home chemotherapy.

If all goes well, the patient is brought home and the treatment begins. The nurse specialist will spend much time here in the patient's home. She will set up the equipment, show the family how it works, explain the nature of the chemotherapy, and have the family watch her while she gives the patient a treatment.

She will be back many times, repeating what she has done, checking on the patient's condition, evaluating the effectiveness of the chemotherapy, and continuing to instruct and educate the family in the procedure.

One aspect of her instruction will be to make sure the family and the patient understand the nature of the drugs being used. The nurse will explain the high toxicity of these drugs, the precautions that have to be taken, and the balance that has to be maintained between the dosage required to destroy the malignant cells and the amount of this medication the patient can tolerate. In time, both the family and the patient will feel less intimidated by the chemotherapy treatment and will more readily accept its adverse aspects along with its benefits.

The greatest benefit, of course, as with all high-tech home health care, is that it's being accomplished in the one place that has the most meaning for the individual—at home.

Guidelines

Because of the complexity of high-tech health care equipment and the special procedures required, both the caregiver and patient should check the following guidelines when considering a home health care agency as the supplier for this type of care:

- Does the agency have twenty-four-hour service seven days a week?
- Are emergency service personnel available at any time of day or night?
- Does the agency have a well-stocked inventory of equipment and medications needed to perform this type of home health care?
- Does the agency offer instruction and supervision for operating the equipment?
- Is a clinical nurse specialist assigned to the patient from the start?
- Does the agency send the nurse specialist to the hospital to start the instruction before the patient's discharge?
- Is the agency licensed by the state—if licensing is required in your state?
- Is this agency recommended by the hospital discharge planner and other health care officials?
- Will the agency give you the names and addresses of other clients as references so you can check what others think of the quality of the agency's service?

These are questions you should ask before contracting with an agency for high-tech home health care. You have to be thorough in your investigation because so much depends on it. The requirements and risks of this type of care do not allow much room for error.

Not every patient can use high-tech home care effectively. For those who can, the benefits are worth all the effort.

12

The Dying Patient

THROUGHOUT THIS BOOK, the emphasis has been on maintaining and improving the quality of life for the individual whose health is being cared for at home. In this chapter, we are still concerned about the quality of life, but this time in preparation for death.

How well this can be accomplished—if both patient and caregiver are "in tune"—is exemplified by a letter I received from Jacqueline Goodrich a good friend and an excellent modern dancer, who temporarily put her career aside while she became the chief family caregiver for her mother, who was dying of cancer.

". . . After the diagnosis of cancer was final, she lived just four more weeks. She was unafraid and ready to die—she had made that very clear. And that helped all of us around her accept her death a bit more easily. None of us could have anticipated all that was to happen during that time. There was so much said, so much humor and genuine happiness, so much anguish, so much resolution, I was continually astonished. There was nothing passive about those weeks—she was not merely waiting to die. In fact, while she continued to bring closure to her affairs and to her relationships with friends and family, she was working very hard to hasten the dying so that those around her—and herself—would be spared a protracted illness. I don't think she was ever in much pain. The only time we couldn't be certain was the last day, when she could no longer speak, so we increased the frequency of the morphine-type drug to the maximum.

"I rarely left the room where we'd set up her hospital bed. By continually caring for her physical needs and by keeping her company through visits from friends, slide shows of our trip to China, partnering in bouts of "Trivial Pursuit" and countless conversations, I attended her dying in a way that helped me live it and accept it a bit more each day. Those days were so full of life that by the time death came, it was a logical part of that day—I don't know how else to describe it. Given her condition at that point—her essential loss of consciousness—or at least her ability to respond to us—there was no way I could want her to live any longer. . . . She did 'go gently into that good night,' and I must say that seems the wisest way to go—if one has a choice."

Death is, of course, inevitable for everyone. However, for the dying patient—for the person who has been diagnosed as "terminal"—the inevitability of death can be a constant and overwhelming presence. In this instance, neither the patient nor the caregiver allowed themselves to be overwhelmed by the presence of death, which was an important factor in how the dying process was handled.

The Stages of Dying

Dr. Elisabeth Kubler-Ross, a renowned psychiatrist and author of the definitive book, *On Death and Dying* (New York: Macmillan, 1969), identified five "stages of dying" the terminally ill patient undergoes from the initial diagnosis until the end: denial, anger, bargaining, depression, and acceptance.

In denial, the person refuses to accept the diagnosis and acknowledge that he is dying. This evasion gives the person time to marshal his emotional defenses against the inevitability of death. It also gives the same opportunity to the caregiver.

Denial eventually erupts into anger—a "Why me?" outcry—the resentment may be expressed against the doctors, hospital staff, health care professionals, caregiver, and even God for what has happened. The patient has to be allowed to work his way through the anger stage without gratuitous advice from the caregiver. The expression of anger and resentment provides a much needed outlet for the extreme emotional turmoil the patient is undergoing at the moment.

Bargaining is a very real matter to the dying patient. Promises to perform some special deed or to change one's conduct and life style if only the wish to go on living is granted represent a clinging to life and an attempt to prolong life in the face of the inevitable. The patient should not be denied this last hope by any admonitions from the caregiver. Realization will set in soon enough.

When the patient finally realizes that death is imminent and that nothing can be done about it, a period of depression can set in. The patient thinks about all that he has left undone and all that he is about to lose. This is likely to be a time of withdrawal. The patient may not want any visitors and may not be very communicative. Sometimes all that will be required of the caregiver is to be there and sit with the patient, perhaps to reach out and touch the patient, if it seems appropriate at the moment, as a reassurance that he is not alone.

With acceptance, the patient shows that he is ready now for death, perhaps even welcoming it. He may be in a detached state (not a coma), remote from what is going on around him, waiting for the final release. There is little the caregiver can do at this time except to stand by with the patient, letting him know that there is someone with him, someone whose hand he can hold if he wants human contact, someone who understands.

As a caregiver, it's important that you understand the emotions, reactions, and behavior patterns of the patient as he or she passes through the stages of dying. Not all dying patients will go through all the individual stages, and not necessarily in sequence, as Ms. Goodrich's letter bears out. But knowing about the stages of dying will help you realize what may be happening to the patient at a particular moment, and this will guide you and help you give the needed support to the patient at the appropriate time.

Relieving the Pain

There is one thought always present for both patient and caregiver during any of the five stages of dying—how to cope with pain. The final stage, acceptance, cannot be the calm "slipping away" that most people desire if pain has been present throughout the dying process. The fear of pain and the inability to control it is perhaps the major concern for the dying patient.

There are, today, many medications available to the physician to alleviate pain and, more important, to prevent it. We'll cover this in more detail later on in the discussion of hospice care for the dying patient, but it should be noted here that the pain prevention techniques employed in a hospice can work at home also. As the caregiver, you should be aware that pain can be managed. You and the physician can work together to keep the patient in your care at home as free of pain as possible.

Should the Patient Be Told?

There is no definitive answer to this question. There are times when it is prudent to withhold distressing news from the dying patient—

for example, not telling someone near death that a beloved relative has just died. In such cases, it's a matter of judgment, and the physician and the caregiver and family members have to consult together and arrive at a decision.

When the bad news concerns the patient himself, however, the decision can be a painful and uncertain one. If the patient does not know he is dying, and has not been told, then obviously he cannot experience denial, anger, bargaining, depression, and acceptance *in relation to his dying*—although these same emotions may well be present in relation to the patient's illness. Some people might not want to know they are dying, and those making the decision as to whether or not to tell will have to take this into consideration. Further, a decision often has to be made as to just how much to tell the patient. Once again, it's a matter of judgment.

There are no hard and fast rules to follow in such situations—except that the decision cannot be an arbitrary one made by one person (the doctor or a family member) based solely on that one person's particular emotional reaction to death and the dying process. Actually, as has been observed, the patient frequently senses that he is dying even before he is told, especially if the telling is delayed while the family tries to reach a decision.

Patient Stress

Chronic illness brings with it many stresses on the patient, but once the patient knows that he is dying, certain stress factors will predominate.

FEAR

Obviously, fear is a major stress factor. We have already mentioned the fear of pain. The patient is likely to dwell on how much pain there will be as the dying process goes on. Additionally, there will be the patient's fear as to whether or not he will have the strength to cope with the pain.

There will also be the fear of the loss of bodily control. The stress that can be generated by such fears can seriously weaken the patient. As with pain, there are ways to alleviate and prevent many distressing bodily control conditions. Incontinence is covered in Chapter 8. Your physician can help you provide the care and necessary medications to keep other bodily discomforts and upsets from dominating the patient's days and nights.

Finally, there is, of course, the fear of the unknown, the fear of facing death and not being really sure of what it is. Religious beliefs, if profoundly held, can be of help here in alleviating the stress brought on by this fear.

The patient may or may not express his fears openly. As the caregiver, you will have to work at understanding what the dying patient is going through and what stresses are acting on him. If you can get the patient to talk about his fears—without pressuring him—the two of you can tackle the problem together. Remember, too, that professional help can be sought if necessary. Your physician or hospital discharge planner can arrange for counseling either from a social worker or a psychiatrist.

GUILT

The dying patient will often have the added stress of feelings of personal guilt. An agonizing thought that may likely occur to the patient will be: "I should have taken better care of myself and this might not have happened to me." If the patient is the type of person who has never been too strong-willed or shown much self-confidence, then he can be very vulnerable to guilt feelings about his present condition, blaming it all on himself.

Guilt can also come with such thoughts as "I'm leaving too much undone," or "I have not provided properly for those I leave behind," or "I am causing too much anguish to those I love."

As the caregiver, you will have to help the patient cope with these guilt feelings (and your own, too, as we'll discuss later). It's a matter of talking it out; unless the patient is absolutely uncommunicative, there will be an opportunity to draw him out, and help him deal with his guilt feelings.

The goal is clear: to keep the patient as free as possible from the debilitating effects of harmful stress. Achieving this goal requires effort, and there are no real shortcuts.

Caregiver Stress

You, the caregiver, along with the heavy responsibility of caring for the dying patient, also will have to cope with the stresses constantly acting on you as you go about your task. The stress factors are almost the same as those on the patient.

FEAR

There are many fears that can beset a caregiver. Chief among them is the fear of the patient experiencing a sudden attack while you stand there helpless. The answer to this fear is to be as prepared as you possibly can be for such an occurrence.

First consult with the physician or the health care nurse. Have them identify for you the possible emergency situations that can arise—and, most important, what you can do about them. Don't hesitate to ask questions; the patient's life (even though now limited) is in your safekeeping. If you know what to expect and what to do in a particular situation, you are not likely to panic.

A similar fear is that of not being able to get needed medical help in time. As before, the better prepared you are, the better you'll be able to function. Keep a list of emergency phone numbers handy. Rehearse in your mind who you will call first in a given situation. It may even be helpful, if (and only if!) the patient expresses concern or fear about emergencies, to discuss with the patient the course of action you will take. You will not only be reassuring the patient but also reassuring yourself.

Unless the patient is bed-bound and completely dependent on constant care, there will be times when you will have to leave the patient alone. Avoid developing any fears about this. Patients are left alone in hospitals, too, don't forget. If you have to go out and leave the patient for a while, make sure that he has everything he'll need for the time you will be away and that he knows how to summon help in an emergency.

It's important, also, to recognize your own fears and emotional reactions to the thought of death. Being so close to a dying person will make you more aware of your own mortality. Do not pull back from thinking about death or the knowledge that you will have to deal with the patient's death in the near future. If you need help in assessing and coping with your attitudes and fears concerning death, talk to the physician or the health care nurse. They can advise you and can, if it's needed, get you additional professional help and guidance.

DOUBTS

Fears and doubts go hand in hand. It will be normal for you to experience doubts about what you are doing in undertaking the care of a dying patient. You will have to learn to cope with your doubts as well as with your fears.

You can probably expect, at some time in the course of caring for the dying patient, to ask yourself, "Am I really capable of handling this?" There's no pat answer here. If you've reached the stage where you have to ask this question, the answer will not be swift and simple. The best way to cope with this doubt is to review all that you have done so far and have handled well. An honest assessment of your capabilities and your limitations will help you deal with any doubts that may come up.

GUILT

The patient is not the only one who can be plagued by guilt feelings. These feelings are just as likely to occur in the caregiver because of the added responsibility of caring for someone who is dying.

If, as is often the case, the patient is a close and loving relative (a wife, husband, mother, or father), guilt can overwhelm you as you think of possible ways you might have been able to prevent or perhaps put off for a time what has happened, thus giving the patient the chance to enjoy a better quality of life as well as a longer life. Such speculation is pointless, even if there is a bit of truth in it. What's past is past, and by dwelling too much on the past and your feelings of guilt about it, you will not be able to function effectively in caring for the patient— who needs your help now.

ANGER AND RESENTMENT

Another stress factor acting on the caregiver is the unwanted and often unexpected reaction of anger and resentment—especially against the patient. When this happens, the caregiver can experience deep shock that such thoughts could possibly be harbored against the patient.

If this happens to you, be assured that you have not suddenly become an evil person. Often anger is a natural result of the stresses and strains pressing in on you every day, and if your anger is directed against the dying patient for "causing" the situation, it's time to step back, take a deep breath, and think things through as calmly as you can.

Usually, this sort of anger is never openly expressed to the patient. It's a suppressed anger that suddenly bursts to the surface of your mind when you are alone and frustrated and somewhat frightened at the enormity of your task. Confront it. Deal with it. Don't push it back into your subconscious. Get it out in the open and examine it and recognize it for what it is—a genuinely human outcry against fate.

Remember, too, that if you allow anger and resentment to build inside you without the safety valve of airing your emotions then you will undoubtedly seriously impair your ability to care for the patient.

Your anger also may be directed against the doctors, hospital staff, and all other members of the health care team for not being able to cure the person who means so much to you. It's an unreasoning anger, as you should realize after some quiet thought, and there is nothing to be gained by allowing it to take control of you or your attitudes toward all those involved in helping you care for the dying patient.

Anger, rage, resentment, helplessness—all these feelings and others like them can engulf you in your role of caregiver. Deal with them as they come up. Your well-being, and that of the patient, is at stake in how you handle these destructive emotions.

Guidelines for the Caregiver

Here's a baker's dozen tips on how to cope with being a caregiver for a dying person, some of them not touched on before and other summarizing what we've already discussed:

- Maintain close contact with your physician and all other members of the health care team. Their expertise and assistance are invaluable in helping you provide home care for the patient.
- Be caring and supportive of the patient.
- Allow the patient to express his doubts and fears—be a good listener.
- Do not initiate talk of death; let the patient take the lead here. Talk to the patient about his dying, if that's what he wishes, and do not try to use elaborate euphemisms in place of the words "death" and "dying." If the patient has opened the door to this type of discussion, do not become evasive either in your answers or your use of language.
- Avoid giving gratuitous advice to the patient. Respect the patient's right to his private thoughts and his desire to think things out for himself. Wait until you are asked for your opinions or advice and, even then, be careful not to "lecture" the patient.
- Do not try to tell the patient that he or she should act or feel a certain way. This is not for you to say.
- Avoid excessive, bubbly cheerfulness—you will not fool the patient. Answer all questions honestly and respond to the patient's expressed concerns the same way.
- Make sure the patient gets the prescribed medications on time and in the proper dosage. This is especially important when administering analgesics (painkillers).
- If the patient talks irrationally or shows irrational feelings, do not get alarmed. It's probably only a temporary burst of emotionalism.
- Search out your own feelings and insecurities about death and dying and confront them. This will help you to a better understanding of what the patient is experiencing.
- Maintain a positive attitude, but don't carry it to excess. It will only appear false then. Keep yourself under calm control, and the patient will likely respond the same way.

- It's all right to grieve for the patient even before death comes, but don't wail and moan and get hysterical in front of the patient.
- If the patient wants to talk about arrangements for the future, such as funeral preparations or settling financial affairs, discuss them calmly and understandingly. Do not try to put the patient off in these matters.
- Be sure to take care of yourself. Good eating, regular exercise and rest will strengthen your reserve and help you cope with the stress of caregiving.

Preparing for Death

In addition to the patient's emotional preparation for death and discussions of such matters as financial arrangements and funeral services, it is important for both the patient and the caregiver to give some thought to one right the patient has—the right to die.

Essentially, what is meant by this phrase is the patient's right to control the manner of his dying when it has become clear that nothing more can be done to cure him or to control the course of the illness, disease, or injury that has struck him down. If the patient is made aware that he is dying, he should also be made aware (if he doesn't already know) that he has the final say on what measures should or should not be taken when death has finally arrived, often heralded by a lapse of consciousness or a cessation of breathing.

If he so desires, the patient can make out, sign, and have witnessed, what is known as a living will, a copy of which is shown.

As is evident from a reading of the sample will, the patient clearly specifies that he does not want "heroic measures" taken to keep him alive when it is clear that he is not going to recover and that death will come.

The legal right to demand a "natural" death is not recognized by all states, and the matter is being resolved by the courts at this time. Those states that do recognize the right of a person to indicate his wishes in a living will have done so by passing legislation known as "natural death acts." Check the laws in your state before taking any action to draw up such a will.

It's important to realize that even where this type of will is legal, it need not be honored under certain circumstances: if it has been revoked; if it has been drawn up so far in the past that its present validity could be challenged; or if the patient himself asks for and

My Living Will
To My Family, My Physician, My Lawyer
and All Others Whom It May Concern

Death is as much a reality as birth, growth, maturity and old age—it is the one certainty of life. If the time comes when I can no longer take part in decisions for my own future, let this statement stand as an expression of my wishes and directions, while I am still of sound mind.

If at such a time the situation should arise in which there is no reasonable expectation of my recovery from extreme physical or mental disability, I direct that I be allowed to die and not be kept alive by medications, artificial means or "heroic measures". I do, however, ask that medication be mercifully administered to me to alleviate suffering even though this may shorten my remaining life.

This statement is made after careful consideration and is in accordance with my strong convictions and beliefs. I want the wishes and directions here expressed carried out to the extent permitted by law. Insofar as they are not legally enforceable, I hope that those to whom this Will is addressed will regard themselves as morally bound by these provisions.

DURABLE POWER OF ATTORNEY (optional)

I hereby designate _____ to serve as my attorney-in-fact for the purpose of making medical treatment decisions. This power of attorney shall remain effective in the event that I become incompetent or otherwise unable to make such decisions for myself.

Optional Notarization:

"Sworn and subscribed to

before me this _____ day

of _____, 19_____."

_____
Notary Public
(seal)

Signed_____

Date _____

Witness _____

_____
Address

Witness _____

_____
Address

Copies of this request have been given to _____

_____   _____

(Optional)   My Living Will is registered with Concern for Dying (No. _____)

Reprinted with the permission of Concern for Dying, 250 West 57th Street, New York, NY 10107.

authorizes medical treatment that contradicts what he has requested in his living will.

Physicians are trained to save, preserve, and protect life. Hospitals see their task as that of healing patients and sending them home as soon as possible. These goals are, of course, diametrically in opposition to the stated purpose of a living will. The resulting conflict in philosophies of life and what to do when it is about to end has resulted in living wills sometimes not being honored. Physicians and hospital administrators have obtained court orders allowing them to use heroic measures to keep patients alive. (A recent case in California was decided by the Appeals Court in favor of the patient's right to die as he wished— but the patient had already died when the decision was handed down.) As long as the laws of the various states are not uniform in this respect, and as long as legal controversy still exists, vigilance on the part of the caregiver is necessary to make sure the wishes of the patient are carried out. This is especially true if, as is often the case, the patient is rushed to the hospital at the last minute—and dies there.

When Death Comes

A living will (if the patient has had one drawn up) is only one of the matters that you, as the caregiver, will have to deal with when death inevitably comes. It's one thing to anticipate it and to know that it's coming soon, but it's another matter when it is finally here.

If you have other family members to help, the task will be somewhat easier because the burdens and the responsibilities can be shared. There's no real advice that can be given on how to handle death. Each of us will react emotionally in our own unique and personal way. In time, though, grief does ease and, even though it's a cliché, life goes on.

Hospice Care at Home

In taking care of a dying patient at home, you have a major resource available to you in the hospice program, now being used more and more frequently all over the country.

Hospice care may not be available in your community, or you may not be able to use it for other reasons, or the patient may not desire it. Nevertheless, it will be very helpful for you, as the caregiver, to know how hospice functions. The procedures and techniques used in a hospice can be applied to home care with excellent results. Also, as will be discussed, a hospice program makes provisions for sending patients home when feasible, and hospice care continues at home with the caregiver being aided by the hospice staff.

The goal of hospice care is to make the inevitable death of a terminally ill person as painless and as restful as possible for both the individual and the family. Hospice programs can be carried out in special units in the hospital or nursing home, in a free-standing facility (sometimes affiliated with a hospital), or at home as part of home health care. It's important to understand, though, that hospice is a *concept* more than it is a building or a place. The hospice program, no matter where it is located or what its administrative ties are, is based on the philosophy of giving care, compassion, and support to those who have entered the final phase of illness and are days, weeks, or, at the most, some months away from death.

Hospice is an affirmation of life, not an abandonment of hope. Dying is recognized as a normal and inevitable process, but it is neither hastened nor fought off with curative procedures or futile heroic measures. A hospice is not where people are sent to die but rather where they are encouraged and helped to live out whatever time is left to them in comfort and dignity with caring family, friends, and staff around them.

"Caring" is the operative word here. The hospice staff is specially trained in the kind of caring the patient needs, and they are allowed the time to do so—time to sit and talk, or maybe just to listen, time to show compassion and understanding, time to help ease the pain, time to provide support for the family.

THE HOSPICE PROGRAM

While our main interest here is in home health care, it is not possible to separate how a hospice program works in a hospice from how it will work in the home. The family caregiver (or caregivers) cannot work independently of the hospice team. There has to be constant interaction between the hospice team and the caregiver and patient at home. Hospice care at home is actually an extension of the care provided in a hospice. For this reason, hospice home care first has to be approached from the standpoint of how a hospice program functions in providing the care needed by the patient and the family.

Basically, hospice care has four main concerns:

- Controlling and alleviating pain and debilitating symptoms in the patient.
- Providing holistic treatment (physical, emotional, spiritual, and social) for the patient and the family as a unit.
- Effectively using a multidisciplinary team—physicians, nurses, therapists, social workers—to treat the patient and family.

- Providing bereavement care and follow-up for the family after the patient has died.

Patients who are accepted for hospice care have to meet certain requirements, which are generally the same for most hospices. First and foremost, the patient must be at the stage where competent medical opinion has determined that attempts to effect a cure or to prolong life would be of no avail. The determination has to be clear: the patient is terminally ill and is dying.

Next, both the patient and the family must be aware of the hospice concept and want to accept the care provided by the hospice program.

The selection process is designed to ensure that the patient and family accepted will benefit from the hospice program. The patient must first be referred to the hospice by his or her physician (usually while the patient is still in the hospital), although referral requests can also initiate with family members, the clergy, or a hospital discharge planner.

Careful evaluation and consultation by the hospice physician, the head nurse at the hospice, and the patient's personal physician follow the referral. All aspects of the case care are considered before acceptance. No one is forced to accept hospice care, of course, and the patient can change his mind and leave the hospice program at any time.

Once accepted into the program, the patient will find a considerable difference from the hospital setting he or she may have just come from. There is a homelike atmosphere in a hospice that is not found in hospitals (even though the hospice may be a unit within the larger hospital). Bedding is often colorful, with colored sheets and bedspreads, usually made by volunteers. Nurses may not be as stiffly and starchly dressed, often wearing brighter colors than the standard white. Patients can wear their own clothing, and while most rooms are semiprivate, each room is cheerfully decorated and made as homelike as possible. To anyone who has spent time in a conventional hospital, the uplifting effect this kind of ambiance can have—even for the terminally ill patient—will be readily apparent.

Generally, around-the-clock visiting is allowed, and children and even pets can come. (In one hospice in Oregon, a cat lives in the hospice and associates freely with patients, families, and staff.) Children, of course, have a wonderful therapeutic effect on the elderly, especially grandparents, and they are always welcome in the hospice.

Although there has to be some kind of routine established, it is flexible and is geared to the needs of the patients and the families. Patients can have meals in bed, in a lounge, on a patio, or sometimes in the kitchen, depending on the physical layout of the hospice. If a patient wishes to sleep late, breakfast can be had later, if so desired. There are always special activities planned (and even unplanned) going on in the hospice: potluck suppers, with food brought in by families; television watching, of course; games for those who want to play; entertainment provided by staff, patients, and families.

This is not to say that everyone tries to forget with wild abandon that all the patients are terminally ill. There is no attempt to escape or hide from that fact. However, life (with the emphasis on life rather than its termination) is made as comfortable and as normal as possible for the patients and families.

CONTROLLING PAIN AND SYMPTOMS

The alleviation and control of pain and symptoms take precedence in hospice care. Medications to relieve and control pain are always available and are given on a regular schedule, usually every four hours. This is known as preventive scheduling, the purpose being to prevent pain from occurring rather than wait for the pain to appear and then try to medicate it. It's a method that works very well, as is evident to anyone who visits a hospice. A patient who is pain-free is a person who can concentrate on living a full life for as much time as is left.

A common medication given in hospices to prevent pain is known as the Brompton cocktail, named after the English physician who first used it before the turn of the century. Generally, it consists of a mixture of morphine (sometimes replaced by heroin), cocaine, alcohol, and a syrup for flavoring. It is taken orally, the dosage being adjusted to the level of pain that needs to be controlled in the individual patient.

Other pain medications are available, including tranquilizers and antidepressants. No one is oversedated, as the goal of hospice care is to keep the patient pain-free and functional. Medication requirements are constantly being reviewed and evaluated to ensure that pain is prevented before it has a chance to affect the patient.

Once a patient knows that he does not have to worry about pain, a tremendous burden will have been lifted from his mind. The predominant fear of most people—especially when there has been a diagnosis of terminal cancer—is how painful the end will be. This fear is alleviated in hospice care.

Undesirable and debilitating symptoms are another cause of fear and anxiety in terminal patients. No one likes to think of endless days and nights of nausea, vomiting, labored breathing, diarrhea, insomnia, depression, incontinence, and the like. Hospice care doesn't magically eliminate these symptoms, but through medication and good nursing techniques, it does ameliorate and control these conditions and allow the patient to be free from extreme discomfort.

COMPASSION AND AFFECTION

The nurses, therapists, and all other staff members in a hospice are specially selected and trained for their tasks. Since the emphasis is not on curative measures, laboratory tests, and invasive procedures, there is time available for the compassion, understanding, and unabashed demonstrations of affection that make life worthwhile to the hospice patients and their families.

A lot of touching goes on in a hospice. Someone who is dying—no matter how comfortable and pain-free he or she may be—will have moments of fear, of deep anxiety, of depression. At such times, often what is needed is the chance to reach out and hold someone's hand, to touch and to know that understanding and compassion are there. Hospice nurses realize this and will extend the needed clasp or touch, letting the patient silently know that someone does care.

In addition to the simple act of touching, the nurses and others on the hospice team often will just sit and listen as a patient or one of the family talks out his or her fears and anxieties. Listening is another way of rendering compassionate care—and so is responding when appropriate. A conversation with someone who cares and who listens and responds helpfully is as important as medicine in helping a person who is ill and troubled or anguishing over a loved one who is going to die.

On other occasions, the hospice nurse may have to try to draw out the uncommunicative patient who has pulled back and has withdrawn from contact with others. In such a case, gentle questions or understanding comments ("I know you must feel sad right now") will often help a patient to open up and give expression to what has been troubling him.

All avenues of help are explored by the hospice team. It's a vital part of their work—just as important as providing medical attention. Obviously, the work of the hospice staff involves much more than listening, touching, talking, and counseling. They are, after all, health care professionals, and they minister to their patients and provide medication and other types of medical attention where and when needed.

The patient, too, takes part in the treatment provided by the hospice program. Decisions as to the nature of the care are made with the full participation of the patient. It is the patient who decides whether or not to accept the preventive scheduling of pain medication. It is the patient who determines the extent of physical therapy, the amount of exercise, or the need for counseling. It is the patient who is the primary decision maker in most aspects of hospice care.

This approach to hospice care allows the patient to take control of his or her own life right up to the end. Along the way, family amd members of the hospice team join in both the joys and the sorrows the patient experiences. Laughter and tears are shared by all.

GOING HOME

One goal of hospice care is to enable the patient to go home and be cared for by family for as long a period of time as possible. It's recognized that there will be times when the patient has to return to the hospice, either for medical care or to give the family a respite. The hospice is always there, ready to welcome back the patient whenever needed.

Special arrangements are made when a patient goes home. As has been mentioned, home hospice care cannot be accomplished by the family alone. The work of the hospice team is needed just as much when the patient is at home as when the patient is in the hospice itself. Thus, visits by the members of the team are arranged in advance, with the home care hospice nurse coordinating everything.

The coordinating nurse has, in many respects, a more difficult task than the nurses in the hospice. She has to handle almost all situations by herself and, in effect, takes over the full hospice duties for the patient and family at home. Often, she has to act as the buffer between the family and the patient when the emotional load gets too heavy for either of them.

The same fears, anxieties, and doubts plague the patient and family members at home as when in the hospice. The nurse has to counsel the family caregiver how to respond to the questions and emotions of the patient. Understanding and compassion have to be the guidelines for the family caregiver, as they are for the hospice team.

Medications and treatment of symptoms will continue at home for the patient. The nurse will assist with this as much as possible, visiting the patient at home and checking on his or her condition, offering advice and guidance, and answering all questions as they come up.

Home hospice care is not an easy task, but help is always there from the hospice team.

FINANCIAL CONSIDERATIONS

Hospice care costs money. Until recently, hospices were supported by private donations, government grants, and nominal fees paid by patients and their families. In 1982, laws were passed by Congress that permitted Medicare payments to help with the financial burdens of hospice care, both in a hospice and at home. A total of 210 days of Medicare benefits were made available, and former restrictions on reimbursement for certain equipment and supplies were waived, as were some medical and hospitalization requirements.

Medicare now requires that a person cannot become eligible for hospice benefits unless a physician certifies that the person has six months or less to live. If the hospice accepts the patient and the patient lives longer than six months, hospice care cannot be discontinued and the hospice must bear the additional cost until the patient dies.

It has been shown that physicians cannot accurately predict a six-month life span with any degree of consistency. Therefore, some physicians are understandably reluctant to make such a prognosis, and some hospices are understandably apprehensive about accepting borderline cases. (There have been occasions when a hospice patient entered a period of remission or clung to life longer than had been expected.)

The rules and regulations of Medicare are complex, and private insurance carriers have not yet fully accepted the need to provide hospice coverage. It's important, therefore, that careful and thorough inquiries be made when hospice care is required to avoid future financial problems.

AT THE END

The time does come when death arrives, and this can happen either at the hospice or when the patient is at home. In either case, the hospice team is there to console the family, to grieve with them (attachments are often formed betweeen patients and the hospice team), and to give what assistance they can.

The hospice concept recognizes the importance of bereavement care and follow-up. Since the patient and the family have been treated as a unit, the loss of one part of that unit (the patient) leaves the other part of the unit (the family) requiring perhaps even more care and compassion than before.

When the patient dies, the hospice team draws together with the family, sharing their grief and offering comfort. The team also helps with funeral arrangements if family members are too stricken to manage, and members of the team will attend the wake and the funeral. The family is encouraged to contact the hospice team any time they feel the need. Thus, the feeling of family and community engendered during the hospice care of the patient carries over and continues even after the death of the patient.

Increasing numbers of hospices will undoubtedly come into being to fill the need for this type of care. One hopes that funds will be made more available to help ease the financial burden for those requiring this special care. Many individuals and organizations are working toward this goal. Success, as always, will require much work and hard effort.

It would be wonderful, indeed, if in addition to providing more hospices, some way were to be found to bring the hospice concept to conventional hospitals. The medical care requirements may be different, but the need to give compassionate human care is as important to a hospital as it is to a hospice.

IV

The Gamut of Health Problems

In this part we'll be covering a variety of diseases, disorders, chronic illnesses, and health problems that are most likely to require and respond to a home health care program. Each of the health conditions covered here is defined and identified, with a discussion of how it affects the quality of life at home for the patient and how that quality of life can be maximized and improved.

There are guidelines for coping with the various health and emotional problems that may arise; a discussion of treatments in current use, and referrals to resources you can turn to for support and help in the task of managing a home health care program.

In many of these cases, you'll be dealing with a chronic illness, which means that it will continue for a long time, slowly progressive, or with frequent recurrences. Additionally, multiple health problems can arise, all of which will add to the task of providing health care at home.

The caregiver has much to prepare for, and this part is meant to help with that preparation.

13

The Aging Person

GING IS NOT a disease.
Growing old is not a chronic illness, although age does bring with it a certain amount of aches and pains and physiological and emotional changes. These changes are not always minor, of course, and the aches and pains can sometimes be debilitating. Also, as we grow older, there is undoubtedly an increasing potential for serious disorders of body and mind.

Aging does have its problems, therefore, and we should not make light of them—but growing older can also be a pleasant time of life. It depends on how well we have prepared for it and in what frame of mind we approach aging and whatever difficulties it may bring.

It's been said that you don't start to feel old until your health goes bad, and then you realize that you are not just sick, but old and sick. This is what can happen in a home health care situation. The elderly person being cared for at home, for example, begins to feel that both age and illness have combined forces against him (or her). It is this perception that can, in some cases, add significantly to the damage wrought by the disease that brought about the need for home health care in the first place. It's a double-barreled attack on the elderly individual, an attack that can be fought off and conquered with a good mental attitude.

Since it's mostly the elderly whose health has to be cared for at home, it's appropriate that we examine aging and some aspects of it that relate to home health care.

The Aging Couple

Home health care for the aging can involve a son or daughter caring for a widowed mother or father, a situation in which an older husband or wife has died and the remaining spouse is alone and being cared for by a younger person. There can also be the case where both of the elderly parents are alive and both in such poor health that they have to be cared for by sons or daughters.

In these situations, there is the common factor of a comparatively younger person (or persons) available as the caregiver. But what about the aging couple who have to take care of each other? Here, we do not have a younger person taking care of an older one, but one elderly person acting as a caregiver for another elderly person. It can create problems in that both the caregiver and the one being cared for may have age-induced vision or hearing difficulties, for example, in addition to one of them having the more serious health problem that necessitated home health care.

The pages that follow, dealing with health problems of the aging, assume a younger caregiver. An aging couple in which one of them is the caregiver will, of necessity, have to apply the particular advice and techniques discussed in the rest of this chapter, as the case warrants. As mentioned, a good mental attitude and a positive approach to problems will be very helpful.

Hearing Loss

The trouble is that the elderly often cannot hear clearly what is being said to them.

Hearing loss is covered in detail further on in this section, but it's important here to realize that difficulty in hearing, which afflicts many older people, can hamper the effectiveness of home health care. If you are the caregiver and the elderly individual in your care is having hearing problems that cannot be completely corrected by a hearing aid, you will have to make allowances.

Not everything you say is going to get through all the time. The older person may nod and smile, but he or she will not have heard or completely understood everything you've just said. This difficulty takes on importance if you are trying to convey some information about medication or other necessary detail about the health care of the individual. You have to be sure you've gotten through, and you have to be tactful about it—no exaggerated lip movements, no shouting, no exasperated expression, no obvious irritation, no patronizing attitude. You're dealing with someone who needs your care, but more importantly, who also needs your understanding.

If the shoe is on the other foot and you're the one receiving the care and you have a problem hearing well, bear in mind that your caregiver is not a mind reader. He or she will not know you've understood unless you make it clear that you have. Your own health is at stake here, so it's vital not to be vague.

Not all elderly people will have a hearing problem. It is, however, something that can develop with age—and both the caregiver and the patient should be aware of this.

The Memory Lingers On

Sometimes it does, . . . sometimes it doesn't.

There have been more than enough jokes about the forgetfulness of the elderly. It makes for lots of laughs on some TV sitcoms, and it's always good for a chuckle or two around the office mail room, or in the health club locker room, or wherever folks get together to swap stories.

It isn't so funny, though, when you have to cope with it while trying to provide home health care for an older person, more often than not someone close to you.

A certain amount of memory loss can occur with aging. It's nothing to get alarmed about, and it doesn't inevitably lead to a serious neurological disorder such as Alzheimer's disease. More often than not, the so-called memory loss is merely the result of confusion on the part of the older person, sometimes caused by momentary disorientation after returning home from a hospital stay.

Whatever the reason, though, memory difficulties have to be taken into consideration in any home health care program involving an older person. This is particularly important in the matter of taking medications on schedule.

In hospitals and other institutions, medications are handed out by a nurse. The patient doesn't have to be concerned about remembering when to take which medication. At home, though, it's another matter. Even with a devoted caregiver on hand, it isn't always possible to give the required medication at the specified time each and every day. Thus, the cared-for individual is often responsible for taking his medication on his own at some time during the day.

If memory is not to be fully trusted, there are ways to get around this problem. Some people have tried writing the medication schedule out on a sheet taped to the refrigerator. Others have used large numbers marked on the caps of the medicine bottles or containers. Also, there are commercial medication scheduling aids available—usually a rack or other device for holding the medications, labeled in the order to be taken—and these can be purchased through your local pharmacy.

You can use whatever method works best for the individual who has to take the medication. With a regular routine to follow and a clearly indicated medication schedule, the cared-for individual will feel more secure and will not worry about any possible forgetfulness. This will help reduce confusion and uncertainty.

This same principle applies to any aspect of home health care dependent upon memory—when to visit the doctor, in which dresser drawers certain articles of clothing are stored, what day of the week to expect the therapist or the nurse, and so on. An established routine, with important schedules written down and prominently posted, will do the trick.

Don't go overboard on this. Too many memory aids can have a "backlash" effect, causing the older person to lose confidence and rely too heavily on artificial devices.

A Little More Light, Please

You won't find many older people who do not have to wear glasses. Reduced visual acuity is part of the aging process. In most cases, this presents no real problems. With many corrective lenses available, and with special low vision aids (telescopic glasses, for example, or video magnification devices) for those whose vision has seriously deteriorated, elderly people can continue to enjoy reading, people watching, and looking at sunsets and whatever other sights give them pleasure.

Elderly vision is not perfect, however. One of the first signs of aging eyes that will be noticed is a decrease in night vision. Older people generally need more light, especially at night. The loss of good night vision isn't too serious, though, unless night driving is a normal activity for the older person.

For reading, cooking, sewing, woodworking, or any other activity in which the eyes are used, the older person will usually need brighter lighting than when he or she was younger. Dimly lit restaurants may have a relaxing ambiance, but they present difficulties for reading the menu to many older people. (One solution practiced by a resourceful senior citizen is to carry a pocket flashlight in her purse and use it to peruse the menu.)

Serious eye problems that may beset the elderly (cataracts and glaucoma, for example) are discussed later on in this section. Regular eye checkups with an opthalmologist will allow early detection of any eye disorder or disease that may develop.

Watch Your Step!

"Old people have a habit of falling."

This rather thoughtless statement was made by a bystander when a small crowd gathered around an older woman who apparently had lost her balance when alighting from a bus and had fallen to the sidewalk. (There are significantly many broken hips resulting from falls by elderly women.)

The person who made the remark thought he was proclaiming an accepted fact, to which everyone would agree, but the truth is that while older people are much more susceptible to falling, it's by no means a "habit" with them.

An older person can fall for a variety of reasons—momentary dizziness, poor vision, confusion, disorientation, drug or medication reaction, poor balance, or muscular weakness in the legs, to name a few. One way to reduce the possibility of falling is to carry a cane. Many elderly people assume that you carry a cane only if you are disabled or lame. This is not necessarily true. A cane can help maintain balance and will provide a steadying force for the elderly person.

Falls inside the home can be even more harmful than ones that occur outside. In the home, the individual is less careful because he or she is in a known environment, a safe place. Thus, a loose scatter rug, dimly lit stairs, a cat or dog sleeping near a doorway, furniture a little out of place—any of these and others—can cause a fall in the home.

Carrying a cane in the home isn't always necessary, but the home should be made as safe as possible for the person whose health is being cared for in that environment. There's no point in adding to the already existing health problems by precipitating a fall.

Heat

Older people usually prefer the warmer weather. Clothes are less bulky. Movement can be freer without the weight of heavy coats. Fingers will not develop splits or skin cracks from cold; noses will not run; lips will not get chapped. Also, the whole outdoors beckons, and leisurely walks can be taken without fear of slipping on the ice.

However, you can get too much of a good thing. In the summer of 1980, a vast heat wave struck many states. Temperatures were abnormally high, with no relief for many days. It was estimated that 1,600 people died of heat stroke, many of them elderly.

Research has now shown that many more deaths were probably due to the heat than just those occurring from heat stroke. Excessive heat and humidity place a tremendous strain on the heart and circulatory system. For an elderly person whose health is already compromised by chronic disease, this form of heat "stress" can be fatal.

Many of the elderly who died during the 1980 heat wave were not aware of the danger to them posed by the high heat and humidity, and they did not have sufficient knowledge of how to protect themselves against the devastating strain that heat stress would place on their bodies.

It may be difficult to picture how, in a normal home health care situation, an older person could succumb to the heat. It can happen, though, if proper precautions are not taken.

If the home (or at least the room in which the elderly person will stay) is air-conditioned, then most of the problem is solved. If air conditioning is not available, other measures have to be taken.

First, use should be made of any electric fans that are in working order. Setting the fan to circulate air across the top of a bowl of ice cubes is a good, temporary cooling device. Fans can also be used to pull cooler nighttime air into the house.

Next, drink lots of liquids. Fruit juices and water are the best. (No alcohol, of course, since it can impair a body's temperature control.)

Eat lightly and avoid hot foods.

Wear loose clothing, preferably cotton.

Take cool baths or showers. If this isn't feasible, a cool sponge bath will do.

If you are the caregiver and have to leave the house for any length of time during the extremely hot weather, make sure the cared-for individual is in a cool room with good ventilation. Heat can build up very fast in a closed room, and an elderly person can sometimes weaken very fast in excessive heat with no air circulation.

With proper precautions, and with the elderly person informed as to what to do to avoid heat stress, there's no reason why a heat wave should cause anything worse than discomfort.

Don't Stay Cool Too Long

The opposite to heat stress is hypothermia. This is the condition when the internal body temperature is abnormally low—95° F or below.

Accidental hypothermia can occur from prolonged exposure to cold. It doesn't necessarily have to be freezing cold. For example, in a poorly heated room, the nighttime temperature might go down to 45° F and not rise above 60° F during the day. An elderly person, living alone, staying huddled in bed without much in the way of protection against the cold, can lapse into hypothermia if exposed to this temperature for a prolonged period.

Hypothermia can lead to kidney and liver damage and can bring on an irregular heartbeat, which can be fatal.

The one sure way to prevent hypothermia, of course, is to stay warm. In a well-heated house with a caregiver nearby, there is no danger to the elderly individual at home. Unfortunately, not every older person receiving home health care lives under such ideal conditions. There are many elderly people who are receiving home health care but who live alone, with a relative or a social worker or a nurse looking in occasionally to make sure everything is all right. This type of person risks hypothermia if subjected to continued exposure to even mild cold temperatures.

Again, proper precautions taken well in advance, along with making sure the older person is informed of what to do to protect himself, will significantly reduce the possibility of hypothermia.

Mental Calisthenics

It's a myth that senility is the inevitable outcome of living too long.

There are changes in the brain as one gets older, but only disease or disuse can keep an elderly person's mind from functioning with clarity and effectiveness. It all comes down to the old saying that can be applied to almost all bodily functions: "Use it, or lose it."

Researchers have found, through a series of tests, that people who stay mentally active stay mentally functional. Playing chess, doing crossword puzzles, playing cards, reading the papers, writing letters—anything and everything that keeps the mind active will help ensure a healthy mind.

Social involvement is still another way of keeping your mind healthy and active. Some older people have a tendency to withdraw from active contact with others. This can be harmful since they will have only their inner thoughts and silent memories of the past to occupy their minds. Taking an active part in what's going on around you and in other people—whether relatives, old friends, or new acquaintances—will provide the spark that will keep your mind going.

Elder Abuse

A seven-year-old child and a seventy-year-old adult—the one unfortunate thing they often have in common is that each can be subjected to physical and emotional abuse. Elder abuse has not received the media attention usually given to child abuse and battered wives, but awareness of abuse of the elderly is growing.

Most of the time, this is an insidious development. It's hard to picture anyone deliberately setting out to abuse an elderly mother or father or other close relative being cared for at home. Our intentions are always just the opposite—to provide the required care and attention to the health needs of the individual entrusted to our care. Why, then, should we even think the unthinkable and talk about elder abuse?

Because it can, and has, happened.

Elderly people sometimes use devious tactics to try to manipulate their adult children who have become the caregivers. Refusing food or medication is a means of drawing attention, as is withdrawal, dropping or throwing things, crying, screaming, and other such behavior. That elderly people being cared for at home can be difficult is an undeniable truth. However, it's no excuse for inflicting abuse on someone who is helpless and vulnerable.

Although actual physical abuse of the elderly is not as prevalent as verbal or emotional abuse, it is, nevertheless, a sociological problem that cannot be overlooked. Older people have been found with severe bruises, broken bones, cuts, burns, scaldings, frostbite, puncture wounds, and many other serious physical injuries. Police officials, social workers, emergency room physicians, and all other who deal with the elderly have seen these repugnant results of elder abuse.

Physical abuse does not necessarily have to involve actually striking the older person. Tying an old man or woman to the bed so they can't wander off is physical abuse. So is ignoring their need to be helped to the toilet until they "have an accident," or letting them wait for their food, or forcing them to take medication, or any other form of neglect or indifference that physical hardship causes the older person.

Verbal abuse involves emotional and psychological factors that can have just as devastating an effect as outright physical abuse. Yelling at older people, berating them, ridiculing them, taunting them—all of these and more represent forms of mistreatment. Sarcasm, irritation, exasperation, and threats all have been used on the elderly with telling effect. Ironically, most of the time the abusers are not really aware of what they are doing to the elderly one in their care. Stress on a caregiver can result in this type of abusive behavior. Caregivers have to be on their guard against this.

It's a crushing blow when an older person has to face the fact that he or she has become incontinent or, as is often the case, just cannot move fast enough to get to the bathroom in time (see Chapter 8). It strikes hard at a person's self-esteem and can make any of us feel that we are reverting to the helplessness of an infant. Even being forced to use a commode chair next to the bed, or the awkward bedpan while propped up in bed, can be an agonizing experience to which hardly anyone ever becomes accustomed. Imagine, then, the feelings of an older person when the caregiver ridicules the older one for not being able to use the bathroom like everyone else.

Ridicule is sometimes resorted to by a caregiver in a misguided attempt to jar the older person into more "normal" behavior. What is not being considered here is that the elderly individual is not doing this deliberately. He or she is already suffering a great loss of self-respect and independence, and to have someone use sarcasm or ridicule in an attempt to correct the situation is humiliating.

Can there be anything more demeaning than a person well along in years being told he or she cannot watch television until all the food is cleared off the plate or the medication taken as ordered? Yet this is not an uncommon tactic used by some exasperated caregivers, not realizing that by treating the older person like a child they are only encouraging more childlike behavior.

Caregivers are not the only ones guilty of elder abuse. Home health aides and others employed to assist in the care of the elderly at home have been both physically and verbally abusive. Often, this abuse occurs when members of the family are not present, and the older person doesn't report it out of fear of reprisal from the abuser. Or, if the patient does complain about it to the family, it's not unusual for family members to listen and not believe. The assumption is that the older person is just being cantankerous or trying to make trouble. Worse still, there are times when the family will believe the older one but will hesitate to take any positive action because it's difficult to find people to assist with home health care. It's easier to try to smooth things over than to look for new help. This, incidentally, is another and more subtle form of neglect that constitutes elder abuse.

Abuse of the elderly is not an easy subject for most of us to think about. Nevertheless, we must recognize that the potential for elder abuse is always there. Home health care is a very stressful situation, bringing on conditions that can get out of hand when least expected.

Understanding is the key here. As the caregiver, you have to make an extra effort to understand what the older person is feeling and fearing. You have to remember that you are dealing with someone who has lost a lot—good health, independence, self-esteem, confidence in the future.

The one receiving health care at home, also has to strive for an understanding of what the caregiver is going through—a pressing sense of heavy responsibility, self-doubts about his ability to perform the tasks required, concern over the future health of the one being cared for.

Mutual understanding and appreciation of each other's problems is important. Both the caregiver and the one being cared for must constantly work at that goal.

14

Cancer

ACTUALLY, cancer is not one disease. It's a general term that refers to the over one hundred different diseases. The symptoms and treatment for lung cancer, for example, are different than those of stomach cancer, pancreatic cancer, and breast cancer. What all of these diseases have in common, however, is that they are characterized by an uncontrolled growth of abnormal cells.

Today, cancer researchers and specialists are developing and using treatment regimes that destroy cancer cells and keep them from spreading. Also, victims of cancer are finding the physical and spiritual strength and the will to live that enables them to cope with the disease.

If you or someone close to you is diagnosed as having cancer, you will want to seek actively the best possible medical care. Although your internist or family physician may have made the original diagnosis, he or she will probably recommend that you see a cancer specialist (an oncologist), since the latest advances in treatment of cancer are now taking place in the specialized areas in which the oncologist works.

You and your doctor can work together to select a specialist who is qualified and whom you will trust. The oncologist will probably be located at a cancer center where patients with your type of cancer are examined and treated. It is in the cancer center that you will find the staff and resources to provide any form of treatment that may be needed.

Before beginning treatment you may wish to obtain a second opinion from another specialist, perhaps one located in the same cancer center or, if you wish, in a different health care facility. Talk it over with your physician and with the specialist also, discussing your questions, concerns, and wishes. It is important that you find and work with a doctor you can trust, one who you feel will give you the time and attention you need. Make sure you ask all the questions that have come to mind about your disease, the planned treatment, and the results that can be expected, including possible side effects and their duration.

The Cancer Information Service of the National Cancer Institute can assist you in your task. If you call their toll-free number (1–800–4–CANCER) you will be connected with staff members in the office serving your area. The staff members will attempt to answer all your questions and will refer you to local resources for further help. (In Alaska, call 1–800–6070; in Washington D.C., and its suburbs in Maryland and Virginia, call 636–5700; on Oahu, call 524–1234; and in New York City, call 794–7982.)

Spanish-speaking staff members are available (daytime hours only), serving California (area codes 213, 714, 619, and 805), Florida, Georgia, Illinois, northern New Jersey, New York City, and Texas.

Once you have selected your specialist, he and your primary care physician will become your major medical advisors. Other specialists—radiologists, surgeons, and others—may be called in, but your oncologist and your primary care physician should be involved with you in the decision-making process for all aspects of your medical care. Your oncologist will coordinate all your cancer treatments, and your primary care physician—who knows you and your home situation—can function as a much needed resource, helping you interpret the recommendations of other doctors and answering your questions.

If you do not have a family doctor to act as your primary care physician, then the oncologist will become your primary physician as well as your specialist.

As you progress in your treatment, do not assume that all of the health care professionals involved in your case talk to each other routinely—even doctors working in the same hospital. To make sure that all of your care is properly and effectively coordinated, it would be best to remind each of the doctors involved to contact your primary care physician.

For example, a surgeon may suggest that, in a particular case, a simple surgical correction of a stoma would offer greater comfort for the patient, enabling better ostomy management and care. (Refer to the section on managing an ostomy in Chapter 18.) With chemotherapy in progress, a decision will have to be made as to whether the surgery takes precedence over the chemotherapy regime (both cannot be undertaken simultaneously). By involving the oncologist in the decision-making process, a decision can be made that will be in the best interests of the health and comfort of the patient.

Many people, physicians included, look upon the fight against cancer as being in the nature of a continuing war against the killer disease. The battle is not yet won; the war goes on. Surgery, radiation therapy, and chemotherapy are the three main weapons (or methods)

Table 21 ▪ Types of Cancer and Their Treatment

Type of cancer	New cases per year	Treatment	5-Year survival rate
Lung	144,000	Surgery usually treatment of choice; radiation and chemotherapy frequently used	40% if localized 13% all stages
Breast	119,000	Depends on person's medical situation • Surgery ranges from local removal to total mastectomy • Also use radiation, chemotherapy, and hormone manipulation • New surgery techniques permit breast reconstruction after mastectomy	96% if localized 70% if cancer has spread
Uterine cervical	52,000	Surgery and/radiation	80–90% for early diagnosis of cervical cancer; 65% all stages
endometrial			91% for early diagnosis of endometrial cancer; 84% all stages
Colon	96,000	Surgery treatment of choice; sometimes used in combination with radiation and chemotherapy	87% for early diagnosis 47% later stages
Rectal	42,000	Surgery treatment of choice; sometimes used in combination with radiation and chemotherapy	78% for early diagnosis 38% later stages
Prostate	86,000	Surgery or radiation; sometimes hormone manipulation	65% for localized and early diagnosis
Bladder	40,000	Surgery and/or radiation	72% all stages

Source: Cancer Facts and Figures, American Cancer Society, New York: 1985).

used in fighting this war and treating cancer. In many cases, doctors will use a combination of these methods to achieve a better result than could be obtained by employing just one of the choices. Table 21 lists types of cancer and the weapons that may be used in fighting them.

Surgery

When a tumor is localized and the location is operable, surgery can usually provide the best results. The surgeon will seek to remove the tumor as well as any nearby tissue that may contain cancer cells.

During surgery, the surgeon may take tissue samples for a biopsy from the surrounding tissues or lymph nodes and send them to the pathology laboratory for examination. If the pathologist's report is "all clear," the surrounding tissues do not have to be removed. If, however, the pathologist identifies cancer cells in the surrounding tissue, the surgeon may become more aggressive in the surgery and also may plan to follow up with additional therapy (radiation or chemotherapy, or both) to attack the remaining cancer cells.

The decision to operate—as well as the type of operation to be performed—may offer the patient options for consideration. Obviously, the type of cancer and its site in the body will dictate the surgical procedures to be considered. For example, with breast cancer, the surgical procedure can allow for subsequent breast reconstruction. Depending on the extent of the cancer, total mastectomy (the breast and all of the axillary lymph nodes are removed) may be preferable to the radical mastectomy, which also removes the pectoral muscles. This newer and accepted procedure permits breast reconstruction within a few months. (In breast reconstruction a plastic implant is used to replace the now absent breast tissue and offers a superior cosmetic result over the former procedure of using special built-up brassieres.)

There are numerous studies underway that seek to document the risks and benefits of less invasive surgery with follow-up radiation. By checking out the surgical choices, the expected results, and the alternative therapy options available, you and your doctor can develop a treatment plan that will increase the odds of recovery and also offer the most acceptable quality of life afterward.

The more you know about a surgical procedure, the anticipated results, and the postsurgery plan, the more you can actively work with your doctor to maximize that plan. For example, many people believe that an operation for colon cancer means they will be forced to have a permanent colostomy (an abdominal opening through which to eliminate body wastes). Permanent colostomies are rare in colon cancer; in operations for rectal cancer approximately 15 percent require a permanent colostomy.

There may be a need for a temporary colostomy to permit healing following surgery, but once the healing is complete, the colostomy is surgically repaired and normal bowel function is restored. By clarifying your understanding of the surgical procedure, you will have time to adjust and come to grips with the anticipated recovery process, thus reducing your anxiety about the unknown.

Radiation

X-rays and other forms of radiation are used to destroy a cancer when it is located in an area that is not operable, or when previous surgery has been unable to reach and remove all of the cancerous tissue. For some forms of cancer, radiation therapy is the main choice. Cases of bladder cancer, cervical cancer, and skin cancer may be treated with radioactive substances such as cobalt and radium.

Your doctor, in collaboration with the radiologist, will individualize your course of radiation therapy. The dose rate (larger doses and fewer treatments or smaller doses over a longer period of time) will be determined, and the area of body exposure will be prescribed.

A thorough discussion of possible side effects should take place so you'll know what to expect. In some cases, depending on the type of treatment and the location of the cancer, there may be a temporary loss of hair, a general feeling of malaise, diarrhea, a dryness in the mouth, a loss of appetite, or nausea. These reactions can be treated. If they are planned for in advance, the discomfort can be lessened.

Special attention may be given to the diet and to other medications taken. Prescriptions for antinauseants or for diarrhea control can be written. Other precautions, such as avoiding talcum powder because it contains heavy metals that can irritate the skin, should also be discussed by you and your doctor.

Since a better-nourished person is more responsive to radiation exposure than a malnourished individual, the nursing team and dietition will work with a patient to maintain a high level of nutrition during the course of treatment. They will also caution the patient not to eat any foods that may irritate the stomach lining.

A nutritional supplement may be recommended, usually consisting of a simple, high-calorie, nutritious liquid that can be easily swallowed. If the nature of the cancer is such that swallowing is impossible, the liquid can be administered through a nasogastric tube inserted through the nose and into the gastric tract. If normal digestive routes are not possible, total parenteral nutrition (TPN) may be used. (Further details on cancer and nutrition are given later in this section. Parenteral and enteral nutrition are covered in Chapter 6.)

Chemotherapy

Although the five-year survival statistics cited in Table 21 are better than ever, the very fact that 440,000 cancer victims died of the disease in 1983 demands that better measures must be found. Over the past forty years, chemotherapeutic agents (some of them products of the development of chemical warfare) have been added as weapons in the war on cancer. In the last ten to fifteen years, oncologists have had some positive results fighting some forms of cancer, especially leukemia and Hodgkin's disease. Where a cure has been elusive, doctors have tried to lessen the pain or the severity of the invading cancer.

Numerous studies and protocols using chemotherapeutic agents alone or in combination have attempted to produce regression of a tumor or its metastasis. In some cases, the agents are used to reduce or slow the appearance of secondary growths following surgical removal of the primary tumor. Doctors and medical researchers feel that chemotherapeutic agents, when successful, may improve the quality of survival for the cancer victim.

Chemotherapy introduces potent mixtures into the body that are capable of destroying young, rapidly multiplying cells. Often, in addition to inhibiting the growth and reproduction of cancer cells in the body, the chemical agents may also affect other cells that normally grow rapidly, such as those in hair follicles, gastrointestinal tract lining, and bone marrow. This may result in side effects that can range from hair loss, nausea, and vomiting to bone marrow depression.

More than fifty anticancer drugs are in use today, many of them with unpleasant side effects. However, the curative and palliative results achieved by these drugs have encouraged many patients to endure the unpleasant—and temporary—side effects stoically.

Because of the toxic nature of these chemical agents, large doses given at one time can produce extreme side effects. To alleviate this, doctors have used a procedure called continuous infusion chemotherapy, in which the drug is administered in small, continuous doses over a long period of time. This procedure has worked well in helping to decrease some of the untoward side effects of chemical agents.

With this approach, the patient can be admitted to a hospital and receive intravenous treatment over a period of time. In certain circumstances, it will also be possible to have chemotherapy in the familiar surroundings of home. If the particular cancer can be treated by continuous therapy and the patient and family are sufficiently motivated, arrangements can be made for home therapy. The patient and the family are prepared and counseled during a hospital stay, and special suppliers are contacted to deliver the medication and monitor the patient at home. Thus, the patient and the family are enabled to manage continuous infusion therapy in the home.

Although the cost savings of home chemotherapy are significant when compared to the cost of a prolonged hospital stay for the same treatment, the procedure does place added responsibility on the patient and the caregiver. However, the drive to remain in the comfort and familiarity of home often outweighs the anxiety and responsibility of managing home chemotherapy.

If home chemotherapy is planned, be sure to arrange in advance for insurance—either Medicare Part B or private insurance—to provide for reimbursement and to avoid any subsequent billing surprises. (If paid for privately, home chemotherapy can be expensive.) Representatives from the companies offering home chemotherapy are often quite knowledgeable about the nuances of insurance coverage for this medical procedure and can be of much help to you in this respect.

Questions to Ask

Before beginning a course of treatment, be sure you know the following:

What is the treatment being done?
How often will the treatment be given?
How long will each treatment session be?
What are the anticipated results of this treatment?
What are the alternatives to this treatment?
What are the possible side effects?
How long will the side effects last?
How can these side effects be treated?
How long after treatment has been completed will these side effects last?

Often, it is helpful to speak with other patients who have successfully received the same treatment. Ask your doctor if he can put you in touch with such people, or contact the local chapter of the American Cancer Society. Sharing information can help reduce the stress of treatment by making you better informed and allowing you to participate actively in planning and implementing your own cancer treatment.

Maximizing Cancer Treatment Through Nutrition

Good nutrition, although important for everyone, is of considerable importance for the cancer victim. The better nourished person will withstand the stresses of the cancer and its treatment better than the poorly nourished individual. In fact, poor nutrition may weaken the body's defenses so dramatically that, even if the disease could be treated successfully, the patient could not survive the treatment!

Weight loss is the most common nutritional problem and can be the simple, direct result of not eating enough. Cancer treatments can reduce appetite, change the way food tastes, or cause nausea or other gastrointestinal symptoms. The end result is that eating becomes unpleasant and less food is eaten. Less food means a weight loss, weakening the individual, and this can be dangerous.

It is important to note any changes in eating habits and nourishment status of a cancer patient and try to identify why this is occurring. If you learn that the patient has found that sweet foods have become difficult to taste, for example, or that cooked chicken or meats taste quite bitter, you can then work to change the way food is prepared and served so as to encourage the patient to return to normal eating. Bitter tasting meats may taste better when marinated in a sweet (orange juice) or salty (teriyaki) sauce. Experimenting with seasonings may help to improve the flavor and aroma of the food, or you can try serving the food at room temperature rather than piping hot.

Even when the cancer patient is obviously nauseated, it is possible to prepare simple carbohydrate foods (baked or boiled potatoes or rice) and serve them in small portions throughout the day. If the nausea is particularly severe and persistent, bring this to the attention of the doctor so that he may prescribe medication to alleviate the problem.

Mouth dryness or soreness sometimes results from cancer treatment. Try cooling ice cream, popsicles, or juicy fruits such as watermelon and cantaloupes, or fruit drinks such as fruit nectars or apple juice. (Citrus juices may be irritating to the stomach.) Once again, if the symptoms persist and interfere significantly with eating, bring this to the attention of the doctor. When mouth soreness is considerable, medication to numb the mouth and throat may not only relieve the pain but also encourage better eating.

Because the cancer patient is fighting a many-sided battle, the caregiver may need to become more actively involved in assuring that the patient is receiving adequate nutrition. (This may involve special shopping and cooking chores.) The assistance of a trained nutritionist can be sought to help create a menu plan and recipe base that will provide good nutrition and promote adequate food consumption.

There may be times when the doctor will present a list of foods to avoid because of their known side effects following a chemotherapy treatment. Here, flexibility and creativity can be a real help.

If undernutrition cannot be adequately treated with regular food, nutritional support may be needed. Whether prepared in a blender or purchased as a special formula, these products are very useful for patients who need added nutrients in their diet. The homemade mixtures can combine and liquefy foods that could not normally be eaten otherwise, adding calories and nutrition in an easy-to-drink beverage.

Added nutrition can also be obtained from one of the medical "nutritionals" manufactured by the pharmaceutical industry. These products come in milkshake form and contain basic nutrients, vitamins, and minerals normally found in a balanced diet. Special formulations are available that can boost your calorie intake or add special nutrients to the diet. If necessary, these enteral formulas can be tube-fed, assuring adequate nutrition when the upper gastrointestinal tract is compromised.

When there is a gastrointestinal obstruction, or some other problem that rules out using the gastrointestinal tract, adequate nutrition can be assured by infusion of nutrients directly into the bloodstream. Called total parenteral nutrition (TPN), it provides, in solution form, the amino acids, fats, vitamins, and electrolytes necessary for good nutrition (see Chapter 6).

Recent advances in formulas, infusion pumps, and delivery systems now make it possible to arrange for nutrition programs (enteral or parenteral) while the patient remains at home. Patients who may have previously been compromised nutritionally can now be helped to fortify themselves as they battle against cancer.

Pain Management

In doing battle against cancer, there may be greater concern and anxiety about dealing with pain and the possibility of suffering than in dealing with the possibility of death itself. (See the section on hospice care in Chapter 12 for a discussion of the management of pain in a hospice, where death is a certainty rather than a possibility.)

For people living at home while undergoing cancer treatment, the fear of pain is increased because the hospital staff is not readily available to provide medication. This concern, although real, is not reality-based. The reality is that, in or out of the hospital, your doctor must be involved in developing a pain management program. The nurse will not dispense painkilling drugs without an order from the doctor. In fact, you have greater control at home over when and under what circumstances the medication will be taken.

The kind of pain, its location, and the duration of the pain must be discussed with your doctor as the two of you work together to develop a pain management program. Withholding information or assuming that "the doctor should know" will not be productive. Open communication between you and your doctor will help you understand the reasons behind your pain and how to control it.

Local pain can sometimes be alleviated by using analgesics, although intervention in the form of a nerve block or use of transcutaneous electrical nerve stimulation (TENS) may be helpful. (See on pain in Chapter 9.)

Narcotics can be used for acute pain, and powerful narcotics such as morphine and even heroin have been used. Although the possibility of addiction because of prolonged use of narcotics has to be considered, the respite from pain may outweigh any other considerations. However, some knowledgeable patients may interpret the prescription of powerful narcotics as a tacit admission by the doctor that "all hope is gone." Even though this may not be true, it is more important for these patients to manage the pain with lesser narcotics than to give in to morphine or what they consider "painkillers of last resort."

Each person experiences and deals with pain in his or her own way, and this choice should be respected.

Activity

Home care for the cancer patient provides the opportunity for a better quality of life when surrounded by familiar faces and belongings. Lying inactive in bed just waiting for rest to repair the body may be more harmful than helpful. Inactivity promotes further weakness, and boredom can bring on depression.

The cancer patient needs to be an active participant in home life. Painting, collage, clay modeling, drawing, gardening, household chores, a structured exercise program—all of these are productive activities that can be life-affirming. Making them part of each day at home can enhance the quality of life for the cancer patient.

Often, new hobbies that have been explored as part of occupational therapy during a hospital stay can be continued at home. The home health care team—nurses, therapists, and aides—can help by suggesting and organizing various activities. Family members can also help by reminding the patient of hobbies or projects that had been put aside or left incomplete during the fight against cancer.

Massage as a form of passive exercise and a way to stimulate circulation should not be overlooked. For the person who has to spend a lot of time in bed, massage can be one of the most soothing of treatments. Massage can relax the patient and will help reduce pain by stimulating circulation. Licensed massage therapists can be engaged to visit the patient and provide massage therapy treatment. Family members wishing to supplement verbal communication with the patient may find that massage provides a form of nonverbal communication that can be reassuring and comforting for both the patient and the caregiver.

Coping with the Cure

Courage, stamina, strength, and determination are basic to winning the fight against cancer. The patient's active participation in the diagnostic and treatment processes is critical, and continuing support from a caring physician who will coordinate all aspects of hospital care is mandatory.

Of prime significance—and perhaps of even more importance than what has already been mentioned—is the support, encouragement, and love of spouse and family. The strain on a husband, wife, or child during their loved one's battle with cancer can be, in some ways, even more stressful than the pressures on the patient. The spouse has to stand by and watch a loved one suffer—and cannot remove the pain.

A loving and caring wife or husband often can make the difference between despair, depression, and death for the patient and hope, determination, and recovery.

Medically, there is also hope. Today, surgeons, oncologists, and radiotherapists are becoming increasingly optimistic about achieving a "cure" for many kinds of cancer—and the survival statistics confirm their optimism.

More and more patients are now dealing with problems that become apparent only when they have won the fight against cancer. Although there continues to be the ongoing fear of recurrence, especially during the first five years, cancer victors find they have to deal with a barrage of new feelings. Although many find a greater appreciation of life and a greater intensity in their personal and family relationships, some actually feel a letdown because a goal so vigorously strived for has finally been accomplished.

Fatigue and lethargy may set in, and just getting on with life may take a period of readjustment to the idea of being declared "cured." The therapy that had been so successful may leave emotional scars to match those left by surgery and radiation.

Sexual problems, for example, may now become apparent. Sexual counseling and reassurance following successful cancer treatment is not infrequent. Dysfunction may arise not only from the readjustments required to a new body image following a mastectomy or a colostomy but because of changed attitudes in both the patient and the spouse.

Attitudes, biases, and fears of contagion of co-workers must be confronted and employment choices considered. If a leave of absence has been taken from the job, for example, the individual may find there now is no room for him at his former place of employment since he had been away so long.

The support groups and resources available from local chapters of the American Cancer Society and other organizations (see the section on cancer in the Appendix) can provide the psychological support and factual information needed to overcome this added battle. Other cancer survivors represent an affirmation of the success that has been won by the individual, and their experiences may provide comfort and renewed confidence for the new victor.

Winning the battle against cancer is not an easy victory. In winning this battle, the victors deserve to enjoy to the fullest this second chance at living.

15

Eye and Ear Problems

Eye Problems

MOST OF US take eyesight for granted. Even if we have to wear glasses, we usually accept the fact that we can see and absorb sight and sensation through our eyes, and we think no more about it—until, unfortunately, something significantly affects our vision.

Elsewhere we cover two of the major eye problems that can develop—macular degeneration (chapter 8) and diabetic retinopathy (chapter 16). In this chapter, we'll discuss three other eye problems you should know about: cataracts, glaucoma, and detached retina.

CATARACTS

A cataract is a gradual clouding of the lens in the eye, which most commonly comes about because of the aging process. The lens in the eye becomes opaque, and vision diminishes over a period of time. If a cataract has developed in one eye, chances are one will develop in the other eye also.

An ophthalmologist can often detect the formation of a cataract even before the person is aware of it. The beginnings of the clouding of the lens will be apparent to the ophthalmologist. The patient may have thought that all that was needed was a stronger pair of glasses, or that his eyes were becoming "tired," or that maybe there was some kind of film over his eyes that drops would clear up.

A cataract cannot be cured or removed by drops or any other medication. If allowed to remain, the cataract will get more and more opaque until virtually all vision will be lost in that eye. And since cataracts often come in pairs, both eyes will be affected.

Cataract removal (yes, this involves surgery) is the one sure way to overcome this problem. Doctors used to say the patient had to wait until the cataract was "ripe" before it could be removed. The cataract was considered ripe when it was totally opaque. This is no longer considered necessary by ophthalmic surgeons. The cataract can be removed whenever it interferes with vision to the extent of causing problems on the job or in every day living. In other words, unless there is a medical emergency, the doctor will let the patient tell him when he is ready to have the cataract removed.

The clouded lens can be removed by one of several methods. (Laser surgery cannot remove cataracts, since lasers burn tissue.) Conventional surgery involves cutting an opening in the cornea with a scalpel, removing the lens, and then stitching up the cornea. Another method uses cryoextraction—applying extreme cold to the lens and freezing it to enable it to be lifted out. Still another technique, phacoemulsification, uses an ultrasound probe emitting high frequency sound waves, which soften and liquefy the lens and allow it to be removed by suction.

The ophthalmologist will discuss with the patient which method of cataract removal he considers to be the best for this particular case. The success rate for cataract removal survey is about 95 percent, that is, 95 percent of those operated on will have their sight restored.

By the time the patient is ready for cataract removal, he'll almost certainly have cataracts in both eyes. The ophthalmologist will suggest that the most advanced cataract be removed first. The reason for this is that, after surgery and until the operated eye heals (which can take several weeks), the patient will have to rely on the untreated eye for vision.

No matter which cataract removal method is used, the hospital stay will be brief. There's no longer any need for long periods of immobility with the patient's head held steady by sandbags placed around it. Instead, the patient will be advised to observe simple precautions as the eyes heals. He will be told not to bend over, not to rub the eye, not to lift anything heavy or strain too much, and not to sleep on the same side as the treated eye. He will also be taught how to apply the eye medication (eye drops) and how to bandage the eye.

While the operated eye is healing, the patient will be using his other eye for vision and will have to get used to this, but it won't be difficult. The doctor will probably advise the patient not to do too much reading, because this involves a lot of eye movement, but watching television will be all right.

Since the surgery involves removal of the lens, the restoration of sight in the treated eye will depend on one of three lens replacement methods: (1) wearing special thick-lensed cataract glasses; (2) wearing a contact lens to replace the missing lens; (3) having a special lens implanted in the eye during the surgery.

Cataract glasses are the oldest of the three methods, also the safest and the least expensive. However, they can be hard to adjust to especially until the second cataract is removed from the other eye.

When the treated eye is healed, the patient is fitted for the cataract glasses—and should expect some difficult moments at first. For one thing, the lens for the untreated eye (the one the patient has been using while the treated eye was healing) will be deliberately blurred. The patient will not be able to see out of this eye while wearing the cataract glasses.

The reason for this is that one of the eyes is missing a lens (the treated eye), which is being replaced by the cataract glasses, while the other untreated eye still has the natural lens in place (a lens somewhat clouded by the second cataract). The cataract glasses will magnify the image in the operated eye about 25 to 30 percent. Also, the lens in the cataract glasses will tend to distort everything. Vertical lines may appear curved and peripheral vision will be extremely limited. The patient will have to learn to look through the center of the thick lens to see anything. It will be similar to tunnel vision.

The untreated eye, on the other hand, will not magnify anything, will not distort vertical lines, and peripheral vision will be as it was before. If the patient tries to look through both eyes at the same time, his brain just won't be able to combine the two images into one. The patient now has a condition known as monocular aphakia, meaning one eye without a lens, and it's for this reason that the cataract glasses are made to blur the vision deliberately for the untreated eye.

When the second cataract operation has been performed and the eye has healed, the patient will then lack lenses in both eyes, and the cataract glasses will allow him to see out of both eyes. The monocular aphakia condition will be gone.

Until then, though, the patient will have to adjust to using the cataract glasses with just one eye (the treated one) functioning. It won't be easy and will require patience, but it can be done.

If the patient chooses to use a contact lens on the operated eye after it heals and it's determined that he can wear a contact lens (some people can't), then he will have no problem with monocular aphakia. The contact lens fits right on the eye; the magnification factor is low; and peripheral vision will be normal. Therefore, the patient will be able to see out of both eyes (treated and untreated) with no difficulty, although he will probably have to wear glasses for reading and close work.

A permanently implanted plastic lens will work even better than a contact lens. The implanted lens, called an intraocular lens, is placed in the eye at the time the cataract is removed. This will be the closest to natural vision possible, and once the eye is healed, the patient should be able to adjust very quickly to this method of seeing. As with a contact lens, ordinary glasses will probably be needed for reading and close work.

Not everyone can adapt to an implanted lens, and not everyone will be able to use one. But for those who do, the benefits are tremendous.

Cataract surgery is quite common today, and if a person has to undergo it, he will find it was well worth it when his vision is no longer clouded and he can see well again.

GLAUCOMA

Glaucoma is an eye condition in which fluid in the eye builds up in pressure, causing eventual blindness if not treated.

The fluid, known as the aqueous humor, is produced in the eye and circulates there to provide nourishment to the eye tissues. If the circulation network should become impaired, as it does in glaucoma, the aqueous humor builds up in the eye, creating pressure inside the eye and on the optic nerve. If the pressure continues unchecked, the optic nerve is gradually destroyed and blindness results.

Glaucoma can be detected during a regular examination by an ophthalmologist. Using a testing method called tonometry, the doctor measures the pressure in the eye. Above normal pressure indicates glaucoma.

Treatment of glaucoma is usually with eye drops or oral medication used both to enlarge the drainage passageway for the fluid and to decrease the production of the fluid, thus reducing the pressure. This medication has to be taken for the rest of the patient's life.

Surgery can also be used to treat glaucoma when the use of eye drops and oral medication fails to keep the pressure down. The surgical procedure creates a passageway for the aqueous humor to flow through.

Marijuana or THC (tetrahydrocannabinol), has also been tried experimentally to treat glaucoma, and good results have been obtained. It is still under study (and illegal, of course, except for special research), and opinion is divided on whether it is more or less effective than the conventional medication.

Glaucoma tends to be hereditary and usually apears after age forty. Chronic glaucoma is the most common type and usually is painless and insidious. Peripheral vision is destroyed so gradually that the individual is not aware of what is happening. By the time vision damage has progressed to where it can be seen, glaucoma has been at work on the optic nerve and normal vision cannot be restored. It's for this reason that regular checks for glaucoma are recommended for everyone from the age of forty on.

A second form of glaucoma, called acute glaucoma, is much more severe than chronic glaucoma. Acute glaucoma comes on suddenly, causing pain in the eye, sharply decreased vision, often nausea and vomiting, and halos appearing around lights.

Acute glaucoma is extremely dangerous. It's considered an emergency condition because if not treated, eyesight can be lost in a few hours. Surgery is the method used to open the blocked passageway and relieve the acute buildup of pressure.

Glaucoma is a leading cause of blindness, but regular eye checks can catch it in time. Keeping one's sight is worth any inconvenience in scheduling visits to the ophthalmologist.

DETACHED RETINA

A detached retina is a serious and dangerous condition. The retina is the lining at the back of the eye, and it contains many blood vessels and the optic nerve. If the retina is detached from the back of the eye, blindness can result.

A detached retina can be caused by scar tissue formed by ruptured blood vessels in the eye in diabetic retinopathy. A more common cause, though, is any sharp blow or shock to the eye—which is why a detached retina can happen to professional boxers. Also, shrinkage of the vitreous humor (fluid) in the back chamber of the eye can allow a pulling away and tearing of the retina. The loose edge of the tear can start a progressive peeling effect.

Symptoms of a detached retina may come on gradually or, in some cases, very suddenly. The first indication will usually be flashes of light or the appearances of moving spots (not the common "floaters" that many people have). This will be followed, days later, by a loss of central vision or a sensation of cloudiness in the eyes.

Retinal detachment is treated surgically, and it can be done on an outpatient basis. In one method, a laser beam (usually argon or xenon) is used to seal the retina to the back of the eye. In another method, cryosurgery is used. A freezing probe accomplishes the reattachment of the retina to the back of the eye.

Retinal detachment is a serious matter, and repairing the damage requires skilled surgical techniques. If any of the symptoms appear following a blow or shock to the eyeball, the individual should see an ophthalmologist immediately. Quick action may save his sight.

Hearing Loss

Close your eyes for a few moments.

Concentrate.

Did you hear the sound of a car driving by? Or the whir of the refrigerator? Is there a radio or television on somewhere? Is there a dog barking?

All these sounds—the pulse of our environment—help keep us tuned into, and in touch with, the world around us. Without them, as the expression goes, the silence would be deafening—or, even worse, frightening.

Almost 20 million Americans have hearing disorders, which the Better Hearing Institute (BHI) in Washington, D.C., calls the "nation's number one handicapping disability."

Hearing loss affects more than our ability to hear the spoken word or the activities around us. The impact of a hearing impairment can be devastating. A world without sound or, at best, with muffled and incomprehensible sounds, becomes an alien and frustrating world. Often, people with hearing impairments will curtail their activities or limit attendance at social events rather than venture out and place themselves in a situation where they will not know or be able to understand what is going on around them. Feelings of loneliness and alienation are common, even among close friends and associates. Hearing difficulties can slice through a person's life, separating him from others and setting him apart from every important aspect of his environment.

The added tragedy here is that, as BHI reports, about 90 percent of people with hearing loss suffer needlessly because help is possible.

Medical or surgical treatment is available and in some instances can help restore a hearing loss. However, when this type of intervention is not possible or beneficial—for example, when the hearing loss has been caused by an irreversible injury or damage to part of the hearing apparatus—excellent results can often be obtained with the use of hearing aids and associated training. This holds true only if there is some residual hearing. If hearing is completely gone and cannot be restored medically or surgically, a hearing aid will not help. However, even for the "profoundly deaf," hearing aids, rehabilitative therapy, and training can be of great benefit.

For most people, hearing loss occurs quite gradually over a period of many years. This gradual change from the ability to hear clearly to hearing mostly muffled or muddled sounds has no clearly delineated threshold to mark the line between understanding and not understanding speech. It doesn't show; it doesn't happen overnight; and it doesn't hurt. Frequently, the last person to realize that there is a hearing problem is the very person who has the problem.

Although the hearing loss itself cannot be seen (it has been called the invisible handicap), the behavior of the person with the hearing loss can provide clues to its existence. One way to uncover the existence of this loss is to ask the individual involved the following questions:

Do you often miss hearing words or phrases?

Do people always seem to be mumbling to you?

Do you have difficulty following conversations in a group setting such as at a party, a family gathering, or a business conference?

Do you prefer the TV turned up louder than the rest of the family?

Do you find it necessary to look at people's faces when they talk to you?

Do you understand what is being said when someone talks to you from a distance?

Do you often ask people to repeat what they have just said?

Do you find yourself frequently accused of not paying attention?

Do you sometimes not hear the ringing of your telephone or the whistling of a teakettle?

If the answers to many of the above questions are yes, it would be a good idea to bring this to the attention of the family physician. He may refer the patient to an otologist (a doctor who specializes in medical-surgical treatment of ear diseases) or to an otolaryngologist (a doctor specializing in diseases of the ear, nose, and throat). The specialist will explore the possibility of medical causes for the hearing problem. A hearing test will probably be included, conducted by an audiologist (a licensed specialist in the testing, rehabilitation, and counseling of people with hearing disorders). The audiologist, through the use of special test sounds and words, will create a graph of the patient's hearing ability, called an audiogram. The audiogram will serve as a valuable tool for understanding the type of hearing loss present and for working out a treatment plan, including what type of hearing aid will probably work best for the particular hearing problem.

CAUSES AND EFFECTS

The human ear is a complex mechanism that converts air movements into neural impulses that the brain then perceives as sound. There are three stages to this conversion process, corresponding to the three parts of the ear: the outer ear, the middle ear, and the inner ear.

The outer ear is the most familiar, since it's the part we can see and touch—to a certain extent. The fleshy part of the ear collects and channels sound waves, which are simply movements of the air caused by a sound-producing stimulus—the ringing of a telephone, for example. The sound waves are channeled into the auditory canal and travel the short distance to the eardrum, which is a tightly stretched membrane across the end of the auditory canal.

The eardrum begins to vibrate in resonance with the sound waves, and these vibrations are transmitted to three small bones linked together in the middle ear. (Most people will remember from their high school biology class that these bones are commonly called the hammer, the anvil, and the stirrup because of their shapes). The three bones vibrate and move back and forth with the motions of the eardrum, reducing the movements of the eardrum into shorter and more forceful motions and, in a sense, giving the original sound wave a boost in energy.

The final bone, the stirrup, in connected through what is called an oval window to the inner ear. Here, in the inner ear, is the fluid-filled cochlea, a delicate structure that coils around itself in a spiral, somewhat resembling a snail's shell. Inside this spiral are thousands of tiny nerve cells with microscopic hairs immersed in the inner ear fluid.

The movement of the stirrup bone causes the fluid in the inner ear to move back and forth across the hair cells in an exact reproduction of the sound waves that first struck the eardrum. This movement of the fluid stimulates the hair cells, generating neural impulses that travel along the auditory nerve to the brain. In the brain, the neural impulses are perceived as sound. The process is now complete, and we "hear" the sound of the telephone ringing.

Hearing difficulties can result from problems at any point along the path that the sound waves or neural impulses travel. When there are blockages or an injury to the outer or middle ear, the result is what is known as a conductive hearing loss.

Wax buildup in the auditory canal, a ruptured eardrum, or other blockages can muffle sounds. Recurring middle ear infections can also cause a conductive hearing loss. Medical attention, with the help of a hearing aid, if necessary, can usually restore normal hearing.

An impairment either in the tiny hair cell nerve endings in the inner ear or in the transmission of impulses along the auditory nerve results in what is called a sensorineural loss. Prolonged exposure to loud noises, infections caused by viruses or bacteria, strokes, or reactions to certain drugs or medications can damage the nerve cells, resulting in a hearing loss.

In addition, as we grow older, deterioration of the hair cell nerve endings seems to take place. This is known medically as presbycusis, which refers to changes in hearing associated with aging. Certain sounds are poorly transmitted, and other sounds may not be transmitted at all. The hearing loss over the years is gradual and progressive. By the time an individual is in his sixties or seventies, the hearing loss can amount to as much as 25 percent.

Elderly people on home care may find that their hearing will grow less acute as time goes by. This development probably will have nothing to do with the original ailment that caused them to require home health care. More than likely, the hearing changes will have been caused simply by aging.

This doesn't happen with all elderly people, of course, but it is frequent enough to require that both the caregiver and the one receiving care at home should be familiar with hearing loss and what can be done about it.

According to Dr. Ralph Rupp, professor of education and audiology at the University of Michigan, writing with Ada Z. Heavenrich, M.A., in the journal *Hearing Instruments,* (Vol. 33, No. 9, 1982), "Over 95 percent of adult hearing impairments fall in the category of irreversible hearing loss, i.e., not amenable to medical or surgical intervention." This does not mean that the individual who develops a hearing impairment will go deaf or that nothing can be done about the hearing loss. Rehabilitative services are available.

As Dr. Rupp states: "Most hearing-impaired persons can be helped to listen more effectively." If you have a hearing loss, you can compensate for this not only with a hearing aid, if feasible, but also be learning how to listen to what is being said to you or to what is going on around you.

The benefits from using proper rehabilitative measures in a hearing loss are many. First, the patient will obtain an improved understanding of what has happened and what effect it can have on his hearing. Next, if he is a good candidate for a hearing aid, he will learn how to make the most effective use of this device and how to keep it in good working order. He will also learn what its limitations are so he won't expect too much from the hearing aid when using it in certain environments.

Good rehabilitation and training will help the patient to differentiate among various types of sound and to distinguish words and phrases as they are spoken. The patient will learn how to use the speaker's lip movements, facial gestures, and body movements to enhance his listening ability.

Listening efficiently will extend the "auditory reach," a term Rupp and Heavenrich define as "the degree of effectiveness by which a person maintains communicative interaction."

If, as the caregiver, you are dealing with someone who has developed a hearing loss, there are certain guidelines you can follow to ease the task of making yourself understood and establishing good communications with the person in your care:

> When speaking to a hearing-impaired person, try to speak from a distance of about three to six feet. This will provide a good visual contact between the two of you.
>
> Speak slowly, allowing time for the hearing-impaired person to process what you have said, aurally and visually. If he has missed any words, your facial expression or the movement of your lips may clue him in to what you have said.
>
> Speak in a tone slightly louder than normal. This amplification of your voice may help get certain words and phrases through. However, if you speak too loudly, or shout, you may only distort your message.
>
> Do not overarticulate. Speak clearly, but do not exaggerate your lip movements as this will only distort the visual clues you are trying to give.
>
> Do not attempt to speak directly into the listener's ear. It may not help, and you will be removing any opportunity for the listener to look for visual clues.
>
> Don't talk with your mouth full. Avoid chewing, eating, drinking, or talking with a cigarette or anything else in your mouth. Also, do not cover your mouth with your hand or any other object. Your face must be in full view of the listener at all times, and your lip and mouth movements must be related only to what you are saying.
>
> Try to speak in an environment where there are no background noises, such as a TV or stereo. A hearing-impaired person will have enough difficulty concentrating on what you are saying without being distracted and confused by other sounds going on in the background.

HEARING VS. UNDERSTANDING

In most cases, a sensorineural hearing loss cannot be cured medically or surgically. However, the audiologist's examination will help to pinpoint the exact nature of the hearing loss and to identify the proper treatment. With treatment, there can be a significant improvement in function.

The audiologist may try fitting the individual with a hearing aid to determine whether amplifying the sound to a higher level will help the individual to understand better what is being heard. For some people, a hearing aid helps; for others, it doesn't.

Whether the individual is fitted with a hearing aid or not, the audiologist will work with him to improve functional hearing.

A hearing test by a trained audiologist measures the ability to hear pure tones in an absolutely quiet environment. Under these ideal conditions, the level at which the individual first hears low-, medium-, and high-pitched sounds can be identified and plotted on a chart called an audiogram. Although this test will reveal the hearing level of an individual, it will be the hearing level of that individual in a laboratory situation and is not indicative of the hearing level outside the laboratory in a normal listening situation.

To calculate a person's ability to understand the spoken word further, the audiologist uses a speech discrimination test. By asking the individual to repeat single words spoken at a comfortable sound level in a quiet room, a measure of the ability to understand speech is established.

The sounds of speech have varying frequencies. Most vowel sounds are lower-pitched sounds; many consonant sounds—for example, "s" and "sh"—are high-pitched sounds. Linking speech sounds into words results in the mixture of many frequencies.

The speech discrimination test can provide a more functional look at the person's ability to put his level of hearing to work effectively. In this test, the individual's ability to differentiate between a "th" sound and a "d" sound can be accurately measured. A variable ability to understand the spoken words of speech may become apparent. Some high-pitched sounds may not be heard, and many of the speech sounds may lack clarity. This type of difficulty will affect the hearing-impaired person's ability to function.

The speech discrimination test helps the audiologist identify which sounds are missed, and he can measure the percentage of spoken words that are misunderstood. This listening test can also be used to measure the improved listening benefits of using different hearing aids in a quiet room. The improvement in function serves as one of the key criteria to determine whether or not a hearing aid will help and, if so, which aid will help the most.

SELECTING A HEARING AID: CAN ONE REALLY HELP?

Because hearing aids work like miniature sound systems (with microphone and speaker components), hearing aid design and capabilities have improved dramatically with the recent advances in electronics and miniaturization. Hearing aids are available in all shapes and sizes, including a tiny "all-in-the-ear" model. Once the doctor and the audiologist have confirmed that a hearing loss cannot be medically or surgically corrected, the benefits of using a hearing aid are usually explored.

Since improved function is the goal, it is important that the individual work closely with the audiologist to test out a selection of hearing aids to determine not only whether an aid will help, but also which one will do the job most efficiently. Manufacturers make a wide variety of hearing aids, and each model is different.

After narrowing the choices to two or three hearing aids that have produced an improved functional hearing, the ultimate choice then rests with the individual to select the one that "sounds" best to him. Most audiologists and certified hearing aid dealers (often called dispensers) will encourage a thirty-day trial period for the hearing aid. For many people, this is a time of adjustment to see how well the hearing aid works in everyday life. Basically, all a hearing aid does is to amplify sound and direct it into the auditory canal. The proper level of amplification can aid in hearing better without distortion. However, there is another aspect of this amplification that must be considered. Many sounds and noises that were not previously heard must now be tolerated, since a system that increases the sound level for speech will also increase the level of other environmental noises as well.

Everyday conversations often take place under less than ideal conditions. Background noises of every sort further confuse and distort conversation. Automobiles, trains, and airplanes operate with a great deal of related noise, which often makes conversation difficult in busy travel areas. Conversations can take place in a doctor's waiting room or in an office or in a restaurant—locations that are not always quiet. Even in a living room at home, where one would expect some quiet to prevail, the telephone may be ringing, other people may be talking, and the ever-present television set may be on. It's understandable to find that situations such as these result in higher anxiety and lower hearing function for the hearing-impaired person.

According to Dr. Rupp, unwanted sounds or "noise" are the leading deterrents to effective listening for the hearing-impaired. To further help hearing aid users in problem listening environments, there are commercially available devices that can serve either as an alternative or a supplement to a hearing aid. These devices help the listener by reducing outside noises and creating a "closed circuit transmission" between the speaker and the listener. In effect, these special devices help deliver the sound directly from the mouth of the speaker to the ear of the listener.

By using other special equipment, it is possible to lower the unwanted noise level and improve the speech signal in such hard-to-hear places as automobiles, churches, lecture halls, theaters, and other public gathering places. Telephones can be equipped with devices to raise the sound volume. There are also special devices to allow the hearing-impaired person to plug directly into the television or radio, allowing him to hear at the required amplified level through special earphones, while the sound level in the room will be at a normal level for others watching the TV or listening to the radio.

Many physicians, audiologists, and other health care professionals are suggesting use of these and similar devices to their hearing-impaired patients. When the devices are designed to aid one-to-one conversation, the result has been better communication between the patient and the health professional—and between the individual and others in his environment.

16

Diabetes

ABOUT 11 million people in the United States have diabetes, and it has been estimated that half of them are unaware they have the disease. Diabetes is the leading cause of death by disease, and long-term diabetics are especially at risk for heart attack, stroke, eye problems leading to blindness, nervous system disorders, and kidney disease—health problems that often lead to the need for intensive home health care.

This is not as forbidding a picture as would appear at first sight. Although there is no cure at present for diabetes, if it is properly diagnosed and a sensible treatment program followed, diabetes can be controlled to a great extent and diabetics can live active and close to normal lives.

Diabetes is a chronic metabolic disease in which insulin, a hormone normally produced in the pancreas, is either not produced at all or, if produced, is not used effectively by the body. Insulin is essential in aiding the body to extract energy from glucose, a natural sugar created by the breakdown of carbohydrates (sugars and starches) in the digestive system. Glucose provides energy needed by body cells; without insulin to regulate and control it, glucose cannot be used effectively by the cells and an excess of glucose builds up in the blood and accumulates in the urine.

It's this excess of glucose, this high blood sugar level known as hyperglycemia, that causes the damage wrought by diabetes.

There are two main types of diabetes: insulin-dependent diabetes (type I); and non-insulin-dependent diabetes (type II). Previously, type I diabetes was referred to as juvenile diabetes (and still is in many cases) because most of its victims become diabetic as children. However, no matter what the age of the person, if the diabetic is insulin-dependent—meaning the body does not supply the required insulin—the disease is called type I diabetes. Type I diabetics must take insulin injections daily in order to survive.

Type II has also been called adult-onset diabetes because it generally strikes later in life, but the deciding factor here is that the body supplies natural insulin and the individual is not dependent on insulin prepared by drug manufacturers. Type II diabetics usually can control their diabetes by diet, exercise, and oral medication.

About 5 to 10 percent of all diabetics are type I; 90 to 95 percent are type II. Additionally, about 80 percent of type II diabetics are obese. For either type, symptoms that should alert the individual to the possibility of diabetes are frequent urination, excessive thirst, genital itching, and slow healing of cuts or other wounds. A physician, with one or more simple tests, can confirm the presence of diabetes.

Treatment

Treatment of diabetes breaks down into three major categories: diet, exercise, and medication. All three of these should be part of the treatment program to ensure the most effective utilization of the benefits of each method.

DIET

Volumes have been written on the best type of diet, or diets, for diabetics. We'll cover just some essentials here.

An effective diet for diabetics follows the general rules of good nutrition: avoid fattening, high-calorie foods with high sugar content; eat foods low in fat and high in carbohydrates and fiber; and for protein stick to lean meats, poultry, and fish. This will enable the diabetic to keep weight within normal limits while still obtaining necessary nutrition.

Together, the diabetic and the physician can work out a diet that will provide the required nutritional benefits while also avoiding foods dangerous to those with diabetes.

For more severe cases of diabetes, stricter dietary control will be required, and the size of food portions will be very important here. To simplify the procedure, an "exchange list" has been prepared by the American Diabetes Association and the American Dietetic Association. The list allows the individual to exchange a specified portion of one type of food for another, as long as the various food types indicated for each meal are not changed. With this list, obtainable in many books or directly from those organizations, the individual can select from a great variety of foods.

The daily diet is made up of selections from fruit, bread, vegetable, meat, fat, and milk exchanges. The quantity of each exchange (usually one, one and a half, or two exchanges) is listed on the diet for each meal. The individual can select, say, any two fruit exchanges, two bread exchanges, two meat exchanges, two fat exchanges, and one milk exchange to make up the breakfast for a 1,500-calorie diet. Translated into food portions, this will provide the following breakfast: a cup of orange juice, two slices of whole wheat bread, one teaspoon of polyunsaturated margarine, one egg, one slice of crisp bacon, and one cup of skim milk or black coffee with no sugar.

Many variations can be worked out for each meal, and meals can be planned in advance, depending on what is in the refrigerator or what foods are going to be purchased later on. Of course, if an individual's diet has restrictions on cholesterol or other substances or food products, the diet can be adapted to whatever has to be avoided or restricted.

It's of great importance, especially when taking insulin, that the proper amounts of food be eaten at specified times during the day. The type I diabetic, who is insulin-dependent, has to match the consumption of food to the dosage of insulin to avoid insulin shock or the possibility of diabetic coma (explained later). Sometimes breaking up the day's food intake into several small meals, or arranging snacks between meals, ensures that the proper amount of food is eaten.

The type II diabetic, who is non-insulin-dependent, also has to follow the diet plan with great care. The physician, when prescribing oral medication, balances the effects of this medication against the amount and type of food to be eaten. Deviations from the planned diet can cause trouble.

Using the exchange lists along with some common sense should allow the diabetic the opportunity to eat well while still sticking to the dietary requirements of the disease.

EXERCISE

Exercise is not just for the hale and hearty who want to "stay in shape." As explained in Chapter 8, a program of regular exercise is important no matter what your age or condition. As long as some parts of your body can move, you need to exercise.

For the diabetic, exercise provides the added benefits of increasing the use of glucose by the body, thus cutting down on excess glucose in the blood, which is the goal of diabetes control. Also, exercise helps keep weight down (obesity has a direct relationship to type II diabetes), while at the same time helping to maintain good muscle tone and an overall feeling of well-being.

One precautionary note: Diabetics have to be careful to regulate their exercise. Unplanned, strenuous exercise can cause the body to use up too much glucose, and this can bring on a low blood sugar (hypoglycemic) reaction. (The effects of this reaction and the effects of too much glucose—hyperglycemia—are explained later.)

The medication for type I diabetics is insulin, which has to be taken daily. Insulin has to be injected because if taken orally the digestive system would destroy the insulin before it could have any effect.

Several types and strengths of insulin are available. Insulin is usually made from the pancreas glands of cattle or hogs and is labeled either pork or beef insulin, or pork and beef combined. Purified versions of these insulin types are available for those individuals who may be sensitive to either type. Human (recombinant DNA origin) insulin is also available, but the majority of insulin now on the market is of the pork or beef variety.

In addition to source, insulin is also rated as to speed and duration of action. Rapid-acting, intermediate-acting, and long-acting insulin may be obtained, depending on which the prescribing physician considers most appropriate for the patient. Each type of insulin has a different time (in hours) of onset of action after injection, of peak action, and of duration of action. Thus, the physician can match the type and action time of insulin to the needs of the patient.

The strength of the insulin is another factor the physician will consider. Insulin strength is measured in units of insulin per milliliter (ml) or cubic centimeter (cc) of solution. U-40 insulin has 40 units per cc, and U-100 has 100 units per cc.

The syringe used for injection of the insulin has to match the strength of the insulin being used. For example, a U-100 syringe must be used with U-100 insulin. If a U-40 syringe is used with U-100 insulin (or the other way around), the markings on the syringe will not correspond to the strength of the insulin being used and the wrong dosage may be injected. These syringes are usually made of plastic with disposable needles, although glass syringes and reusable needles are also available. The latter have to be thoroughly cleaned after each use to maintain sterility and avoid infection.

Insulin is injected subcutaneously—under the skin. The procedure for performing this injection is not complicated and can be quickly learned. Since giving an insulin injection is an important part of home health care—whether done by the patient himself or by the caregiver— the physician or the nurse will usually go through the procedure with both the patient and the caregiver until they can perform it without assistance or supervision. The steps on pages 348–349 will give you a general idea of what's required. However, *do not attempt this procedure on your own before consulting with your physician or nurse.*

1) Wash your hands. The need to do this should be obvious. Injections of any kind require cleanliness and sterility.

To avoid damage to skin and tissues, the injection site is changed each time. This is done by marking off imaginary sections on the parts of the body where the injections will be made (the front of the thighs, for example) and rotating the injection sites. If desired, a chart can be drawn with the sections marked and a record kept of the location of each injection. Your physician or nurse will help you set this up and will show you other injection sites—upper arms, flanks, and upper buttocks.

2) Mix the insulin in the bottle. Do not shake it. Roll it gently in the palms of your hands.

3) Remove the protective cap from the bottle, but do *not* remove the rubber stopper. (You would have to pry up the metal ring to do this.)

4)Wipe the top of the bottle with an alcohol swab. (Sterility and cleanliness again.)

5) Hold the disposable plastic syringe in one hand (your left hand if you're righthanded) and grasp the end of the plunger with your other hand. Remove the protective plunger cap. Do *not* remove the needle cover at this time.

6) Pull back on the plunger, draw air into the syringe equal to the amount of your insulin dose, and leave the plunger in that position. For example, if the dosage is 35 units, pull the plunger back until the edge stops on the 35 mark.

7) Remove the needle cover. Holding the bottle on a table top with one hand, hold the barrel of the syringe with the other hand and place the syringe in a vertical position with the needle tip directly above the center of the rubber cap on the bottle.

8) Gently but firmly push the needle through the rubber cap and into the insulin.

9) Holding the barrel of the syringe between the thumb and last three fingers of your hand, push the plunger down all the way with the tip of your index finger, injecting the previously drawn-up volume of air into the insulin. This amount of air inside the bottle will make it easier to withdraw the insulin into the syringe.

10) Lift the insulin bottle and the syringe as a unit from the table top and turn them upside down. Hold the insulin bottle between the sides of the index and middle fingers of one hand and clasp the barrel of the syringe with the tips of the thumb and ring and little fingers of the same hand, leaving your other hand free.

11) Using your free hand, slowly pull the plunger down, drawing insulin into the syringe until the edge of the plunger reaches the correct dosage mark.

12) Still holding the insulin bottle and the syringe, check the syringe for air bubbles in the insulin. The presence of air is harmless, but a large air bubble will reduce the dosage. If you see air bubbles, push the plunger in, inject the insulin back into the bottle, and withdraw the dose again.

13) Check again to make sure the dose is correct and remove the needle from the bottle.

14) Hold the syringe up and gently flick the barrel with a fingernail. This will serve to eliminate any air bubbles you may have missed.

15) Push the plunger in just a bit to see if insulin will spurt out of the end of the needle. (If you wish, you can draw just a bit more insulin into the syringe than the required dose in step 11 to allow for this test.)

16) Lay the syringe down so that the needle will not touch anything.

17) Using an alcohol swab, clean off the area of skin where you are going to make the injection.

18) With one hand, pinch the skin and pull up a large area of skin and hold it.

19) Hold the syringe with the other hand as you would hold a pencil and insert the needle into the pinched-up skin. Insert it at a right angle and push it in all the way. Do not jab the needle. A steady insertion push will be sufficient.

20) After inserting the needle, pull back on the plunger and check for blood to ensure that the needle has not pierced a blood vessel. If blood appears after drawing back the plunger, do not complete the injection. Pull the needle straight out and discard the needle and syringe and insulin. Repeat steps 2 through 19 with a fresh syringe and needle. If there is no blood this time, inject the insulin by pushing the plunger all the way in, injecting the insulin in one smooth motion that should take no more than five seconds.

21) Hold an alcohol swab near the needle and pull the needle straight out. Press the alcohol swab over the injection site for a few seconds, then discard it.

22) Bend the tip of the needle so it cannot be used again and destroy the syringe and needle before disposing of them.

ORAL HYPOGLYCEMICS

In type II diabetes, insulin injections are usually not required, except in special circumstances, and the medications normally prescribed are known as an oral hypoglycemics. There are four types of pill medication from which the physician can select the one most appropriate for the patient. There four types are Orinase (Tolbutamide), Diabinese (Chlorpropamide), Tolinase (Tolazamide), and Dymelor (Acetohexamide). The purpose of all hypoglycemics is the same: to stimulate the secretion of insulin in cases of moderately severe adult-onset diabetes. Their possible side effects are itching, skin rash, hives, indigestion, nausea, diarrhea, and headache. If taken in excessive doses, low blood sugar (hypoglycemia) may result.

Oral hypoglycemics are not prescribed as a substitute for insulin. The pancreas of the diabetic individual does produce insulin, but it usually isn't sufficient to do the full job of regulating the body's glucose use. The action of these medications improves or supplements the natural action of whatever insulin is produced by the body.

As with insulin, it's important that the patient follow the prescribed diet and also perform the exercises worked out by the doctor or nurse. The medication may be different, and most people are happy not to have to deal with a daily injection, but the effects of ignoring any aspect of the full treatment program can be just as damaging as with insulin use.

THE INSULIN PUMP

A fairly recent development in the treatment of type I diabetes has been the use of the insulin infusion pump. The pump is a portable device (usually worn at the waist) that delivers insulin at a predetermined rate into a needle inserted beneath the skin in the patient's abdomen a short distance from where the pump is located.

The pump delivers insulin at what is known as the basal rate, which is the constant amount of insulin required by the patient when not eating. The basal rate is usually one pulse of insulin every eight minutes, although the pump can deliver much more than this.

Before eating, the patient adjusts the pump to deliver an increased dose of insulin to provide the additional insulin that will be needed after eating. Some pumps will automatically reset to the basal rate after this extra dose; others have to be reset manually.

The capability of the pump to provide this additional insulin on demand allows the individual greater freedom in eating a meal when desired. Without the pump, the diabetic individual has to eat meals and snacks at certain times of day so as to maintain the balance of insulin injected earlier with the food being consumed in set quantities at set times.

The insulin pump is not a miracle device, nor does it relieve the individual of responsibility for maintaining proper control of the diabetes. In fact, it adds to the regimen the diabetic must follow. Blood glucose levels have to be measured frequently to make sure the proper dosage of insulin is being maintained. There is the constant danger of getting too much insulin into the body, leading to a hypoglycemic reaction, which can be quite dangerous.

The pump cannot be worn while showering, swimming, or playing contact sports. Also, it can be quite uncomfortable to wear during sleep. Many individuals, however, are willing to put up with these difficulties for the freedom afforded by use of the pump. This is especially true for those who have problems maintaining steady control of their blood glucose levels.

The pump, although in present use, is still being perfected. Research is continuing, and future pumps will probably be smaller and present fewer problems than those now in use.

Dangerous Reactions

There are two very dangerous reactions to too much or too little insulin in the body: insulin shock and diabetic coma.

INSULIN SHOCK

Too much insulin leads to what is known as insulin shock or insulin reaction, or, to give it its medical terminology, hypoglycemia, that is, too little sugar in the blood. This condition can have a number of causes. An overdose of insulin could have been taken, upsetting the balance of insulin and glucose. A meal may have been skipped or too little food eaten during the meal, reducing the amount of sugar ingested. Or unplanned, vigorous exercise may have been indulged in, resulting in using up extra glucose.

Whatever the reason, there is now not enough sugar in the blood, and the patient is hypoglycemic. Insulin shock can follow, and the onset can be sudden and sometimes without warning. Symptoms of insulin shock are:

cool, pale, moist skin	tremors	headache
dizziness	mental confusion	belligerent behavior
rapid pulse	extreme hunger (sometimes)	nausea

If not treated, insulin shock can lead to convulsive seizures and loss of consciousness. Treatment requires getting some sugar into the system as soon as possible. If the individual can swallow, give him or her sweetened orange juice, several small hard candies, or sugar cubes in water. Do not force food or liquids on an unconscious person. Call for an ambulance.

Many diabetics carry sugar or candy with them at all times in case of sudden insulin shock. Be prepared to recognize the symptoms and to act quickly and appropriately should such an emergency develop.

Too little insulin leads to too much sugar in the blood. This condition is known as hyperglycemia and can result in a diabetic coma. An excess of sugar can be caused by failure to take insulin when required; illness or infection; eating too many sweets; or severe stress, such as undergoing surgery, sustaining injury in an accident, or experiencing great emotional upheaval.

Unlike insulin shock, hyperglycemia comes on slowly over a long period of time, and there usually is sufficient warning. For this reason, diabetic coma is not nearly as common or as frequent as insulin shock. Symptoms of hyperglycemia are:

dry, hot skin, sometimes red	stomach cramps
tiredness and lethargy	nausea and vomiting
dizziness	deep, labored breathing
blurred vision	breath smells "fruity" (acetone)
excessive urination	acetone (ketone bodies) in the
excessive thirst	urine

Since hyperglycemia is an excess of sugar in the blood, which is one of the main symptoms of diabetes, you can see the similarity here to symptoms displayed by a diabetic individual. Bear in mind, though, that the above symptoms—especially the last five—represent what happens when hyperglycemia goes untreated.

Loss of consciousness—a diabetic coma—is the end result of not treating the excess of sugar (or the lack of insulin) in the individual. If this happens, immediate medical attention is needed.

Complications of Diabetes

The course of diabetes in an individual, even with treatment and control of blood sugar, can eventually lead to complications involving the blood vessels, the eyes, the kidneys, the feet, the nervous system, and the heart. It's important for both the diabetic being cared for at home and the caregiver to be aware of these possible complications. All of them are serious, but let's start with the one that most people seem to fear most—the possible loss of vision.

Perhaps the most devastating long-term complication of diabetes is diabetic retinopathy, a disease of the small blood vessels in the retina of the eye and a leading cause of blindness in adults in this country. The longer a person has diabetes, the more likely it is that diabetic retinopathy will develop. After ten years, 50 percent of those diagnosed as diabetic will show some indications of retinopathy. The figure rises to 85 percent for those who have had diabetes for twenty years.

Diabetes damages the retinal capillaries, the extremely fine blood vessels that supply nourishment to the retina, the light-sensitive lining at the back of the eye that contains millions of nerve cells, many small blood vessels, and the optic nerve. Tiny bulges (microaneurysms) develop in the capillary walls, swell outward, and begin to leak fluid and particles of fatty material called exudates into the retina. This is known as background retinopathy, and the fluid leakage can cause blurring of vision if the central portion of the retina—the macula—is affected. However, about 80 percent of people with background retinopathy do not have serious vision problems, and the disease never gets beyond this initial stage.

If, however, the disease progresses, as it does in a small number of cases, it can lead to what is known as proliferative retinopathy. In a process called neovascularization, new blood vessels begin to grow out from the surface of the retina, extending into the vitreous humor, the clear gel that fills the inside of the eye. These new vessels are abnormal and weak and can rupture and cause blood to flow into the vitreous humor, clouding it and obstructing vision because light cannot get through to the retina. Additionally, scar tissue may form near the retina. Contraction of this scar tissue can pull the retina inward, detaching it from the back of the eye. If proliferative retinopathy progresses to the extreme, it can lead to severe loss of vision and possibly permanent blindness. However, total blindness is relatively rare; severe visual loss from retinopathy affects about 3 percent of diabetics.

Diabetic retinopathy can be detected and diagnosed by an examination usually conducted by an ophthalmologist, a doctor who specializes in treating disorders of the eye, or by a retinal specialist. The doctor will use an instrument called an ophthalmoscope to look into the eye and study the retina for the tiny microaneuryisms that indicate background retinopathy.

If this examination is not conclusive, further checks for retinopathy can be made by a procedure known as fluorescein angiography. A special dye is injected into the patient's arm. As the dye moves through the circulatory system and into the blood vessels of the eye, a camera is used to take a series of photographs of the back of the eye. When the film is developed, the pictures show whether any of the dye is leaking out into the retina, indicating the presence of retinopathy.

Treatment of diabetic retinopathy usually involves photocoagulation—using laser beams to seal off the hemorrhaging blood vessels. The laser beam is focused on various spots on the retina and a series of "burns" (in the hundreds and sometimes over a thousand) are made. The heat from the laser coagulates, or "welds," the leaking blood vessels, stopping the flow of blood, fluid, and exudates.

Studies have shown that photocoagulation can reduce the possibility of severe visual loss by about 60 percent in individuals with advanced retinopathy. Additional studies are now being conducted to determine whether this type of laser treatment can be effective in keeping background retinopathy from progressing to the proliferative stage.

Photocoagulation may not be an appropriate procedure for all individuals with retinopathy. When there has been extensive bleeding inside the eye, the doctor cannot see the retina and thus be able to focus the laser beam. The same holds true if a cataract has formed in the lens of the eye, obscuring the retina.

Cataracts can be removed, of course, and there is also a surgical procedure called a vitrectomy for removing the bloody vitreous humor and replacing it with a clear substitute fluid. In some cases, a vitrectomy will restore some useful vision to the individual, but there are risks involved with this surgery that may make it unsuitable for certain people. The decision will have to be made by the eye surgeon and the patient after due consideration of all factors involved.

Another aspect of photocoagulation that may keep it from being used on many patients is that the treatment with laser beams can cause a loss of some central and peripheral vision. If there has already been a severe visual loss because of damage done by the retinopathy, it may not be productive to add to this loss by the extensive use of lasers. This is another situation in which potential risks and benefits have to be weighed against each other before a decision can be made.

There is presently no known way of preventing diabetic retinopathy, nor of curing it, although its progress may be retarded by the methods explained. Experts presently disagree as to the extent that good diabetes management and very tight control of blood glucose levels can be effective in combatting diabetic retinopathy. Answers are still being sought.

KIDNEY PROBLEMS

The kidneys are two small bean-shaped organs, about four and a half inches long and two and a half inches wide, located in the lower back, that filter the blood, regulate the blood pressure, maintain the body's acid–base balance, regulate the sodium–water balance, and excrete waste matter in the urine. Each kidney contains over a million microscopic filtering units and many millions of capillaries. The kidney can filter a quart of blood a minute. It is one of the most remarkable and hardest-working organs in the body.

Unfortunately, the kidneys can be severely damaged by diabetes. As with retinopathy, diabetes attacks the small blood vessels, the capillaries, in the kidneys. Since the capillaries play such an important part in all the functions of the kidney, damage to these tiny blood vessels invariably leads to severe kidney problems.

The small blood vessels of the kidneys, when damaged, can leak protein into the urine (proteinuria), which can lead to hypertension and eventual kidney failure. The changes brought about in the capillaries can result in a hardening of the kidney (nephrosclerosis), inflammation of the kidney, and a host of other disorders that can cause the kidneys to fail.

Treatment of kidney disorders can involve dialysis, when the damage is severe, or a kidney transplant. Both of these methods have been in use for a long time, and there has been much success with them, especially with kidney transplants. Dialysis is, in a sense, a temporary, holding action. A machine takes over the kidney function of cleaning the blood and eliminating waste, but the procedure is tiring and emotionally and physically exhausting to many patients.

As with retinopathy, there is presently no way known to stop the damage done to the blood vessels in the kidneys. For now, good control of blood glucose levels has to be the only answer.

DIABETIC NEUROPATHY

In addition to affecting the blood vessels, diabetes attacks the nervous system, the diabetes causing a demyelination of the peripheral nerves. Normally, the myelin sheath around the nerves insulates the nerves and aids in conducting nerve impulses and signals. Damage to the nerves in the lower extremities causes a tingling sensation in the feet (peripheral neuropathy), which later can increase to the point where the diabetic's feet "feel like stumps." There is hardly any sensation, and walking and moving about becomes extremely difficult.

Nerve damage can also extend to the autonomic nervous system, the "caretaker" of the body and its organs. Involvement of the autonomic nervous system can lead to double vision, nocturnal diarrhea, male impotence, and orthostatic hypotension (a sudden drop in blood pressure that causes dizziness and fainting when rising to a standing position).

Diabetic neuropathy can also affect the hands, causing the same sensations in the hands and fingers as in the feet. In severe cases of diabetic neuropathy, the individual has great difficulty and much pain in moving about and in using the hands.

There is no cure for this form of neuropathy and very little treatment that can be offered, except the use of analgesics such as aspirin.

FOOT PROBLEMS

One of the consequences of diabetic damage to the small blood vessels in the body is the development of impaired circulation in the feet. Poor circulation, coupled with peripheral nerve damage, can bring on a loss of sensation in the feet. Cuts or blisters may develop, and the person will not be aware of them.

The diabetic has to give special care to the feet. If a cut occurs and is not noticed or treated, infection can set in. Moreover, because of the impaired circulation, there will not be the normal blood flow to help heal the wound. Gangrene can develop, resulting in the unavoidable amputation of toes or in the entire foot, and often part of the leg.

The diabetic should check her feet every day, looking for cracks, cuts, blisters, calluses, and bruises. If, as is the case with some diabetics, there is poor vision, regular visits to a podiatrist will be necessary. Even with good vision, it's wise to use the services of a podiatrist. He can keep a careful check on the condition of the patient's feet and take corrective action when needed.

For the diabetic, it's important that the feet be kept clean and the skin smooth and well tended. It has been said that a diabetic should spend as much time and care on her feet as she would on her face. Wash the feet with soap and warm water, pat dry, then use oils, creams, or lotions as necessary to ensure that the skin does not dry out or crack.

Toenails should be kept trimmed. If vision is good, the patient may do this herself. If not, the podiatrist should perform the task. Nails have to be cut straight across, not too short, and with the corners left intact. Some people want to cut into the corners of the nails in an attempt to shape them like fingernails. This must not be done under any circumstances.

Proper shoes are also important. If necessary, style will have to be sacrificed to good fit and solid support. Even a small amount of walking in a poorly fitted shoe can result in calluses, corns, or bunions, all of which are unhealthy for a diabetic. Furthermore, where calluses and corns are concerned, no attempt should be made to cut them or to use foot medications on them. If the condition becomes serious or painful, consult your physician or podiatrist.

Taking good care of the feet is a must for all diabetics.

Diabetic Testing at Home

Diabetics soon get used to testing for blood sugar at home. It's a necessary part of dealing with the disease, and it's the only way to keep a careful check on your own condition.

Urine testing is the simplest and oldest method used for home testing. Various urine-testing kits are available, with different techniques involved. The individual takes a sample of his or her urine at various times of the day and tests for the presence of sugar and its concentration, usually by dipping a test stick (a piece of chemically impregnated heavy paper) into a few drops of urine (diluted with a certain amount of water) and comparing the color change on the paper with a chart supplied with the kit. Matching the colors gives the concentration of sugar in the urine. Other test kits employ tablets that are dropped into the urine, but the goal is the same—to determine the percentage of blood sugar in the urine.

Careful and consistent records have to be kept so both the patient and the physician can chart progress and keep informed on the effectiveness of the treatment plan.

Urine testing can be very useful and, in fact, is the one way to check for the presence of ketone bodies, which indicates a potential diabetic coma. However, sugar in the urine does not indicate the exact blood glucose concentration at the moment of taking the test. The urine has been collecting in the body for some time, and the blood glucose content may have changed in the meantime.

A much more effective way of determining blood glucose concentration is testing the blood itself, as when a laboratory test is performed. Now, however, the test can be performed at home with near-laboratory accuracy. State-of-the-art devices are available that will allow the patient to take a drop of blood from the tip of his finger, place the blood on a test strip, and insert the strip in the device, which then gives a digital readout of the blood glucose content.

Less elaborate devices are also available, some using the color comparison method, and these can be equally effective.

The main advantage of home testing of blood glucose—called self blood glucose monitoring (SBGM)—is that the percentage of glucose in the blood can be determined at any desired moment and the insulin dosage changed on the spot as required. Of course, the patient doesn't set all this up on his own. SBGM is done in cooperation with the physician, who will instruct the patient in the proper response, if any is needed, to the various readings obtained.

Use of the SBGM method allows "tight" control of the diabetes. A well-motivated patient—one willing and able to maintain the self-discipline needed—will be able to check his blood sugar at various times and see for himself just how it changes with the consumption of certain foods or beverages or by participation in certain athletic activities. A balance can be achieved and maintained that will allow the patient to keep near-normal, if not completely normal, blood sugar concentrations.

It's not a method everyone can use successfully, but for those who can, it means better control of the diabetes—and certainly better health.

The Elderly and Diabetes

Latest estimates indicate that about 4 million Americans over age sixty-five have diabetes. Half of these have had the disease diagnosed; the other 2 million are not aware that they are diabetics, usually because the symptoms have not been pronounced enough to send them to a doctor.

Older diabetics who have had diabetes for several years and who are now being cared for at home have usually established, with the help of their doctors, a life style and a medical regimen for dealing with their diabetes. Consequently, some doctors will advise against elderly longtime diabetics attempting "tight" control of blood sugar levels through self blood glucose monitoring (SBGM) with the new self-testing devices or by using the recently introduced insulin pump.

There are three reasons for this. First, it's difficult to motivate older people to change the patterns and habits of many years of dealing with diabetes and adopt the strict regimen and complex new techniques required for such tight control. Second, if the complications that generally appear with long-term diabetes—diabetic retinopathy, neuropathy, and nephropathy—are already present, it will be too late to institute preventive measures, and although it's necessary to minimize any further harm to the patient, strict control will not necessarily make any appreciable difference as compared to the conventional therapy program the patient has been following for so many years. Finally, home monitoring involves careful and regular checking of blood glucose levels, with the attendant risk that unless insulin dosage adjustments are promptly and accurately made, the patient may suffer insulin shock if blood glucose is too low, or run the risk of diabetic coma if blood glucose is too high.

This does not mean no elderly diabetic should attempt tight control through use of the new methods available. A major factor will be the individual's motivation. There are many elderly people who are active and who energetically seek new interests and outlets and continue to work or to keep busy even in retirement. On the other hand, some older people welcome the pleasures of retirement and prefer a more easygoing life style. For either type of individual (and those in between), a main consideration will be how well the diabetes is being managed with the present regimen.

As always, the final decision should be made by the diabetic person and the physician.

Tips for the Diabetic

Here are some tips* that a diabetic, regardless of age, should follow for better management of the disease:

- If taking insulin, eat extra calories when unusual physical activity is anticipated.
- Eat a bedtime snack when taking insulin (if permitted).
- Rotate the sites of insulin injections in a systematic manner.
- Keep syringes and needles in one special place.
- Keep the bottle of insulin in current use at room temperature.
- Know the conditions that produce an insulin reaction: omission of a meal; unaccustomed or strenuous exercise; too much insulin.
- Know how to combat an impending insulin reaction: take orange juice, sugar, or candy when symptoms first occur; test urine; carry extra carbohydrates (sugar lumps or candy) at all times.
- Know the conditions that bring about diabetic acidosis (lack of insulin in the blood—can lead to diabetic coma): nausea and vomiting; failure to increase insulin when urine sugar is increasing; failure to take insulin; stress; infections.
- Know how to combat impending diabetic acidosis: test urine for sugar and acetone and report results to physician; take additional insulin as advised by physician; go to bed and keep warm; alert someone to be in attendance; drink a glass of liquid hourly, if possible.
- Follow good health practices for diabetics: avoid tobacco; take only prescribed medications.
- Carry a diabetic identification card or wear an identification bracelet.

---

*Adapted from *The Lippincott Manual of Nursing Practice,* 3rd ed. (Philadelphia: Lippincott, 1982).

17

Neurological Problems

Alzheimer's Disease

A DIAGNOSIS of Alzheimer's disease marks the beginning of a long and agonizing confrontation with irreversible dementia. "Dementia" means "deprived of mind." It's the word physicians and other health professionals now prefer when describing diseases that affect cognition—the ability to perceive, to think, and to remember.

Alzheimer's disease produces an insidious loss of memory, intellectual deterioration, personality changes, and a progressive decline in the ability to perform the normal activities of daily living until the victim can no longer function as a sentient human being. It tragically alters the lives of both patients and their families, inflicting heavy emotional damage before bringing on the inevitable death of the victim. Not everyone will experience all symptoms of Alzheimer's; however, when the disease strikes, the results are devastating.

Robert R. was one of the last men you'd ever expect to suffer from any mental or emotional problems. He was a successful businessman, running his own factory, where he made an excellent living manufacturing small electronic parts for industry and the military. He was outgoing, cheerful, always ready with an appropriate joke, and he had a vast number of friends who were genuinely fond of him. He never forgot a name or a face or a joke, this was his proud boast.

Shortly after his sixtieth birthday, Robert became just a little forgetful. Every now and then he drew a blank when he tried to fit a name to a familiar face, and there were times when he fumbled with the punch line of a joke he had told for years. He paid little attention to this, telling his wife he was getting older and naturally everything was slowing down for him—even his fabulous memory reflexes. Unfortunately, it wasn't that simple.

By the time Robert reached sixty-five, he would look at his wife when she greeted him in the morning and ask who she was. No matter how many times the incident was repeated, and no matter how often his wife patiently told him they were married and that she was Ruth, his wife, it never seemed to make any difference. Robert could not recognize his wife after nearly forty years of marriage.

And then came the day when Robert stared into the mirror and didn't know who he was looking at.

Some loss of memory is not unusual as people age. It happens to many individuals, and usually all concerned take it good-naturedly, perhaps even humorously. It's only when this expected slight memory difficulty becomes more pronounced and progressive that it is no longer perceived either with good nature or with humor. Unfortunately, a progressive loss of memory is one of the clear symptoms of the form of dementia known as Alzheimer's disease.

In the early part of this century, the disease, named after the German physician who first described the condition in 1907, was considered to be "presenile" dementia. It was widely assumed that some form of dementia was to be expected as part of the aging process. We know today that this is not true. There are many examples of people living into their eighties and nineties with full command of their faculties and a vigorous life style.

There are, of course, changes that occur in the brain as our bodies age, but under normal conditions, these changes will not affect mental capacity or functioning. Dementia is a group of symptoms brought on by a disease. It is not a normal outgrowth of aging, and it is now realized that many cases that were referred to as "hardening of the arteries in the brain," "senile dementia," or "organic brain syndrome" were actually cases of the most common irreversible dementia—Alzheimer's disease.

Estimates of the prevalence of this disease vary, but the general consensus is that about 5 to 10 percent of people over sixty-five have moderate to severe dementia and about 10 to 20 percent of those over seventy-five are so afflicted. Further, it is estimated that more than half of the dementias occurring in elderly people are cases of Alzheimer's disease. Although we can look on the brighter side and say that about 80 to 85 percent of the elderly do *not* have any significant dementia, the statistics, when converted into actual figures, show that about 3 million older people in this country suffer from some form of dementia.

Despite what we have learned since Alzheimer's was first recognized, there still is a prevalent conception that dementia and aging go hand in hand. Perhaps this is due to the greater public awareness of

Alzheimer's and the other dementing illnesses, or it may be caused by the frightening fact that Alzheimer's is irreversible and leads to a tragic loss of the quality of life before ending in death.

At present, research shows that Alzheimer's disease is the fourth or fifth leading cause of death in this country. From the time the first symptoms are noted, the disease can progress at different rates in each individual. Death can come in three or four years or sometimes not for as long as ten or fifteen years. No matter how long it takes, though, these are not easy years, either for the victim or for his family.

The diagnosis of Alzheimer's disease is a difficult one. The only certain way to confirm the presence of Alzheimer's is after death. An autopsy that includes microscopic examination of the brain tissue is, at present, the one positive way of identifying Alzheimer's.

In its early stages, Alzheimer's is often missed completely. Frequently, the reason for this is that the person does not see a physician, accepting the initial slight memory loss as nothing to worry about—and the family goes along with this. This does not mean that every time you or someone close to you seem a bit forgetful you have to hurry to the doctor. However, although memory lapses are not uncommon, it would be a good idea to check with your family physician and a neurologist if someone starts to forget things with increasing frequency over a period of more than a year (especially if this is not characteristic of him) and also requests, on several occasions, that you repeat something that has been recently discussed at length. Another clue would be if the signs of forgetfulness and memory problems appear in unfamiliar surroundings, such as when taking a trip. Being away from familiar sights and sounds can trigger anxiety and cognitive difficulties in someone in the early stages of dementia.

It's important that the individual be given a thorough physical examination, not only to determine his present state of health but also to rule out any physical causes of the memory difficulty, such as a head injury. After this, a neurological examination can be conducted, and this will probably include what is known as a mental status examination. This is a test in which a series of questions are asked on fairly simple subjects such as the current date, the age of the patient, his date of birth, and who the president is. If moderate dementia is present, the patient will make several conspicuous errors, more than would be statistically expected.

From this point on, neurologists can establish the presence of Alzheimer's disease only by a careful process of elimination. There are a number of ailments called pseudodementias that can give the impression of dementia. These include depression (with many symptoms very similar to dementia), drug intoxication or adverse interactions (many elderly people take several prescription drugs, along with over-the-counter drugs such as aspirin and laxatives), chemical imbalances in the body, head injuries, brain tumors, chronic lung disease (producing oxygen shortage to the brain cells), lead poisoning, alcoholism, nutritional deficiencies (nutritional anemia, for example, or a vitamin B_1 deficiency), meningitis, and excessive exposure to carbon monoxide, pesticides, or industrial pollutants.

It is crucial to determine whether the patient's cognitive difficulties are being caused by these pseudodementias or similar ailments, since many of these conditions will respond to treatment. If treatable, the symptoms of dementia often can be reduced or eliminated, whereas with Alzheimer's there is at present no such possibility. If the diagnosis of Alzheimer's is made prematurely, it may turn out to be the wrong diagnosis, and the patient will not have received the treatment that may have helped him.

After all possible other ailments are ruled out, the diagnosis of Alzheimer's disease can be made on the basis of a complete history of the patient's symptoms and how they have progressed over a period of time. This history is usually taken from both the patient and family members. The patient himself is not a good source for the type of information needed. He will often appear cooperative but will not be able to answer the questions because of memory difficulties. He may even become irritated and resort to sarcasm. He may be unaware of his cognitive difficulty, or he may tend to minimize it, making his answers unreliable. The family members, on the other hand, can give a more objective and factual history of the patient's symptoms and behavior over an extended period of time.

The examining neurologist will question both the patient and the family and correlate the results in a search for symptoms indicating Alzheimer's disease. Some characteristic symptoms the neurologist will look for are a significant loss of recent memory (what has happened in the immediate past, as opposed to remote memory of incidents and people far back in the past), any history of getting lost or wandering around, a slacking off in attention to personal hygiene and cleanliness (especially if this is counter to the patient's usual habits), a clinging to and a dependency on a spouse or close relative, and most important of all, incidents that show a decline in the ability to conduct routine matters that involve abstract thinking, such as paying bills or balancing a checkbook.

Because of the seriousness of this disease and the way it can ravage the lives of all involved—patients and families alike—much attention and research is being devoted to the study of Alzheimer's disease. It will be helpful for you, as the caregiver, to know as much as possible about the symptoms of Alzheimer's at its various stages, preparing you for what to expect and how to deal with the conditions and problems that will arise.

Barry Reisberg, M.D., an expert in the field of geriatrics and a specialist who has studied Alzheimer's disease for many years, has listed seven levels of cognitive decline to help define the progress of Alzheimer's. These levels are:

Level 1) Normal • At this level, there would be an absence of any serious cognitive difficulties or problems with intellectual functioning. For those remaining at this level, there would be no significant impairment as they age.

Level 2) Normal Aged Forgetfulness • Most people as they reach age sixty-five and go beyond it will have some episodes of forgetting names and dates and where they put things, but none of these are serious complaints. As long as there is no impairment of the ability to work and socialize, there is no need for concern. However, it's understandable that those who fear that this normal forgetfulness may be the beginning of Alzheimer's may become apprehensive at the appearance of some of these memory difficulties. The passage of time should help to allay these fears, as the person begins to realize that his memory difficulties are actually slight and are not getting any worse.

Level 3) Early Confusion • We reach the borderline of Alzheimer's disease at this level. Memory deficits begin to hamper the individual and also are more apparent now to family and friends. The individual may find that he cannot remember something he has just read or has just been told. He may forget someone's name moments after being introduced. He often cannot find the right word or words to express his thoughts. His concentration is decidedly faulty; his job suffers; his social life is strained.

There is an awareness on the part of the person that something is definitely wrong with his mind. He is sure he's starting to lose it. Anxiety takes hold of him—and grows with each new incident. Frequently, he will deny that anything is wrong and will try to cover up his cognitive difficulties.

At this time, it's imperative that a physician be consulted. A thorough physical examination, followed by a neurological examination, is mandatory if the underlying cause of the problem is to be discovered. It's well to bear in mind here that the symptoms bringing on the anxiety in the individual can be caused by conditions other than dementia.

Many people with these symptoms show no further significant decline for many years, and sometimes not at all. Alzheimer's is not the inevitable diagnosis. All the pseudodementias previously mentioned must be considered and ruled out, if possible. It's only when physical illness, trauma, depression, and other possibilities have been definitely eliminated that dementia has to be considered.

Whatever the diagnosis, it's important that the individual continue with social activities and with the activities of daily living. It might be helpful to consider a change to a less stressful job and a more relaxed life style, perhaps even retirement. The family's support and understanding is of great value at this time.

Level 4) Late Confusion • When this level is reached in the course of an individual's cognitive decline, the symptoms displayed are the same as those of early Alzheimer's disease. Memory loss is more pronounced and there is the additional loss of the ability to deal with routine tasks such as shopping in stores, managing money, and running a household.

However, in many cases, the individual still retains the ability to recognize familiar faces and places and is aware of where he is and what is going on around him. Denial of his condition now becomes an active defense mechanism, with the person refusing to acknowledge his problem recalling current events and even some facts of his own personal life. Concentration has deteriorated, and a complex task becomes an impossibility. As a further defense, the individual will avoid situations and tasks that demand an ability he no longer can command. He withdraws, physically and emotionally.

It will still be possible for the person to function—with some assistance. Someone in the family has to take over financial tasks, as well as making sure that the individual is watched and cared for a little more closely now. There's a tendency for him to wander and perhaps get lost and forget where he lives. It sometimes becomes necessary to use devices such as an identification bracelet or labels sewn into clothing to make sure the person will be able to return home with some help from outsiders or the police.

Level 5) Early Dementia • We're at the stage now where the dementia can be properly considered "moderate" Alzheimer's disease. Cognitive decline has progressed to the point where the person can no longer manage without constant help and supervision. Memory loss varies unexpectedly. On a "good day," the person may remember his address and what day of the week it is; on a "bad day," he may not remember any of this but will be able to recall where he went to school or some other fact from his personal life. To the family, these memory twists and turns can be quite upsetting, since the person seems to be gaining ground, then losing it.

Denial is even stronger now. The individual will not face the truth of what is happening to him and can have sudden emotional outbursts when things get to be too much for him. The family will have to learn to deal with these outbursts, as well as with displays of anger and tearfulness.

Personal care will begin to be affected by the course of the disease, although usually the individual will be able to manage to use the toilet without assistance and to eat meals with no trouble. At times, however, there may be some confusion and difficulty with dressing, and help will then be needed, especially with selecting clothes to wear. Also, it may be necessary to remind the person to bathe—and to repeat the request patiently when the person insists that he has already bathed.

At this stage, the family will begin to realize the extent of the task facing them. Constant supervision of the individual becomes a full-time task. Part-time help will probably be needed, unless the core family is large enough to provide the help needed by themselves. If the patient (we can start considering him in that light now) lives alone, the problem is compounded. Outside help will definitely be needed, and family and friends will have to set up and oversee the care being given.

Guidance for the family will become essential now. Health professionals—the family physician, social workers, and therapists—will have to be consulted as to the best way to handle emotional outbursts by the patient and how to avoid stressful situations that will only confuse and anger him. Urging him to participate in various activities will not "keep his mind active." If the activity is too complex or is perceived as threatening by the patient, he will resist.

The caregiver will have to strike a balance between keeping the patient from withdrawing from almost all activities and, at the same time, not pushing him into stressful situations. Often going to the movies or the theater or similar social activities that do not demand too much from the patient may prove helpful and calming.

Level 6) Middle Dementia • Cognitive ability of the patient, at this stage, continues to decline. Assistance is now needed with almost all everyday activities, especially toileting and bathing. Actually, the patient will have forgotten the mechanics of using the toilet and will have to be shown, time after time, how to use the toilet and how to accomplish wiping and washing.

In many cases, the patient will not even realize that he has to use the toilet, and urinary or fecal incontinence will occur. This is perhaps the most unpleasant aspect of providing care for the Alzheimer's patient.

The caregiver will find it a difficult task to clean the patient after an incontinent episode, and the patient, whose memory is not completely gone, may realize what is being done for him and to him and will feel shame, humiliation, anger, and resentment. Professional guidance will be useful here. A health care professional will be able to show the caregiver how to deal with this situation—the type of incontinence underclothing that may be helpful, the use of bed pads, and how to set up a schedule for getting the patient to the toilet in time to avoid "accidents."

Bathing will be another problem. The patient will often have a strong fear of the tub or shower and will have to be gently persuaded to bathe. He cannot be left alone during this time, as he may inadvertently change the temperature of the water and scald himself. Statistics show that the bathtub or shower is the site for many home accidents and injuries—for nonimpaired people. The hazard potential will be even worse for someone with Alzheimer's.

Memory loss will be much greater at this stage. The patient may forget his wife's name, although he will know his own name and will generally be able to distinguish between strangers and family and other people he knows. His recent memory will be diminished or even gone, but he may retain some of his remote memory, being able to recall isolated incidents from his past.

By the time the patient has reached this level of cognitive decline, the chemical balance in his brain will have changed. It will no longer be possible for him to hide from the reality of his situation through denial. He will not be able to perform this mental feat, and this will result in increased anger and emotional turmoil. He can, at this stage, become paranoid, delusional, and violent. He may talk to someone who isn't there; he may imagine dead relatives have come to visit him; and he may become agitated and react violently to any situation he perceives as threatening.

This is the stage at which the caregiver (or caregivers, if several family members are involved) will experience feelings of being overwhelmed with the enormity of the task of providing care for the Alzheimer's patient. Help will be needed—full-time if possible, part-time at the very least. Moreover, not only will there be the difficult task of locating people who will be capable as well as willing to undertake such a responsibility, but the matter of finances will have to be considered. Insurance policies, government or private, usually do not cover this sort of "maintenance" or "custodial care" for a patient.

There is an immense emotional burden on the family, and thoughts will naturally turn to the possibility—no matter how distasteful—of placing the patient in an institution. Most often, episodes of incontinence or violence cause the family to think of institutionalization, perhaps because these are situations that most people feel incapable of coping with on a regular basis. Realistically, competent staffs in well-run institutions can often provide better care than the family at this stage of the patient's functional and cognitive decline.

Level 7) Late Dementia • At this stage of Alzheimer's disease, the patient loses the ability to talk or to move about. He cannot communicate verbally. Screams, grunts, facial grimaces, and what seems like gibberish will become a means of expressing himself. It would be well not to ignore these outbursts. The patient may not only be in emotional distress but may also be trying to tell you that he has pain in a particular part of his body. Watch what he does with his hands, perhaps pointing to or covering up a part of his body. It may be an indication of something wrong internally.

Denial once again becomes possible as a defense mechanism for the patient, and it may work to his benefit—and the families'. In some cases, denial works so well that the patient will appear to be happy and contented and will be able to sit with the family and seemingly enjoy the activity going on around him. When this does happen, a small portion of the burden on the family is lightened.

There will still be problems, though, and one of the major problem areas will be in eating. Food will have to be carefully cut up for the patient, who will be incapable of handling a knife and fork to do this. Later on, if the ability to chew is lost, a soft food diet will be necessary. And, if the patient reaches the stage where eating is impossible, either because the patient has lost the ability to swallow or because he absolutely refuses to eat, "tube feeding" may be required (see Chapter 6).

As the final stage of the disease approaches and the patient seems to be completely unaware of the world around him or the family who is near him, it should be realized that human contact is still needed. As Dr. Reisberg puts it: "A loving voice, attention and touch are enormously important—they keep the patient emotionally and physically alive."

The final stage of Alzheimer's is death, sometimes preceded by coma. Frequently, the patient succumbs to other illness, such as pneumonia, and this is listed as the cause of death on the death certificate. But in actuality, Alzheimer's disease has claimed another victim.

IS THERE A CAUSE OR CURE?

The answer to both of the above questions is: "Not known at this time."

Research is moving ahead on finding the cause or causes of Alzheimer's disease. Theories of the causes fall into five categories, not mutually exclusive.

Acetylcholine Deficiency • Nerve cells in the brain produce a chemical—acetylcholine—that acts as a neurotransmitter, sending nerve signals from cell to cell. Independent investigators have found that there are decreased levels of acetylcholine in the brains of people who have died as a result of Alzheimer's disease. This discovery is an important development and opens a promising avenue for further investigation.

Genetics • While genetics does seem to be a factor, since the odds of developing Alzheimer's disease are greater if it's in the family, the exact familial link has not yet been determined.

Slow Virus • Researchers are investigating the possibility that a slow-acting virus enters the body and much later brings on Alzheimer's. However, attempts to transmit the disease, which would indicate a viral origin, have not been successful, partly because it can take as long as thirty years for some viruses to act—and laboratory animals do not live long enough to make the determination. Research in this area is continuing.

The Autoimmune Phenomenon • Sometimes, the body's immune system, which protects against outside infection or disease, turns on itself and starts to destroy the tissues in the body. When this happens, tissues in brain cells can be destroyed. However, research has not yet proved a link with the development of Alzheimer's disease.

Aluminum • Autopsies have disclosed aluminum in large amounts in the brains of Alzheimer's victims, but research is still inconclusive on this.

CARING FOR THE ALZHEIMER'S PATIENT

Although no cure has been found for Alzheimer's disease, and there is no known way of preventing it, much has been done in the area of providing care for the Alzheimer's patient, both in the hospital and at home. Here are some general guidelines:

1) If the patient is at the stage where familiar faces are not always recognized, make it a point to identify yourself to the patient, even if you are a spouse or other close relative.

2) Always speak in a low, quiet voice. Keep tension out of your voice as this will be conveyed to the patient and cause anxiety and possibly fear.

3) Use short sentences and plain, easily understandable words.

4) If you have to ask questions, ask them one at a time. If there is no response, use exactly the same words and ask the question again.

5) Ask questions that can be answered yes or no.

6) Avoid questions or instructions that require the patient to make a choice or to think out a decision.

7) If you have something you want the patient to do, break it down into short, simple steps and present them one at a time, giving the next step only when the preceding one has been accomplished. (Example: "Here is your toothbrush." "Take it in your hand." "I will put some toothpaste on the brush." "Bring the brush to your mouth." And so on.)

8) Make an effort to interpret the patient's body language and whatever noises he may make.

9) Try playing some soft music. This may be soothing for the patient, who also may remember some songs from the past and even sing them along with you.

10) Touching the patient is a sign of caring and may have a calming effect. Bear in mind, though, that the patient may perceive any sudden touching or holding as a threat.

HELP THE CARETAKER

The family of a victim of Alzheimer's disease may need as much help and care as the patient. Knowledge of resources, such as day care, respite care, and family support groups will be helpful to you as the caretaker. Using any and all of the support services that can be found in the community can help reduce the pressure on you. Day care centers can provide socialization for the patient and respite for you.

The growing burden on you, as the caretaker, cannot be ignored. Pressure is constant, and although an outsider may feel that the patient appears outwardly normal, the stress imposed by the patient's dependency on you is always present. Moreover, when the patient becomes confused, agitated, or paranoid, you will have to cope with this to the best of your ability, and sometimes by yourself.

As the caretaker, you must not feel that you have to bear the burden alone. That attitude can be harmful in the long run. Above all, do not set up unrealistic goals or expectations for yourself. Do the best you can—and do not hesitate to seek outside help.

There are more than 300 support groups in the nationwide organization of the Alzheimer's Disease and Related Disorders Association (ADRDA), with more than seventy chapters in thirty-one states. (Refer to the Appendix, "Tapping the Resources," for more details on this organization.) Call the local chapter and find out where and when meetings are held—and plan to attend.

Support groups provide a forum where caretakers can talk out their feelings of frustration, anger, guilt, and loneliness, feelings that can be overpowering. As a caretaker, you will have to cope with seeing the one in your care slowly decline. Moreover, your patience will often wear thin as the gradual loss of cognitive abilities in the patient, coupled with irrational behavior and a good-one-day-bad-another-day progress, begins to take its toll on you. The future can start to look devastatingly grim, and you will feel powerless to do anything about it.

This is where a support group can help. Join one as soon as you can. Meanwhile, there is much that you can do to "take care of the caretaker"—yourself. Here are some suggestions:

- Try to learn to accept the things you cannot change.
- Take one day at a time. Do not dwell on the future. There are no absolutes; the course of the illness may vary. Find humor where you can in daily activities.
- Talk out your feelings and worries with others—a clergyman, an old friend, or the new friends you've met in the support group. Hearing how others have managed with the same problems you have will clarify the situation for you and give you new insights.
- Be good to yourself. Take care of yourself; eat well; exercise regularly; get enough sleep.
- Find additional help if it's needed.
- Be aware of potential problems that can be brought on by depression, sleeplessness, or drug abuse. Stay alert and active.
- The support group may help you find a counselor who understands your situation, or you may find assistance through one of the agencies listed in the Appendix of this book. If you are selecting a counselor, be aware that just as doctors differ in their approach to patients, so do counselors to their clients. You may need to shop around until you find the kind of help that works best for you.

RESPITE CARE

When Alzheimer's disease progresses to the point that someone has to be with the patient at all times, it is vitally important that you get help in caring for the patient—if you plan to care for him at home at this time rather than send him to an institution. It is not reasonable to assume that you will be able to provide the twenty-four-hour care required without some form of respite.

In finding assistance, you will first have to determine the extent of the patient's cognitive problems. You will then be able to guide your assistant caretaker so he or she will be able to provide the kind of care needed. You will probably need someone who will act as more than just a housekeeper. A confused Alzheimer's patient needs continuing attention, and it's unrealistic to expect someone to clean the house and look after the patient at the same time.

A "sitter" will provide you with the respite you need and the care that the patient needs. You may find this sitter through a newspaper advertisement or by checking with the student placement office of a local college or by word of mouth from someone in a position similar to yours. In hiring the sitter, as with any employee you take into your home, it's necessary to check references and define and describe the duties and tasks of the job. If you can, have the helper visit when you are present so the patient will get used to another person in the house.

DAY CARE

Adult day care centers vary in type of staff, recreation and social activities offered, and clients who are accepted. Finding the right center will provide several hours of respite for you each day, while at the same time providing the Alzheimer's patient with structured activities and association and socialization with others. The patient may feel better and become more manageable at home if he has been involved in an effective day care program.

NURSING HOMES

As the disease progresses, it may become increasingly difficult to care for the patient at home. As cognitive function declines, the care of the patient becomes a twenty-four-hour-a-day job that can best be done by health care professionals.

Although placing a loved one in a nursing home is a difficult and agonizing thought to contemplate, it may ultimately be the most responsible decision a family can make. The thought of a nursing home can conjure up horror stories of inadequate and unfeeling care, but not all nursing homes deserve that bad reputation.

Nursing home care is expensive. You will have to do a good deal of investigating and homework to ensure that whatever insurance coverage or financial assistance you are entitled to is obtained.

Most important, though, you will have to consider what is the best kind of nursing home for your loved one and what kind if impact it will have on all of you. Your lives will change because of this, and you will have to make sure you understand and are prepared for the change. You will also have to do your best to prepare the patient for what is to come.

It won't be easy. But then nothing about Alzheimer's disease is easy.

Amyotrophic Lateral Sclerosis (ALS)

For many people, the words "amyotrophic lateral sclerosis" repre-sent medical terminology that is difficult to remember and hard to pro-nounce. Because of this, the ailment is often referred to as Lou Gehrig's disease (it received wide publicity when it struck down the famous New York Yankees baseball star in 1941) or simply ALS, as it will be here.

ALS is a disease of the nervous system in which, for reasons as yet unknown, motor neurons in the brain and spinal cord are attacked and destroyed. Motor neurons are nerve cells that control the activity of muscles. The destruction of motor neurons leaves the muscles without any control and leads to progressive muscle weakness and wasting.

In ALS, the "voluntary" muscles are affected. These include mus-cles that are involved in the movement of the arms and legs and also the muscles associated with talking, chewing, and swallowing. Addi-tionally, the intercostal (between the ribs) muscles and the muscles controlling the diaphragm are also affected as ALS progresses.

Muscles are "energized" by impulses from motor neurons. These impulses, or signals, cause the muscles to contract, thus moving the arm or leg or other part of the body being controlled by a particular set of voluntary muscles. The motor neurons also supply "nutrient signals" to the muscles to allow proper nourishment and growth.

Motor neurons in the brain ("upper motor neurons") conduct impulses from the brain down along the sides of the spinal cord. In the spinal cord, these impulses are transferred to other motor neurons ("lower motor neurons") that connect to the voluntary muscles. Gen-erally, lower motor neurons in the lower part of the spinal cord control and activate the leg muscles; lower motor neurons in the upper part of the spinal cord are connected to muscles in the arms and hands and fingers; and motor neurons in the brain stem control the muscles used for talking, chewing, and swallowing.

When everything is working normally, the nerve impulses from the upper motor neurons in the brain are transferred to the lower motor neurons in the spinal cord, which then activate the muscles necessary to provide the desired movement. It all works so smoothly and so quickly that we aren't conscious of any deliberate mental or neural processes directing this activity.

When ALS strikes, the nerve fibers of the upper motor neurons in the brain, along with their fatty insulating sheaths called myelin, are destroyed and replaced by hardened *(sclerosed)* scar tissue. This means the nerve impulses cannot be transmitted down the sides (the *lateral* portions) of the spinal cord to the lower motor neurons. The lower motor neurons in the spinal cord also degenerate, leading to a lack of stimulus and nourishment for the muscles (an *amyotrophic* condition). As you can see, the name of this disease specifically describes what is happening.

As the motor neurons in the spinal cord and the brain degenerate, the muscles controlled by these neurons waste away and become useless. Initial symptoms are usually seen in the hands. There is a loss of dexterity; the individual cannot completely control his hand movements; fine finger movements are not possible. This difficulty is often attributed to clumsiness, although the fatigue and general weakness that are also initial symptoms of ALS should alert the individual that this involves something more than simple clumsiness.

About one-third of those afflicted with ALS first noticed symptoms affecting hand and finger movements. Approximately another third of ALS individuals first became aware of something wrong through weakness in the legs and feet. For the final third, the earliest indication was difficulty in speaking and swallowing.

ALS generally strikes people in the forty-to-seventy age range, and men seem to contract it twice as often as women. It has been pointed out that ALS affects more people than muscular dystrophy, although through fund raising and publicity the public seems to be more aware of the ravages of muscular dystrophy. Recently, however, more attention is being focused on ALS because, ironically, it has stricken famous people such as David Niven, the actor, and Jacob Javits, the former senator.

Often, the onset of ALS goes unnoticed. It may be present for some time before any symptoms are observed, as healthy motor neurons take over the work of damaged motor neurons, compensating for their lost function. It isn't until the workload becomes too great that the individual realizes something is wrong, usually because of unexplained fatigue and weakness.

As the disease progresses, more of the muscles controlling the arms and legs are affected, and a form of paralysis develops. The individual is unable to move his arms or legs because the muscles, which are no longer being stimulated by the motor neurons, waste away from disuse and can no longer function.

The disease sometimes progresses rapidly and can even reach a plateau where it momentarily comes to a stop. However, the usual course of the disease is to progress at a fairly steady rate with the person becoming increasingly disabled as more and more muscles are involved. Eventually, the muscle weakness can affect the ability to talk, to chew, to swallow, and even to breathe. The individual may be confined to a wheelchair, wearing a cervical collar to keep his head upright, with braces and other devices to keep his arms and legs from flopping around.

If breathing becomes a serious problem, a respirator can be used, with a permanent opening (a tracheostomy) in the throat for insertion of the breathing tube.

If the chewing and swallowing muscles become useless, the individual will not be able to eat. In such cases, nourishment can be provided through a tube inserted through the nose and into the stomach (nasogastric feeding, see Chapter 6). If this method is undesirable—and many physicians do not prefer to use it on a long-term basis—other methods can be employed.

A tube can be inserted through an opening made into the stomach (gastrostomy), and the ALS individual can be fed in this manner. The opening is permanent and presents problems of gastric leakage and the necessity of removing clothing and lying down to accomplish feeding.

A method often used for permanent long-term feeling is a "cervical esophagostomy." A permanent opening is formed in the esophagus at about the level of the clavicle (collarbone), through which a tube can be inserted when it's time for feeding. The opening is a small one and can be covered with a blouse or scarf when not in use and protected with a small bandage to absorb any leakage or drainage. Feeding can be accomplished with the individual sitting in an upright position.

Nourishment is important for the ALS individual, and the above feeding methods usually are employed only when the muscle weakness and paralysis has spread to the point that swallowing is almost impossible. Before this, the individual can eat small but frequent meals consisting of food that doesn't have to be vigorously chewed and that can be swallowed without difficulty, such as ground beef in broth or gravy, baby food, puræed food, and any food that can be prepared to the proper consistency for the individual's needs.

Difficulty with swallowing also means that saliva can collect in the mouth. This can cause drooling, but, more serious, it can bring on choking. Various methods can be used to control the accumulation of saliva, including suction and drugs that reduce the formation of saliva.

The ALS individual has to be guarded against exposure to others with colds or flu or to any conditions that might bring on respiratory distress. Coughing may be a problem because of muscle weakness in the throat and chest, and the person has to be checked regularly and carefully to make sure his throat is clear.

The bladder, bowels, and sexual functioning are not directly affected by ALS. However, bladder problems may occur as a result of weakness in surrounding muscles, or because of a condition other than ALS. Loss of bowel control in ALS has not been reported. In fact, constipation is the usual complaint. Exercise and proper diet, along with stool softeners, if needed, can help in this respect.

The average course of the disease is said to be three to four years, although the number of persons living with ALS ten or more years is on the rise. When death comes, ALS itself is not directly responsible. Usually, a respiratory problem or heart trouble is the immediate cause. However, recent reports indicate that about half of ALS individuals are living three years after diagnosis of the disease (which probably was present but not in evidence some time before this), and 10 percent are still alive ten years after diagnosis. There have been people who have lived with this disease for ten to twenty years and have still managed to remain productive and enjoy their families and their work.

Since ALS attacks only motor neurons, intellectual capacity is not diminished. The ALS individual remains fully and mentally alert, and the sensory faculites remain unimpaired. Ability to think and reason continues despite the inability to control the muscles so necessary to everyday living. The acute and clearheaded awareness of what is happening increases the ordeal for the ALS individual. Emotional support of the family and friends is, therefore, vital in coping with this disease.

After the diagnosis of ALS the person confronted with a progressive neuromusclular disorder must learn to plan and budget physical activity to conserve strength and avoid stressing the muscles. The goal should be to maintain as active a daily life as possible within the limitations imposed by the disease.

At the onset of ALS, there is always the question of how long to continue working. Much will depend, of course, on the person's financial situation, as well as on the type of occupation, the demands of the job, and whether or not disability or retirement options are available through company insurance plans and other programs. As before, the goal should be to continue an active life as much as possible.

People who stop working abruptly because of ALS may experience anxiety or depression, or both. It's better to arrange a gradual decrease in working hours, if the job is too demanding, rather than stopping work suddenly and losing the stability and emotional reassurance provided by steady work and pride of accomplishment. Of course, employment that involves dangerously stressful or strenuous activity should be avoided. Work hours and rest periods should be planned to relieve the general fatigue and weakness that are so much a part of ALS.

TREATMENT

There is, at present, no known cure for ALS. However, much can be done to help the ALS individual cope with the physical limitations and the emotional problems involved. The goals of the treatment plan should be to assist the individual to maintain useful functioning and a satisfying quality of life.

Rehabilitation therapies and techniques can be of much benefit to the ALS individual. Physical therapy, occupational therapy, and other rehabilitation therapies provide a multidisciplinary approach to helping the person learn how to compensate for losses in strength and function.

Since the nature and degree of impairment will vary with each individual, treatment plans have to be tailored to the type of problems encountered and their severity. The multidisciplinary approach offered by teams of physicians and therapists at a number of medical institutions throughout the country provides a necessary integrated approach, including support for the family and rehabilitation for the patient. Contacting the National ALS Foundation, the ALS Society of America, or the Muscular Dystrophy Association (see the Appendix) will help identify the clinical and therapeutic services available in your community.

In some cases of ALS, there may be minimal impairment in walking with little or no fatigue, unless long distances are covered, or fatigue may appear after only short exertion. The ALS patient and the therapist will have to develop a plan of action that will provide for the maximum of movement and exercise to keep up muscle tone and prevent weakness from disuse.

Combining functioning and fatigue prevention is a major consideration. For example, a person with ALS who tires after walking long distances can take a wheelchair with him when walking. He can push the empty chair until he feels fatigue setting in, then can sit in the chair and rest—or, if the fatigue isn't too great, continue on his journey in the wheelchair. Such a procedure has to be planned with care, especially to avoid the possibility of the ALS individual being stranded with the chair when excessively fatigued and far from help of any kind.

A physical therapist, working with the ALS patient, will assess the needs of the individual and work out a treatment plan accordingly. The goal may well be not to build muscles but to deter muscle wasting and atrophy by a planned series of mild exercises or passive range-of-motion exercises. If muscular weakness is severe, the physical therapist may recommend assistive support devices such as foot braces, hand splints, a back support, or a cervical collar.

An occupational therapist will perform a functional evaluation of the ALS patient and work with him to maximize abilities and compensate for loss. Special grooming aids, utensils, and dressing tips will help to maintain a level of independence for the individual. The occupational therapist will also be able to provide the family members and any home health aides with information and guidance needed to assist the ALS patient.

While the occupational therapist and the physical therapist work to promote muscle tone, prevent muscle contractures, and maintain function in the ALS patient, another member of the team may be a speech/communications therapist working to maintain muscle strength and flexibility in the head, neck, tongue, lips, and other muscles used for speaking, chewing, and swallowing.

When the patient's ability to talk has been affected, other means of communication are introduced. Writing or typing, if manual dexterity hasn't been diminished, is often used as a substitute for speaking. Letter boards will help the patient spell out words or point to phrases. Modern computer technology has produced a talking computer, as well as small computers and printers to print out a message. One ALS individual, who can move only his eyes and his eyebrows, has helped develop a computer and a program that allow him to to operate the computer through movements of his eyebrows.

One important aspect of treatment for the ALS patient is taking all necessary precautions to prevent pressure sores (decubitus ulcers). Since the ALS patient will spend much time in bed or in a chair, unable to move because of muscle weakness, skin care is of great importance.

Turning the patient often is the primary method for dealing with the decubitus problem. Coupled with this are gentle massages to stimulate circulation—back rubs with lotion and rubbing the feet and applying lotion at bedtime. Refer to Chapter 10,"Pressure Sores," for more details on proper skin care in this situation.

RESPIRATORY ASSISTANCE: A CHOICE

Not too long ago, ALS victims often ended their battle against the disease by succumbing to respiratory failure—their muscles were just too weak to sustain breathing. Today, ALS patients can adapt readily to mechanical respiratory assistance at home. This, then, raises the question of whether or not to make use of a home respirator.

This is a decision a competent patient has to make. Knowing the eventual outcome of ALS and the deterioration involved, the patient, in consultation with his doctor, his family, and other advisers, has to decide whether he wants to avail himself of life-sustaining devices such as the home respirator. In other words he has to decide if he wants to invoke the "right to die"—a highly controversial issue, still unresolved legally.

This decision should be made *before* the necessity for it arises. Dr. Walter Bradley of the University of Vermont College of Medicine, writing in *ALSSOAN*, the newsletter of the ALS Society of America, gives a clear and pragmatic presentation of the reasons for making this decision early:

Respiratory impairment develops insidiously in ALS, . . . but terminal failure is almost always acute. Therefore, unless there has been active discussion before this stage, many patients find that the decision of whether to go onto a respirator has been made for them by default. Some who would have wanted respiratory support die before reaching hospital. Others reach hospital in a state in which it is impossible to discuss the question of respiratory support and therefore are involuntarily connected to a respirator.

RESEARCH

With the increasing public awareness of ALS—brought about in no small part by the activities of Senator Jacob Javits and the Muscular Dystrophy Association—there seems to be a renewed interest and activity in research. The National Institutes of Health, the Muscular Dystrophy Association, the Amyotrophic Lateral Sclerosis Society of America, and the National ALS Foundation underwrite studies at major medical centers, including St. Vincent's Hospital in New York City and Johns Hopkins University Hospital in Baltimore.

To date, neither the cause nor a cure for ALS has been found, although there have been inroads made in proving or disproving some of the theories being proposed. One very strong theory concerns the possibility of ALS being caused by a "slow virus," that is, a virus that entered the victim's body years before, remaining dormant until something triggered an attack on the motor neurons. Other scientists are exploring the theory that ALS, like diabetes, involves metabolic or nutritional deficiencies.

A research team at the University of Southern California's Neuromuscular Center in Los Angeles has been able to demonstrate improvement—although temporary and short-lived—in the muscle strength of ALS patients receiving massive doses of thyrotropin-releasing hormone (TRH). This substance is normally present in spinal cord motor neurons but has been found to be deficient in some ALS patients. Research in this area is continuing.

According to the ALS Society of America, symptomatic therapy for treatment of the symptoms of ALS is of great help. However, this is about the extent of what can be done for the ALS patient today, and the society expresses concern over reports of special "treatments" or "cures" and emphasizes that no known cure exists. If patients or physicians have any questions about experimental treatments for ALS, it would be best to contact any of the national organizations dealing with the disease, who will then be able to refer the inquirer to someone knowledgeable about ALS and any experimental treatments presently being explored.

RESOURCES AVAILABLE TO ALS PATIENTS

Treating ALS and caring for the patient can pile up some very heavy financial costs. Private insurance policies can provide some coverage, but policies vary with each insurance carrier, so you would have to check your own policy carefully to see what coverage is available. Medicare, Medicaid, and Social Security disability benefits may help. You will have to explore the eligibility requirements in each one carefully.

The Muscular Dystrophy Association offers free medical and recreational services for all ALS patients. For further information, contact your local MDA chapter or the national office—810 Seventh Avenue, New York, NY 10019—for the location of a chapter near you.

People with ALS may require a great deal of physical care. Home care programs enable the ALS individuals to be cared for in their own home. Local visiting nurses can provide services for patients and their families by explaining the medical orders they are carrying out and by teaching family members and home health aides how to help care for the ALS patient.

In working with home health aides for ALS patients, it is best to specify in detail the activities and duties of the position. If the ALS patient is severely disabled, comprehensive care will be needed, and the job description will be different for each shift of the twenty-four-hour coverage that is needed. Decisions have to be made as to whether the aide/attendant provides only services in support of the patient or household chores as well. The ALS Society of America, in one of their numerous fact sheets, suggests that family members do the household chores and the aide devote full time to the ALS patient.

The society advocates writing out a complete job description for the aide/attendant, including areas in which special training will be provided. The work can usually be broken down into specific treatment and care routines. Here is an example of routines the society considers important for care of a typical ALS patient:

Personal hygiene routine	Lifting and transfer routine
Bowel and bladder routine	Dressing routine
Skin care routine	Feeding routine

Communication routine   Work routines
Tracheostomy care routine   Rest and respiration routines
Suctioning routines

THE SPIRIT OF THE ALS INDIVIDUAL

Each individual is unique, and this applies equally to individuals with ALS as to other members of society. However, in the literature of ALS, especially in the newsletters, such as that published by ALS Society of America, there is such a preponderance of letters and stories concerning spirited, inspired, and outgoing people with ALS that it causes one to think that there may be some element in all the physical and emotional travail the ALS individual has to go through that gives all of them much more than a common bond of suffering. It seems to imbue them with an outlook, philosophy, and inner strength that the rest of us could well use. This is epitomized in the comment made to a group of doctors by Jacob Javits:

If there is anything I can leave with you in terms of the treatment of patients with a terminal illness, it is this: We are all terminal—we all die sometime— so why should a terminal illness be different from terminal life? There is no difference.

Multiple Sclerosis

MS is not a killer disease, and the majority of those who have it can expect to live a near-normal life span. The first manifestations of this disease usually appear in individuals between the ages of twenty and forty. The symptoms of MS they experience range from mild to severe and come and go unpredictably.

Multiple sclerosis is a disease of the central nervous system, which consists basically of the brain and the spinal cord. The central nervous system (CNS) controls how we move and speak and see and hear and sense the world around us. The CNS exercises this control through a network of nerves, which carry impulses and messages to and from the brain. Nerve fibers provide the pathways for these messages and are protected by a fatty substance called myelin that serves as an insulating sheath for the nerve pathways and also helps speed the impulses along.

In multiple sclerosis, small patches of the myelin sheath are attacked, destroyed, and replaced by scar tissues (*sclera*). The myelin insulation becomes uneven and cannot perform its function. When this happens, the nerve signals are slowed down and interfered with, becoming distorted, misdirected, and sometimes blocked completely. Because the messages are not getting through in full strength, various body functions become uncontrollable to varying degrees.

The destruction of the myelin produces scar tissue ('sclerosed' tissue), and since the nature of the disease is to attack the myelin at various (multiple) points in the CNS, the name "multiple sclerosis" is an apt medical description of what has taken place.

Why it takes place has not yet been determined. At present, the cause or causes of MS are unknown. There is no known cure, and doctors and scientists cannot even predict which part of the population is strongly at risk for this disease. Certain facts are known, however, and certain theories have been advanced and are being investigated to determine the cause of multiple sclerosis. Three theories currently head the list of possible causes: the slow virus; the autoimmune reaction; and the combination reaction.

According to the slow virus theory, a slow virus might enter the body and lie dormant for years before having any effect on the CNS. It's also possible that a common virus, rather than some new and as yet unknown type is the culprit in MS. Research is progressing. It has been determined that the incidence of MS is greatest in temperate regions of the world (northern United States, Canada, and Europe) and less prevalent in tropical areas, establishing broad general areas of statistically high and low risk for MS. There are also indications that an individual moving from one risk area to another *after* the age of fifteen will neither increase nor decrease his risk of getting the disease. On the other hand, if he moves from one area to the other *before* the age of fifteen, the degree of risk may change accordingly.

Not enough studies have been done to establish firmly that age is a contributing factor in MS, but the studies so far do suggest that perhaps some event (the invasion of a slow virus?) that occurs before the age of fifteen may be a predisposing factor in MS.

The autoimmune reaction theory of MS focuses on the body's immune system, which acts as a defense mechanism by attacking invading viruses and bacteria. Some "misfire" of this system may cause the body to attack its own cells in what is called an autoimmune reaction. The possibility that this could be a cause of the attack on the myelin sheath is being investigated.

In the theory of the combination reaction, an invading virus lodges in body cells. The body's immune defense system then attacks both the invading virus and the cells it has taken over. This would involve a combination of both the slow virus and the autoimmune reaction theories—and this possibility is also under investigation.

THE SYMPTOMS

Since MS attacks in multiple areas of the central nervous system, the symptoms can vary considerably, depending upon where the demyelination has taken place. Thus, symptoms may vary in different individuals and sometimes even in the same individual at different times. Moreover, many of the symptoms are the same as encountered in other diseases, so we can't say that one particular symptom, or a series of symptoms, definitely indicates the presence of MS. In general, here are some of the symptoms that could indicate MS:

- Seeing double, having incidents of uncontrolled eye movements, or temporary dimming or loss of vision in one or both eyes (Vision problems are often a first indication of possible MS.)
- Tingling sensations, numbness, or pricking in the hands and feet
- Lack of coordination (unable to walk a straight line, for example)
- Speech difficulties
- Feeling unusually tired or weak for no apparent reason
- Lack of balance, causing staggering
- Hand tremors
- Involuntary foot dragging
- Paralysis of any part of the body, partial or complete
- Loss of control over bladder or bowel (incontinence)

Some of these symptoms obviously will appear more serious than others (double vision, paralysis, incontinence, for example), but whatever the symptoms, they should not be ignored—even if they disappear in a short period of time. It's best to consult your family physician if there's any doubt in your mind.

Multiple sclerosis is very difficult to diagnose. Early symptoms may be slight and disappear quickly, so the individual doesn't bother going to the doctor. Even if one episode is reported to the doctor and even if a neurologist is consulted, no definite diagnosis of MS can be made. For one thing, the symptom may be the same as that of another disease. However, if the symptom has disappeared by the time the doctor is consulted, there's not much that can be done.

Today, with sophisticated CAT (computerized axial tomography) scans and MRI (magnetic resonance imaging) equipment, plus other diagnostic tools, it is possible to rule out other diseases—and this may assist in making a firm diagnosis of MS.

There is no laboratory test that can be performed to indicate MS, and all that the family physician and the neurological specialist can do is wait for the possible appearance of other symptoms. Since MS attacks the central nervous system in different areas, only the appearance of symptoms indicating the involvement of two or more parts of the CNS can allow the doctors to start confirming the diagnosis of MS. However, symptoms of MS can come and go without warning, adding to the uncertainty of making a firm diagnosis.

It's this uncertainty and the possibility of having to wait weeks, months, or even years for the appearance of additional symptoms that can cause emotional wear and tear on the individual. It has been pointed out by both physicians and patients that there's often a sudden feeling of relief when a confirmed diagnosis of MS can be made. At least then the individual will not have to wonder and worry at the appearance and disappearance of disturbing symptoms at widely separated intervals.

True, a diagnosis of MS will often bring on a feeling of despair because of the negative image many people have of what MS is and what it can do to you. Visions of people with twisted limbs huddled in wheelchairs abound in the public mind. These are extreme cases. Most people with MS function at a remarkably near-normal level.

A group of MS patients were studied and followed for twenty-five years, and at the end of that time, two-thirds of the group were still able to walk, some with the assistance of walking aids. The wheelchair cases are the easiest to recognize, and this may account for the poor public image. But it's a fact that most MS patients do not have to use wheelchairs. Many of them are free of all disabling symptoms; others may be only slightly handicapped.

MS is not a disease to be treated lightly, to be sure, and there *are* cases of extreme disability, but the situation is far from hopeless and should not be considered as such. According to Marci Catanzaro, Ph.D., assistant professor of nursing at the University of Washington School of Nursing, and a consultant to the Puget Sound Chapter of the National Multiple Sclerosis Society, writing in *RN Magazine* (December 1977),

The first thing to keep in mind is that there's really no such thing as a "typical" MS patient. MS is a complex disease with many, many faces. The nature and severity of symptoms vary widely from person to person depending on which areas of the central nervous system the disease process attacks. Moreover, the progress of MS is so unpredictable that it's impossible to foretell what course it will take. With proper management, the majority of MS patients are able to lead active productive lives within their limitations.

COURSE AND PROGNOSIS

Multiple sclerosis is not a disease that lends itself to neat categorizations. The course it takes is usually different for each individual. However, there is a general progression that the majority of cases seem to follow, and this progression will determine to a great extent the nature and extent of the home care required by each individual.

MS progresses in a series of irregular attacks (exacerbations) and remissions. After a remission, there may be a long period—sometimes years—before the next exacerbation. The intervals between exacerbations and remissions may change over a period of time. Often, the exacerbations will last longer as time goes by, with the remissions progressively less complete each time. It's all rather sporadic and unpredictable.

MANAGEMENT AND TREATMENT

MS is not contagious and is not considered a hereditary disease in that parents do not pass it on to their children. It's also not classified as a fatal disease, although it may reduce life expectancy by about 15 percent. There is no known cure at present, but experience has shown that MS patients can be helped in many ways to lead productive and independent lives.

Treatment for MS consists of a combination of: maintaining overall good health; using drugs as necessary to relieve specific symptoms; employing physical therapy to maintain muscle tone and flexibility; preventing infections, particularly recurrent bladder infections; getting professional counseling when needed; and having regular reevaluations of the patient's condition.

Other methods—some experimental—are also being tried. A significant problem for the MS patient can be differentiating legitimate therapeutic trials from unproven fads. Be sure, by checking with the National MS Society in New York City to provide you with the medical community's opinion about the legitimacy of a treatment program. Often treatments that are too good to be true are unfounded and unproven.

Maintaining Good Health • The general rules of good health apply to the MS patient. This means eating well-balanced meals, getting plenty of rest, and exercising moderately. During periods of exacerbation, all of this may not be possible, but when MS is in remission, the health regimen can be resumed. The family physician should be consulted, of course, and a joint health program worked out—and adhered to.

Special precautions will have to be taken. It's very important to avoid infection—even minor ones such as a cold or the flu—that can cause a fever and perhaps bring on an exacerbation. Heat is not good for those with MS. It has been found that too much warmth can trigger a relapse. So the advice to those with MS is to stay out of the sun and not to take hot baths or showers.

Medications • The physician will prescribe whatever drugs or other medications are needed, especially during an acute exacerbation. Drugs to suppress the body's immune system may be prescribed to inhibit the destruction of myelin. ACTH and steroids may also be prescribed, but these powerful drugs can have adverse side effects and the physician will be the one to judge their effectiveness.

Physical Therapy • Exercise programs will help to keep the patient in condition, maintain flexibility, and promote endurance. Physical therapy can help individuals get the most out of whatever physical abilities they may have. A physical therapist can provide training in how to move about with safety despite any physical disabilities. Also, if required, the therapist may fit the patient with braces and provide training in their use to help promote independence.

Special Diets • People with MS will, quite naturally, pay close attention to reports of new methods, medications, or procedures for treating the disease. One area where caution must be observed is in the matter of proposed new diets that are supposed to help fight MS. It's unfortunate that because of the sporadic and spontaneous appearance of exacerbations and remissions, the individual may attribute the onset of a remission to a new diet that has just been tried. At present, there is no known diet that will do more for the MS patient than the standard, well-balanced, nutritionally sound diet prescribed by trained nutritionists.

Bladder Problems • As has been mentioned, one of the symptoms of MS is problems with bladder control. Sometimes this occurs only during exacerbations, but regardless of when it happens, it can be dealt with in a variety of ways. A urologist should be consulted to make sure the bladder difficulty is not due to some disease or ailment other than MS. Also, the urologist may prescribe medication or mechanical devices (catheters for women or condom catheters for men) or even surgical procedures to correct the problem.

A more simple solution is often just to keep a record of when the patient has to go to the bathroom and then, when a pattern has been established, set up a schedule of visits to the bathroom in anticipation of the need to void. This form of bladder training can be quite effective. In addition, there are a variety of disposable briefs and undergarments which, when worn, can provide effective and discrete protection from the embarrassment of an accident (see Chapter 8).

Constipation • Bowel problems that develop with MS usually involve constipation. This can be a serious as well as an uncomfortable situation. A diet high in fiber content will help, as will an increased fluid intake. Stool softeners, laxatives, and suppositories are also available and can help relieve the constipation.

Skin Problems • MS can affect the ability of the individual to move about freely, especially when confined to a wheelchair or to bed for any length of time, or when mobility is restricted to sitting in the family recliner or easy chair for most of the day. In such instances, the patient must be on guard against skin breakdown and the development of pressure sores (see Chapter 10). Areas of the body requiring special attention are the heels, buttocks, elbows, and anywhere a bone projects near the surface of the skin.

Uncertainty and Unpredictability • This is a very stressful area for those with MS. Since the course of the disease is so unpredictable, uncertainty about the future places a heavy emotional load on the individual. There is a feeling of helplessness when trying to plan for the future—there's no way of telling how things will turn out. The best course to take here is to follow the often quoted advice to take each day as it comes. One day at a time can be the immediate goal when stress or depression take hold. Afterward, planning for the future can be looked at sensibly and pragmatically. MS is not a hopeless life sentence. Plan for the future—with flexibility.

Fatigue • Only an MS patient can know the depths of the fatigue that can be reached with this disease. It's something each individual has to learn to live with. There are times when heavy fatigue will hit, even though the individual has done nothing more strenuous than taking a slow walk or even reading a book. What makes matters worse sometimes is that family or friends will look at the person and remark that they cannot understand why he is so tired when he looks so well—thoughtlessly forcing the individual to feel that others think he is faking it and adding to the stress the person already feels.

Four main causes of this fatigue phenomenon have been outlined by Dr. Robert M. Herndon, director of the Center for Brain Research at the University of Rochester in New York:

- Nerves that have had the myelin sheathing damaged require the expenditure of more energy to get the nerve impulses through to the brain or from the brain. The resulting weakness and loss of coordination for the patient can bring on the fatigue.
- Someone with MS will already have some weakened muscles, which will, in turn, put more of a strain on the other muscles, causing fatigue.

- The emotional strain imposed by the depression and frustration to be expected from those with MS takes its toll in the form of fatigue.
- People with MS can have muscle fatigue just as those without the disease can. However, because of the energy expended in fighting MS, "normal" fatigue will hit the MS patient much harder and more frequently.

Perhaps the best way to handle the problem of fatigue is to follow the guidelines for dealing with fatigue presented by the National Multiple Sclerosis Society:

- Don't fight it—work with it.
- Recognize that it's not you; it's the MS.
- Fatigue usually hits hardest in the afternoon. Arrange to do your strenuous activities in the morning.
- Heat affects fatigue. Don't plan too much activity in hot weather.
- Sometimes fatigue can induce depression. There are drugs to help in such a situation.
- Exercising those muscles not affected by MS can help relieve overall fatigue.
- Educate your family and friends about the fatigue factor. Once they understand, you will have new coping allies.

Rehabilitation • Training in the activities of daily living is an important phase of rehabilitation for the MS patient. Rehabilitation goals need to be realistic, yet work to keep the patient as independent as possible and to preserve his sense of dignity. Whether able to walk independently or wheelchair-bound, the MS patient can be taught the techniques necessary to permit the greatest possible function despite the disabling effects of the disease. There are a variety of devices and techniques for use in every room in the house (see Chapter 5) that can make life simpler for the MS patient and promote independence.

Emotional Changes • A disease such as MS brings with it many emotional changes for the individual and his family. Such disturbances of mood and thought can lead to feelings that range from euphoria to depression. In "normal" circumstances, we deal with emotions every day and can experience feeling cheerful, calm, content, displeased, upset, shameful, scared, hopeful, and happy. Each person with MS and his family will find their own ways of responding emotionally to the limitations and uncertainties of the disease.

Support groups and group therapy can be helpful. The person with MS can listen to other people's perceptions of their life styles, with differing values and reference points than his own. Family members can also benefit from participation in groups of their own. This type of therapy can be of great value to all those closely involved with MS.

Perhaps the best advice and guidance that can be given to someone with MS is contained in two brief paragraphs in a booklet entitled "Emotional Aspects of MS," published by the National Multiple Sclerosis Society. They are repeated here with their kind permission:

It seems that people who manage to 'make it' with MS do so in several ways. First, they look into themselves, digging deep to find strength they did not know they had. They come to realize that the process of attaining satisfaction must start with themselves. Secondly, they reach out. Living with this disease requires significant changes in your life and can be a very lonely task. The task may be less lonely if you can talk, really talk, with your family, friends, other people with MS, and with health professionals.

Real talk can provide understanding, suggestions, feedback, and a way to look at and modify your thinking, when necessary. It can facilitate the knowledge that you are involved with the joys and struggles of others and that your life remains part of the whole, part of the shared human experience.

Parkinson's Disease

It used to be known as the shaking palsy—an apt description of one of its symptoms. Now, however, it bears the name of the physician who first described its various manifestations and symptoms as a separate disease and thus paved the way for it to be studied as such.

Parkinson's disease is a disorder of body movement. It's most obvious symptoms are hand tremors, muscular stiffness or rigidity, slowness of movement, and a masklike facial appearance.

Our bodily movements are controlled by opposing muscles that contract and relax in pairs. For example, when you flex your biceps, the contraction of this muscle moves your arm into the familiar "make a muscle" pose. At the same time, the triceps muscle on the underside of your upper arm relaxes. There's a dual muscular activity here: the contraction (or tightening) of one muscle and the coordinated relaxation of the opposing muscle. Your arm could not move without both muscles working in coordination and opposition.

Parkinson's disease attacks that part of the brain (the basal ganglia) that controls the smooth movement and balanced interaction of muscles. Scientists noted that in patients who had Parkinson's for a long time there was a distinct loss of nerve cells (or neurons) in an area of the basal ganglia containing dark-pigmented cells (the substantia nigra). Nerve signals from the brain to the muscles were thought to pass through the substantia nigra and to be subject to its control. A loss of neurons in this area would, therefore, affect these nerve signals, bringing on the muscular problems of parkinsonism.

It was also found that the area of the basal ganglia in parkinsonian patients was deficient in dopamine, a chemical that acted as a neurotransmitter in the brain, transmitting nerve signals from one cell to another. Dopamine is made by the dark-pigmented cells of the substantia nigra, and the loss of these cells in Parkinson's disease causes a subsequent loss of dopamine and the ability of nerve signals to get through to the muscles.

The first signs of Parkinson's disease may appear to be little more than what some people would call aging—some slight hand tremors and a little difficulty in trying to get up from a deep chair after having sat in it for a while. Since Parkinson's usually strikes those in their sixties or older, it would be natural to dismiss early symptoms as part of getting older.

In time, though, the symptoms become much more pronounced until it becomes apparent that this definitely is not a normal part of aging. The tremors increase, the muscular stiffness gets worse, and other symptoms appear, for example, a lack of balance, a "festinating" gait (taking short, accelerated steps), a loss of facial expression because of muscle rigidity, and an inability to start movements (bradykinesia), causing the individual to "freeze" on the spot.

Physicians can often spot the early symptoms of Parkinson's disease before the individual is aware of them. A young doctor just completing his military service came home on leave to visit his parents. Having just treated several parkinsonian patients in a veterans' hospital, he was more than usually aware of the symptoms of Parkinson's disease. He wasn't quite sure, but he thought he detected just a trace of a shuffling, hurried gait in his father as he walked behind him. To be on the safe side, he arranged for a complete physical and neurological examination of his father. The diagnosis was Parkinson's, and they were able to start early treatment and therapy for his father.

Although tremors had not yet appeared in the doctor's father, they would likely develop in the future, as about two-thirds of those with Parkinson's disease are afflicted with them. Tremors, or involuntary shaking, seem most disturbing to the parkinsonian individual. One peculiar characteristic of these tremors is that they become more severe when attempting to rest the hands. The tremors are not as pronounced during purposeful movements, but when the individual is advised to relax or when there is an attempt made to rest the hands, the tremors increase.

Along with the tremors, the festinating gait seems to cause much difficulty for parkinsonian individuals. It's difficult, and sometimes impossible, to engage in normal activities of daily living—reading a newspaper or window shopping, for example—when your hands are shaking severely and you have to lean forward and shuffle hurriedly along in order to maintain your balance.

It has been estimated that Parkinson's disease affects about 1 person in 100 over the age of fifty. Moreover, since people are living longer and Parkinson's is not usually terminal, the actual numbers of those with this disease will accumulate and increase. Present estimates are that there are close to half a million Parkinson patients in North America.

The cause of Parkinson's disease is yet to be found. Although most cases of parkinsonism fall into the category of "idiopathic" diseases (no known cause), there are illnesses and conditions that "mimic" parkinsonism and have similar symptoms. For example, the use of the tranquilizers Compazine or Thorazine can sometimes cause the muscular rigidity symptoms of Parkinson's disease. These symptoms disappear, however, when the medication is discontinued.

A more puzzling aspect of the appearance of Parkinson's symptoms occurred during the 1920s, when many people feel victim to encephalitis, commonly called sleeping sickness. Some of those who survived the illness later developed Parkinson's disease, usually at a much younger age than was to be expected in the normal population.

Also, in another form of encephalitis that broke out during World War I, some of those who survived had to be placed in insititutions because they were seemingly permanently "asleep," unable to function or communicate. The fact that they showed symptoms of Parkinson's disease was noted, but nothing could be done to help them. Then, in 1969, the newly discovered drug L-dopa, or levodopa, as it's also called, which was being used to treat Parkinson's disease (more on this later), was tried on those encephalitis victims still alive and still in an institution.

The results were nothing short of miraculous—for a time. The administration of L-dopa to the patients brought them out of their decades-long sleep. They began to function, to speak, to walk about, to communicate with others. But then, trouble set in. Emotionally, many of the patients were not prepared for this type of awakening. There was withdrawal into a trancelike state in one instance, and in others there was unrestrained frenzy. Apparently, the reactions were caused by both the L-dopa and the emotional trauma of the sudden reawakening.

These incidents emphasize the fact that research is still ongoing.

Progress has been made in treating the symptoms of Parkinson's disease. The cause—and an eventual cure—still have to be found.

Medication and exercise are the two mainstays of treatment for Parkinson's disease. Physicians and therapists have at their disposal many medications and many therapeutic exercise techniques to aid the Parkinson patient.

MEDICATION

One of the most effective medications used in treating the symptoms of Parkinson's disease is L-dopa, or levodopa, as it's often called. This drug, first used in treatment of parkinsonism in 1967, is a natural substance found in the body. The most common brand names of the prescription drugs containing levodopa are Sinemet and Larodopa.

Levodopa, when administered in large doses, helps increase the amount of dopamine in the brain. With an increased level of dopamine, a significant number of patients experience a reduction of the tremors, rigidity, and immobility (bradykinesia) associated with Parkinson's disease. Before the advent of levodopa, no other medication had been successful in reducing bradykinesia.

As effective as levodopa is, certain precautions have to be taken. Undesirable side effects can include nausea, dizziness, and abnormal involuntary movements (dyskinesia), in which the patient experiences uncontrolled facial grimaces, tongue movements, and involuntary jerky movements of the neck, shoulders, arms, and leg. Since these undesirable effects depend upon the amount of levodopa taken, physicians usually start the patient off on small doses and gradually build up the dosage until the patient's body has become accustomed to the medication.

Researchers reasoned that these side effects were being experienced because the levodopa was stimulating the production of dopamine in other areas of the body before reaching the brain. They found that by adding another drug—carbidopa—the action of the levodopa could be focused more directly on the brain. Carbidopa was added to the levodopa in Sinemet, and the troubling side effects were reduced, especially the nausea.

One of the side effects that may be experienced with the use of levodopa is a darkening of the urine and sweat. Urine will be reddish at first, then turn black when exposed to air. This side effect is not harmful and need not cause any concern.

Vitamin B_6 (pyridoxine) in large amounts can reduce the effectiveness of levodopa. If you are taking vitamins, check with your pharmacist and your physician on how to avoid taking too much of this vitamin.

Although some physicians have recommended dietary restrictions to avoid foods with a high content of pyridoxine (bacon, beans, beef liver, and peas, for example), the general consensus is that a normal, well-balanced, nutritious diet will present no problems in this respect.

Other medications being used along with levodopa to combat the symptoms of Parkinson's disease are known as anticholinergic drugs (drugs that act on specific parts of the nervous system), which help reduce the tremors and rigidity. Trade names for these drugs are Artane, Kemadrin, Cogentin, and Pagitane. Side effects of anticholinergic drugs can include dryness of the mouth, constipation, blurred vision, and an increase in the effects of glaucoma, if already present in the Parkinson patient.

Antihistamines, especially Benadryl, can be of some help in reducing tremors. Also, they can act as mild sedatives where needed.

Amantadine hydrochloride (brand name, Symmetrel), a drug used to treat virus infections, has been found to reduce some of the tremors, rigidity, and bradykinesia. However, the benefits of using this drug may decrease after it has been taken for three to six months.

Obviously, your physician is the best judge of which drugs to use and how to use them most effectively.

Continued use of large doses of levodopa can lead to what is known as the on-off phenomenon. This can occur after about three to five years of successful levodopa medication. The symptoms of Parkinson's suddenly seem to switch on and off, often within a matter of hours. Where the individual may have been progressing and functioning well for some time, the abrupt reversal brought about by the on-off reaction will suddenly plunge the individual into rigid helplessness, or perhaps the jerky, uncontrolled movements of dyskinesia will take over. Conversely, the individual who has been having difficulty reducing the symptoms of parkinsonism may suddenly find himself free of them—only to have them reappear a short while later. The effect on the individual can be highly disruptive and emotionally devastating.

Current thinking holds that the on-off effect is caused by the length of time the patient has been taking medication, rather than by a natural progression of the disease. Accordingly, many physicians now do not prescribe levodopa at the beginning of treatment for Parkinson's disease, especially if the symptoms are not too severe.

Another method physicians use to deal with the on-off reaction is to place the patient on a "drug holiday." In this procedure, the patient is put in the hospital for from three to seven days, during which no levodopa is administered. Hospitalization is necessary because the patient has to be watched closely and monitored on a regular basis to make sure there are no unexpected ill effects from the withdrawal of levodopa. Special attention is given to any breathing difficulties the patient may have if the disease has progressed to the point where the breathing muscles have been affected.

To ease the transition to complete withdrawal of levodopa, the physician might gradually reduce the dosage of levodopa for a period

Table 22 ■ ANTIPARKINSONISM DRUGS

Generic names	Brand names[a]	Usage information / precautions[b]
Levodopa Levodopa and Carbidopa	Bendopa, Dopur, Larodopa, Levopa Sinemet	Take with liquid or food to lessen stomach irritation • Take at same time each day • Takes 2–3 weeks to see improvement from drug • Takes 6 weeks or longer for maximum benefit • Prolonged use may lead to uncontrolled movements of head, face, mouth, tongue, arms or legs *Overdose symptoms:* muscle twitch, spastic eyelid closure, nausea, vomiting, diarrhea, rapid pulse, weakness, fainting, confusion, hallucination, coma
Benztrophine Biperidine, Ethopropazine Procyclidine Trihexyphenidyl	Bensylate, Cogentin Akineton Parsidol, Parsitan Kemadrin Aparkane, Artane, Tremin	Take with food to lessen stomach irritation • Take at same time each day • Takes 1 to 2 hours to work after taken • Prolonged use may cause glaucoma • May cause impaired thinking, hallucinations, nightmares in people over 60 • Don't drive until you learn how the drug affects you • Internal eye pressure should be measured regularly • May aggravate symptoms of enlarged prostate *Overdose symptoms:* agitation, dilated pupils, hallucinations, dry mouth, rapid heartbeat, sleepiness

[a]These brand names are only a sampling. Several generics reviewed are available under additional names not listed here.
[b]Check with your doctor for specific directions and precautions when taking these and any other medications.

of time before finally stopping it completely when the patient is put into the hospital. Whatever procedure is followed, the patient has to be closely followed by the physician.

The drug holiday is not an easy time for the Parkinson patient. During the time the patient is completely without levodopa, there can be an opportunity for rehabiliation therapy (physical, occupational, and

---

Possible side effects[c]

Common: mood changes, uncontrolled
body movements, dry mouth, diarrhea, body odor
Infrequent: fainting, severe dizziness,
headache, insomnia, nightmares,
flushed face, skin rash, blurred vision,
constipation, nausea, vomiting, irregular heartbeat, muscle twitching,
dark urine, difficult urination, tiredness
Rare: duodenal ulcer, anemia, high
blood pressure

Common: blurred vision, constipation,
nausea, vomiting, difficult or painful
urination
Rare: confusion, dizziness, skin rash,
eye pain, sore mouth or tongue, muscle cramps, numbness, weakness in
hands or feet

---

[c]This does not list all of the possible side effects. Check with your doctor regarding safety and possible side effects when taking these and or any other medications.
Source: H. Winter Griffith, M.D., *Complete Guide to Prescription Drugs* (Tucson: HP Books, 1983).

speech therapy) to assist the patient in coping with the withdrawal of the medication. At the end of the period, a new dosage of levodopa has to be worked out with the physician, and in some cases a lower dosage will be found to be effective.

One other problem associated with taking certain medications over a long period of time is what is known as end-of-dose akinesia. When this occurs, the usual dose of levodopa the patient has been taking is effective for only three to four hours. The unpleasant symptoms of parkinsonism return in full force, especially the problem of "freezing" and being unable to move. The drug holiday, involving complete withdrawal of the levodopa, is usually the treatment recommended by the physician in this case.

Bear in mind that medication for Parkinson's disease is "symptomatic" and not "curative." There is no medication required or available to slow down the progress of the disease, as there is for diabetes or hypertension, for example. Levodopa and all the other medications are used to treat the *symptoms* of parkinsonism, and if a particular drug is seen not to be effective, it can be withdrawn and another drug tried. In the case of levodopa, of course, the withdrawal is only temporary to combat the on-off and end-of-dose akinesia reactions.

See Table 22 for a list of the most frequently used medications for Parkinson's disease.

EXERCISE: AN ABSOLUTE NECESSITY

An active physical therapy program, although customized to meet the specific needs of the Parkinson patient, will include therapeutic exercises to maintain the full range of motion in the joints. Active exercises (performed by the patient) and passive exercises (performed by the therapist on the patient) will help prevent stiffness and contractures (shortening of muscles) and will, by stretching the muscles, help overcome any rigidity that is already present.

"Gait training," which emphasizes and encourages the patient to walk with a heel-toe foot placement, coupled with a natural arm swing for better balance control, is an important aspect of physical therapy. Because parkinsonian patients often have difficulty with balance, learning to control the distribution of body weight will help prevent falls (a serious problem, discussed later in this section).

Because of the way Parkinson's disease affects the muscles, it is vitally important that the patient exercise regularly under a planned program. If muscles are not kept in tone through regular exercise, the rigidity that Parkinson's disease produces will soon take over the muscles and render them useless. A muscle that cannot be used means a part of the body that cannot function—the arms, the legs, the breathing muscles, for example. When enough body parts cannot function, the individual can become virtually completely paralyzed.

Exercises do not necessarily involve the kind of conventional "calisthenic" movements most of us are familiar with. In parkinsonism, for example, facial exercises are necessary to prevent the rigid, masklike, expressionless appearance that can result from muscle problems. These facial exercises are simple and can include wriggling your nose, opening your mouth as wide as you can, whistling, puffing out your cheeks, raising and lowering your eyebrows, and wrinkling your forehead. These types of exercises may seem much too easy for "normal" individuals; however they are not always easy for the parkinsonian patient to perform. Nevertheless, they are an absolute necessity—as are all other exercises for the parkinsonian—and must not be neglected.

Other exercises can include neck rotation, simple arm and leg movements from a sitting, standing, or lying down position, coughing exercises, muscle stretching, and flexing of knees and elbows, wrists and ankles, toes and fingers. Using a cane or an ordinary stick, the parkinsonian can perform a number of more vigorous exercises, grasping the cane or stick in both hands and raising it over his head, then lowering it, moving it from side to side, and going through many different motions that will keep muscles flexible.

Many of these exercises are performed as part of a group program. Group physical therapy is an excellent way for the parkinsonian to exercise. He or she is with others who have similar problems and difficulties with the same disease; there's a lack of self-consciousness; a spirit of group cooperation and group endeavor prevails; and the exercise program can become one of pleasurable associations rather than an onerous chore.

OCCUPATIONAL THERAPY

Physical and occupational therapists often work together to help the parkinsonian patient, concentrating on teaching the patient the tricks of the trade to help him initiate movement and foster independence. Activities such as getting in and out of a chair or bed, stepping off a curb and crossing the street, sliding into the front or back seat of a car, and walking up and down stairs are all vital tasks necessary to maintaining independence. These tasks can be made easier and safer under the watchful eyes and practical assistance of both physical and occupational therapists.

The occupational therapist will also guide the patient and provide training for the activities of daily living that require a finer degree of motor coordination—toileting, shaving, bathing, dressing, maneuvering safely around the house. These are all voluntary and purposeful activities, and a better understanding of "body mechanics" will help make these tasks easier for the parkinsonian to perform.

Both the physical therapist and the occupational therapist may set up programs requiring the patient to practice each day at home. Practicing the activities of daily living and performing the exercises designed to allow these activities to be accomplished are necessary tasks if the patient is to maintain independence and prevent muscle rigidity and immobility from developing. The more the patient keeps active, the better will be the quality of life preserved.

SPEECH THERAPY

Muscles are used in generating speech, the primary form of communication among people. Practice and therapeutic exercises that maintain flexibility and mobility of the lips and the tongue can make the Parkinson patient more aware of the muscles of speech.

The speech pathologist may find that special exercises are needed to allow the patient to coordinate breathing and talking. Otherwise, the individual might "run out of air" before completing a word or phrase. Voice practice helps in attempting to increase loudness and to vary the tone of voice. Some people with Parkinson's have difficulty making themselves heard. If the person's natural speech is affected by the disease to such a degree that it is too low for the average person to hear, the speech pathologist may suggest the use of a special electronic device that will amplify the sound of the parkinsonian's speech.

Constant practice of specific words and phrases selected by the speech pathologist will help the parkinsonian patient to maintain the ability to speak and thus effectively communicate with those around him.

COMMON PROBLEMS AND SOME SOLUTIONS

Difficulty in Walking • The Parkinson patient can experience difficulty not only in walking but also in taking the first step. This "freezing" can occur when the person comes to a door or some other "obstacle" or even a line drawn on the floor. Crowds, doorways, turns around corners—all these and similar conditions can cause the parkinsonian much difficulty. Often, no movement at all can be made, not even to get started, and even when some movement is possible, it's slow and uncertain.

Adding to the difficulty will be expressions of undue concern by family or friends accompanying the patient. This only makes the problem worse. A gentle offer of support—often no more than just taking the patient's hand—may be all that is necessary to get the person started moving again.

Parkinson patients are usually reminded to take large steps to maintain balance and to keep the feet apart. Also, they are instructed to use the heel-toe style of walking—hitting the ground with the heel first and then rolling to the toe before lifting the foot for the next step.

Fear of Falling • For many Parkinson patients, the fear of falling is a very real fear—and a justified one. This fear is often a result of a partial loss of balancing reflexes coupled with difficulty in raising each foot from the floor when walking.

By keeping the feet wide apart, the individual will have a broader base of support and should feel more secure. Above all, the person is warned never to cross one foot in front of the other when turning a corner, as this may result in a fall.

As with all other activities, practice is necessary—and then more practice. The parkinsonian can never take movement for granted. It cannot be as automatic as it is for those not afflicted with this disease. The parkinsonian has to develop a way of thinking that will keep the various movements involved in everyday activities always uppermost in his mind. He will have to concentrate on each movement, step by step.

As a further precaution against falling, the home can be set up to make each room as safe as possible for the Parkinson's patient who, because of the disease, will be slow-moving and unsteady on his feet.

The first thing to do is to make sure the patient will have secure footing underneath, and this means getting rid of all scatter rugs, runners, and any other loose rugs on the floor. If the floor is covered with carpeting, make sure it's flat and well secured, with no buckled portions sticking up to trip the patient.

If possible, have all doorsills removed and the space filled in and made smooth and level. A carpenter or a home handyman can do this with little difficulty. A raised doorsill, even one a couple of inches high, can become a major obstacle for the parkinsonian and represents a hazard that might cause a fall. Of course, if you live in an apartment and not your own home, removing the doorsills might not be possible. It might be best, then, to place grab bars alongside each doorway to enable the patient to hold on to something secure while he attempts to get over the doorsill.

Installing grab bars or sturdy wooden rails on the walls adjacent to a door is a good idea for another reason also. If the patient has to reach for a doorknob to open a door, he may be even more off balance than usual. Having a grab bar or a wooden rail on the wall near the doorknob will enable the patient to hold on to the bar or rail with one hand while he opens the door with the other hand. In this way, he can maintain balance and will not be thrown backward if the door should open more smoothly than he expected.

Dangerous furniture should be removed or put out of the way. This means any tables or chairs or other pieces of furniture with sharp edges or projecting corners will have to be removed or relocated in the room to minimize any accidental contact by the patient. The room doesn't have to be bare, of course, but the goal should be to make everything as level and as easy to navigate as possible.

It would also be a good idea to remove or relocate any fragile items that could be knocked over or broken by an unsteady parkinsonian.

If the patient has to use a stairway, make sure it's secure and steady and, if possible, have rails installed on both sides. If the stairway has to be used frequently on a daily basis, it may become necessary to install an elevator chair on the stairs that the patient can use.

Managing a Chair • An ordinary chair that most of us take for granted can represent a trying experience for someone with Parkinson's disease. Sitting down safely and then getting up again requires effort as well as a special technique.

In sitting down, the best procedure is for the patient to approach the chair as closely as possible, then turn so the backs of his knees touch the chair seat. From this position, the patient should bend his body sharply forward while placing his hands on the arms or seat of the chair, whichever is most convenient, and then slowly lower himself to a sitting position on the chair.

In getting up from the chair, it would be helpful if the back legs of the chair could have been extended or securely propped up on a heavy board so that the chair is tilted slightly forward. Such a chair arrangement will be very helpful to the parkinsonian, but it absolutely must be solid and secure.

It's not a good idea to have someone pull the patient up out of the chair. It's better to have the patient push himself up from the edge of the chair. If any help is needed, it will generally involve only placing a supporting hand on the patient's upper back as he rises from the chair.

Getting out of Bed • After a night's sleep, the Parkinson patient may find that stiffness and rigidity greet him in the morning, making getting out of bed a formidable task. One technique the patient can use is to extend his arms and legs to start a rocking back-and-forth motion until he can rock himself to the edge of the bed. Then, rolling to one side and extending his feet over the edge of the mattress, the patient can use his hand on the mattress edge for leverage and push himself into an upright sitting position.

If this type of movement is not possible, there are devices that can be used to help in getting out of bed. A triangular trapeze arrangement over the head of the bed can be used to help the patient pull himself to a sitting position. Or, if the trapeze installation is not feasible, a pull rope with one end fastened to the foot of the bed and the other end clipped to the bedcovers near the patient's hand can be used. The end near the patient's hand should have a strong loop or a sturdy ring for the patient to grasp as he pulls himself upright.

Using the Bathroom • Safety measures are critically important in the bathroom. Chapter 5 of this book covers many devices and techniques that can be used as aids in getting around in the bathroom. For the parkinsonian, who will be fighting against stiffness and muscle rigidity, one of the most important aids will be a raised toilet seat with safety rails around the unit. Sitting down on a toilet seat and getting up again later is a bit different from sitting in a regular chair in the living room. The raised seat and the safety rails will help make the task easier.

In the bathtub, a strategically located grab bar and a tub bench will enable the parkinsonian patient to get into the tub with a minimum of difficulty. A flexible hose with a showerhead (sometimes called a showerall) will be useful in allowing the patient to shower while sitting down on the tub bench. If a stall shower is used, grab bars, a stool, and a flexible showerall will also do the trick.

As mentioned, Chapter 5 lists many devices that can be used by the Parkinson patient in performing the necessary toileting, washing, and grooming activities normally carried on in the bathroom. These devices will aid the patient in maintaining the precious commodity of personal independence—which is especially important in the bathroom.

Clothing • The Parkinson patient's wardrobe should be checked for items that will be very difficult for the patient to put on. Whenever possible, these items should be replaced with something better suited to the needs of the patient. For example, tying shoelaces can be an almost impossible task for someone who cannot bend too far forward or who lacks finger dexterity (people with arthritis will have the same problem). The difficulty can be resolved by wearing shoes that do not have laces or, if laces are desired for the sake of style or fashion, elastic laces can be substituted.

For women, dresses that zip down the front are preferable to dresses that have to be put on over the head. Girdles and other difficult undergarments should be avoided whenever possible.

For both men and women, flared pants are preferable to tapered ones, which can present problems in being slipped on over the feet.

Men can use shirts that do not require a necktie. If one has to be worn, the clip-on type can be used.

In many instances, Velcro closures can be substituted for buttons and zippers. Do not hesitate to make any wardrobe changes that will make dressing easier. Chapter 5 lists many devices that can be used in this respect.

Living in a warmer climate, although it has no influence on the disease, does allow the parkinsonian to enjoy the outdoors with less bulky clothing. A word of caution, though: Patients with heavy tremors expend a lot of energy and tend to suffer in hot and humid weather because of all the physical activity involved. Light clothing is a must in this case, and the best thing, of course, is to avoid going outside on a very hot, muggy day.

Nutrition and Diet • The act of eating—lifting the fork or spoon to the mouth—can be extremely difficult for the Parkinson patient. Caregivers and patients should make sure that enough time is allotted for eating and that proper equipment (knives, forks, and spoons with built-up handles, for example) is available.

Overweight individuals should reduce to the proper weight for their height and sex, since the more weight that has to be carried around, the greater the difficulty in moving about. There's no point in adding to the problem of muscle stiffness by putting the burden of excess weight on those muscles.

Underweight individuals should eat a well-balanced nutritious diet and gain the necessary weight to maintain health and strength. Lack of strength will only increase the difficulty of moving about with stiffened muscles.

People with Parkinson's will tend to eat considerably slower than other people. An aware family will allow enough time together at the table so that the parkinsonian will not feel isolated and shunned as he or she attempts to finish the meal alone. Social companionship, especially that of family members, is important during a meal. At least one, and preferably two family members should remain at the table with the patient until the meal is finished.

Since food will tend to get cold the longer it takes to eat it, an electric warmer will help keep the parkinsonian's food warm throughout the meal.

Constipation • This can be a problem for those with Parkinson's disease. Some of the medications used to treat the symptoms of the disease can cause constipation as a side effect. There are several simple and effective techniques that can be employed to counter constipation.

Drinking at least six glasses of water a day will help maintain a good fluid intake. (This is in addition to the normal consumption of coffee, tea, milk, and fruit and vegetable juices.) Increasing the fruits and fibers in the diet and getting regular exercise will also help. Agents that add bulk to the stool can be taken, as well as a mild laxative (milk of magnesia) or a stool softener.

A daily bowel movement is not a must. Each person will establish his or her own pattern of bowel movements. If constipation becomes a serious problem, it would be best to consult a physician since the cause of the severe constipation may be something other than Parkinson's disease.

Psychological Problems • Patients with Parkinson's disease not only will experience difficulty in moving and communicating with others but also will often find that they have now become heavily dependent on others—especially a wife or husband or other family members. This situation can and often does bring on depression.

Along with the depression can come an aggravation and a magnification of the symptoms of Parkinson's disease. Rigidity, slowness of movement, and all the other aspects of the disease will be intensified. If this happens, professional help should be sought. Consult first with your physician, who will probably be able to recommend a psychologist or other professional who can provide helpful counseling. It's important not to ignore depression when it appears. If not treated it can, in its own way, be much more destructive than Parkinson's disease itself.

Do not confuse depression with the "flattening" of the emotional expression seen on the face of a Parkinson patient. The loss of flexibility and the rigidity of some of the facial muscles create an expressionless appearance on the faces of many parkinsonians. In our society, such a lack of apparent emotion or expression signifies a depressed person, dull and lacking in alertness. This is not necessarily true. The person may not be at all depressed and certainly is alert. What the outside world sees on the Parkinson patient's face may just be his "normal," at rest look.

There may be cognitive problems for some people with Parkinson's disease; however, there is no reason to suppose that the majority of parkinsonians have experienced any decline in intellectual capabilities.

There are intellectual and emotional problems, though. Even with medication, many patients still retain some of the symptoms of the disease and are frustrated by their inability to do all that they would like to do. At best, this can cause the person to be irritable and impatient with himself and the world around him. At worst, it can bring on depression.

It is not uncommon to find that Parkinson patients experience unwanted symptoms and do tend to develop a pattern of dependency. This dependency can grow, creating its own set of problems—and then the whole situation can be turned around if new medication and therapy prove successful in eliminating most of the symptoms of the disease.

In such cases, the patients and their caretakers have to learn new patterns of living together, undoing what may have been years of dependency. Not only does the Parkinson patient have to readjust to renewed capabilities but the family now has to readjust to the appearance of a new and more capable person. In effect, the old person has returned to some extent, which can make the situation even more confusing.

The recent availability of new medications that work to reduce symptoms and, in turn, restore function will cause the patient to require professional assistance in coping with the restored physical ability. With proper physical therapy, muscle tone will normalize gradually and strength will return. It will require concentration and effort, but it will be a happy effort.

Keeping Active • Whether new medication restores function or the Parkinson patient is at a plateau with some symptoms still remaining, it's important to remain as physically active as possible. Inactivity can only worsen immobility.

The activities involved in dressing, preparing food, writing, walking, playing a musical instrument, gardening, seeking out new hobbies, and keeping physically and mentally in tone in general, are all necessary for maintaining flexibility and retaining personal independence.

The more the Parkinson patient can do on his or her own, the better for all concerned. However, this does not mean that assistance must never be solicited or offered. There are times when it's best for family and friends to sit on their hands and let the parkinsonian manage as best as he or she can. At other times, there's nothing wrong in extending a helping hand—or in asking for one.

Keeping busy and active requires effort on the part of the patient and understanding on the part of family and friends. The parkinsonian individual should be included in family activities and outings as much as possible. Where recreation and social activities are concerned, the patient should not hold back for fear of people staring. At movies, theaters, ball games, and concerts, the patrons will be more concerned with the event than with noticing parkinsonian tremors or momentary freezing.

If crowds present a problem, arrive early and leave after the crowd has departed. Look for ways to do what is desired rather than for reasons not to do anything at all.

Of course, not everything can be accomplished. A Parkinson patient with poor balance should not attempt to ski, for example, or to do anything that might endanger his health or safety. Within these limitations, however, the parkinsonian can venture off on his own and seek out new activities and scenes.

Travel is not forbidden. If there's some doubt in the patient's mind about being able to get around without difficulty, he can take along a friend or family member and try a short bus ride around town. He'll soon find that, despite some difficulties, the planned activity is not only possible but enjoyable—and educational as well. The parkinsonian will learn, for example, that when taking a bus ride it's better to sit on the driver's side. Because of the way roads are crowned and then slope to the curb, the bus will be slightly higher on the driver's side when he pulls to the curb. Thus, the parkinsonian will have gravity giving him a slight boost when he has to stand to get off the bus.

Sticking to Routine • There's nothing wrong with a Parkinson patient being adventuresome, but sober reflection will indicate that certain routines and procedures have to be followed. Exercises have to be performed regularly, medications have to be taken on schedule, and doctor's advice cannot be ignored.

Routine is important—and working closely with the doctor is equally as important. The parkinsonian's physician should be kept informed of all developments that might affect treatment. In this respect, it would be a good idea for the Parkinson patient to keep notes, perhaps in the form of a daily journal in which can be noted exercise routines and schedules, progress made, setbacks encountered, problems that have come up, possible side effects of the medication—anything and everything that will record what has happened. This journal will prove to be an invaluable tool for the patient and the physician when discussing the patient's progress and possible new treatments.

Feelings and Resources • After a lifetime of moving at will and with ease, it is natural for the Parkinson patient to become upset when that freedom and control of movement is reduced. Feelings of denial, of anger, of depression may occur. Fearing pity from other people, some parkinsonians may withdraw from social interaction. Others may lose interest in the world around them.

A booklet, *The Parkinson's Patient,* available from the National

Parkinson Foundation (see the Appendix), gives a compelling answer to the Parkinson patient who may be experiencing these negative feelings: "It takes time to accept the fact that you have Parkinson's disease and to learn how best to live with it. Try gradually to take a new view of things—to be flexible in your everyday activities and not make unnecessary demands on yourself."

Support groups and information exchanges can be a real help. The National Parkinson Foundation (1-800-327-4545) has a list of Parkinson's patient support groups throughout the country. The Parkinson's Educational Program PEPUSA (714-640-0218) has been formed to spearhead the effort to form support groups.

These organizations and other foundations, associations, and voluntary agencies publish a number of excellently written and informative booklets and pamphlets concerning Parkinson's disease. Some of them are listed below. Check the Appendix for additional information, addresses, and telephone numbers.

From the AMERICAN PARKINSON DISEASE ASSOCIATION:
　　"Aids, Equipment, and Suggestions to Help the Patient with Parkinson's Disease in the Activities of Daily Living"
　　"Home Exercises for Patients with Parkinson's Disease"
　　"A Manual for Patients with Parkinson's Disease"
　　"Speech Problems and Swallowing Problems in Parkinson's Disease"

From the NATIONAL INSTITUTES OF HEALTH:
　　"Parkinson's Disease: Hope Through Research"

From the NATIONAL PARKINSON FOUNDATION:
　　"The Parkinson Handbook"
　　"The Parkinson's Patient: What You and Your Family Should Know"

From the PARKINSON'S DISEASE FOUNDATION:
　　"Exercises for the Parkinson Patient with Hints for Daily Living"
　　"The Parkinson Patient at Home"
　　PEP Exchange (newsletter)

From the UNITED PARKINSON FOUNDATION:
　　"One Step at a Time"

Spinal Cord Injuries

They are mostly young; their backgrounds are different; the endings of their stories are tragically similar:

- We were driving home from a party off-campus. My date fell asleep at the wheel. I survived the crash . . . as a paraplegic confined to a wheelchair.

- I was a quarterback for a pro football team. During the second half of a big game, I was sacked as I faded back to pass. They had to carry me off the field. I couldn't move. My arms and legs were completely numb.
- My partner and I were working on the thirty-second floor of a new building going up on Madison Avenue. My partner asked me for a wrench. I started walking the beam to hand it to him. A sudden gust of wind hit me, and I lost my footing. I fell and hit the extended boom of a crane three floors below. It saved my life, but snapped my spine.

Each year about ten thousand healthy people, two-thirds of them under thirty, most of them men, have to deal with the sudden and overwhelming problems associated with spinal cord injury. These injuries often result from motor vehicle accidents, are sports-related, or involve accidents around the home or on the job. Their impact is profound and their effects last a lifetime.

THE SPINAL CORD: THE BODY'S COMMUNICATION LINK

The spinal cord, approximately two feet long and composed essentially of nerve cells and long nerve fibers, extends from the brain to the lower back inside the spinal column. Together, the brain and the spinal cord make up the body's central nervous system. Messages—nerve impulses or signals—travel up and down the spinal cord, relaying information to the brain about what is happening to the body and sending messages back from the brain instructing the muscles and organs of the body how to react or how to function in response to a particular set of conditions.

For example, in the case of the football quarterback mentioned earlier, his brain was actively receiving signals telling him what was happening to his body during the attempted pass play. His brain was assessing the positioning of his arms and legs, the feel of the ball in his hands, the way his body was leaning, the tension in his muscles—all the myriad sensations his nerve cells were picking up and relaying to his brain. In turn, his brain was sending back movement messages to muscles all over his body, since the activity he was engaged in affected almost all parts of his body, and messages were also going to his organs, releasing hormones (adrenaline) and other secretions to facilitate his actions.

The sudden onslaught of the opposing defense team accidentally, but permanently, cut off the two-way message traffic in his spinal cord. He was paralyzed.

Normally, the spinal cord is well protected by the bones (the ver-

tebrae) of the spinal column (the backbone), as well as being surrounded by a strong membrane (the dura) and cushioned by a fluid (the
cerebrospinal fluid) that helps absorb shocks. All this protection, however, is sometimes not enough when an accident causes a sharp, sudden, and heavy impact against the spinal column.

Injury to the nerve fibers of the spinal cord—whether cut, bruised,
or otherwise damaged—interrupts the free flow of signals from the body
to the brain and from the brain back to the body. When the messages
of sensation being sent to the brain, or movement instruction messages
sent back from the brain, are blocked from reaching their destinations,
there is a resultant loss of feeling and an inability to move.

WHEN THE SPINAL CORD IS INJURED

The extent of the injury (or how "high," as therapists often refer to
it) depends on the point of injury to the spinal cord. If the injury occurs
at the neck (the cervical area), then most of the two-way communication between brain and body may be disrupted. Paralysis may occur in
both arms and legs, although shoulder and upper arm movement may
be present to some extent. When this happens, the person involved is
known as a quadriplegic. In addition to not being able to move his arms
and legs, he also may be unable to sense whether or not his skin is hot
or cold, or know what his body is actually touching, or be aware of the
position of his arms and legs.

If the injury occurs lower down on the spinal cord, for example at
chest level (the thoracic area), the paralysis and loss of sensation may
affect only the lower parts of his body, including the legs. The individual is then known as a paraplegic.

Although paralysis is instant following a spinal cord injury,
researchers have found that the actual destruction of the nerve tissue
in the spinal cord occurs from four to six hours after the injury itself
occurs. The swelling and bleeding following the trauma are the culprits
that cause the gap in nerve fibers in the spinal cord.

Researchers are experimenting with steroids and other drugs to
determine whether the effects of the spinal cord injury can be contained. Studies are being conducted to explore a variety of treatments
that can be attempted during those first few critical hours after the
spinal cord is injured: use of experimental drugs (to block possible shock
to the spinal cord); cooling the cord (to slow down metabolism and perhaps avoid tissue damage); and surgery (to reduce swelling and relieve
pressure on the spinal cord). Although these experiments may not
directly help the more than 200,000 people now living with spinal cord
injury in the United States, scientists are hopeful that a way may be
found to prevent total paralysis for future victims of this disabling injury.

The break in communications between the brain and the body, below the point of the spinal cord injury, can cause problems and disabilities far beyond the loss of mobility. Voluntary control of bowel and bladder functions often are affected. Sexual functioning can be affected, depending on the extent of the injury and the emotional state of the victim.

Loss of the sensations of pressure and pain removes an important self-protection safety mechanism. Reflexive reactions to discomfort or danger are impaired, and serious injury can result from the individual not being aware of potential harm to his body from, for example, a hot stove or a protruding nail. Skin irritations, pressure sores, and ulcers also can loom as possible problems.

Additionally, individuals with spinal cord injury may be more susceptible to urinary infections, respiratory disorders, and gastrointestinal problems. Genital sensation and sexual function may be impaired.

Overall, the readjustment to the sudden and complete change of bodily ability and function can require massive reorientation of goals, priorities, and emotional responses.

THE LONG ROAD BACK

The resourcefulness and inner strength of the great majority of young people with spinal cord injuries can be seen in the effort they put into rehabilitation therapy and the adjustments they make in their emotional outlook and life styles. They learn to use the abilities they still have to live as independently as possible.

Help for them comes first from special rehabilitation facilities that provide physical therapy, occupational therapy, vocational therapy, and psychological support, once the acute stage of trauma has passed. At these facilities, therapists and patients work together to maintain and build strength in unaffected muscles and to practice the skills needed for independent living, despite the physical limitations with which they have to cope.

Special training is provided in the techniques of getting in and out of bed, using a wheelchair, dressing, grooming, and performing all the various tasks of daily living. (See Chapter 5 for tips on how to manage these tasks.) Special adaptive equipment may be recommended, depending on the task to be performed and the abilities of the individual. Some of the equipment used may consist of simple gadgets; other equipment will utilize recent developments in computer technology and microminiaturization (See Tables 9–15 in Chapter 5.)

Much of the complex technology that is available has been developed in consultation with the major rehabilitation facilities throughout North America. Voice-controlled devices and "sip and puff" units assist the quadriplegic to use specially adapted appliances, telephones, and other devices and aids necessary for daily living, thus removing his dependence on others for assistance.

Before some of these aids can be used effectively, the disabled person has to be trained to live in the so-called normal world. Months of rehabilitation training may follow a spinal cord injury. Depending on the level of spinal involvement and the extent of the injury, as well as the kind of work the patient will have to do and the kind of life he will lead, special training will be provided, for example, in using a car that has had the gas pedal, the brakes, or the steering wheel specially adapted for use by a disabled person. It takes much practice and training for the individual to learn how to use this type of car, as well as how to transfer to it from a wheelchair and then back to the wheelchair again when the destination is reached.

To help the individual muster his inner strength for the task of achieving recovery and independence, the rehabilitation center may offer a one-to-one session with a former patient now living independently. Or support groups may be organized to promote the exchange of feelings and to give the opportunity for members of the recovering group and their families to help each other.

GOING HOME

The goal of the rehabilitation center is to get the patient back home and functioning independently. The staff and the patient work toward this goal with care and with extensive planning. Home visits are sometimes made by the staff to evaluate accessibility of the home (stairs, ramps, doorways) and to suggest modifications that will help the disabled person to move about and function in the house without assistance.

Home visit weekends may also be arranged for the disabled person to test out living at home with the comforting knowledge that upon return to the rehabilitation center there will be expertise and support available to help deal with any problems that may have come up during the weekend visit home.

Once the disabled person leaves the rehabilitation center and comes home to stay, considerable assistance may still be required. The level of independence that can be reached will depend on the extent of the injury to the spinal cord, the remaining level of function, and his motivation to make the most of his abilities. Even the most able paraplegic will need to consider where and how to spend his limited amount of energy each day. Home health aides and housekeepers may be needed to shop, help with personal care, clean, and prepare meals.

Whether assistance will be needed on a full- or part-time basis will depend on the abilities and energy resources of the disabled person. Even if there is a family member available to assist, the part-time involvement of a home health aide will provide the needed care while offering a period of respite to the family member. Also, the part-time aide can help the disabled person conserve his energy for higher priority tasks.

Physical therapy, vocational training, and psychological support usually continue for the disabled person at home. He must now be more vigilant about his exercises, his catheter care (to avoid urinary infections), the techniques for preventing pressure sores and ulcers, and most of all, his spirit and his attitude toward participating in life. Decisions must be made about work, about returning to school (if an education has been interrupted by the spinal cord injury), about socialization, and about all the aspects of daily living.

Involvement in a local chapter of the many organizations devoted to individuals with spinal cord injuries may prove most helpful. Learning the ropes from informed individuals who have similar disabilities can provide much practical information. The National Spinal Cord Injury Association has forty-one local chapters serving individuals and their families and helping them cope with the problems involved in this type of disability. In addition, if so inclined, the disabled person can participate in wheelchair sports as a means of providing exercise and association with other young people with similar problems.

Although career goals may have to be modified because of the individual's disability (you can't become a commercial airline pilot with a spinal cord injury), there are, nevertheless, examples of numerous disabled people working in many fields and professions despite their disability. The lobbying efforts of national organizations for the disabled have opened many previously closed doors. Where once most buildings and transportation facilities were completely inaccessible for the wheelchair-bound individual, today offices, theaters, buses, and other public facilities are incorporating accessibility for the handicapped in their architectural design.

There are physicians, teachers, factory workers, draftsmen, and many others working and earning a living despite the handicap of the disability caused by a spinal cord injury. People with this type of injury have worked energetically to help themselves and to help others in the same situation. Kent Waldrep, president of the American Paralysis Association (APA) and thirty-year-old victim of a football injury that now confines him to a wheelchair, is vigorously working to raise funds for research that he hopes will help him and others like him to walk again someday.

One such research program, which the APA has funded, is looking into the use of laser stimulation in fighting paralysis. This particular research is being conducted by Dr. Judy Walker of the Walker Institute in Los Angeles. Dr. Walker seeks to reduce spasticity, or muscle rigidity, in patients with spastic paralysis through use of laser therapy.

Another energetic individual, Susan Sygall, has combined her interest in travel with the desire to help other disabled people. Her organization, Mobility International USA (MIUSA), with offices in Eugene, Oregon, is involved in expanding opportunities for travel, leisure activities, and educational exchange programs within the United States and abroad for disabled individuals. MIUSA offers low-cost travel ideas for independent travelers and education exchange programs for those seeking to broaden their knowledge.

Researchers in many parts of the country are working on a variety of techniques to help the wheelchair-bound to walk again. Microcomputers using electrical muscle stimulation are the focus of researchers in California and Ohio, in Yugoslavia, and at numerous universities.

Although all of this research is still highly experimental, the hope and the goal of the researchers is to help people with spinal cord injuries to restore part of their lost mobility.

Stroke

Although stroke is the third leading cause of death among adults in the United States (after heart disease and cancer) and produces the greatest incidence of long-term disability, the majority of stroke victims do survive—and many of them, after treatment and rehabilitation therapy, go on to lead productive lives.

A stroke is a frightening occurrence. Speech, bodily movement, sensory perception, the ability to read, to understand—all of these and more can be abruptly affected. A stroke involves a sudden interference in the blood supply to the brain. The flow of blood has been cut off. No blood flow means no oxygen reaching the nerve cells (neurons), depriving them of the ability to function. If the blood supply remains cut off for more than four or five minutes, the cells can be permanently damaged and die.

We have about 10 billion neurons in the brain, and this is a lifetime supply. Once a nerve cell dies it cannot be regenerated or replaced. Cells depend for their survival on oxygen and nutrients supplied by the blood, and when this vital supply is cut off and the cells die, that portion of bodily function controlled by the dead cells is affected.

Various parts of the brain have specialized functions. One area of the brain controls the voluntary movements of a leg; another sends impulses to the muscles controlling the tongue and lips; and still other areas are responsible for the ability to think and speak. Collectively, the nerve cells of the brain control not only our bodily movements but also the way we receive and interpret sensory inputs and other information conveyed from the outside.

CAUSES OF STROKE

Interruption of blood flow to the brain—commonly called a stroke and medically referred to as a cerebrovascular accident (CVA)—can be caused in a number of ways. A prime cause is blockage of an artery in the brain, or in one of the neck arteries leading to the brain, due to the formation of a blood clot, or thrombus. Blockage of this type is known as cerebral thrombosis. Thrombosis can have its start when blood begins to clot around projections of thick, rough deposits on the artery wall. These deposits, called plaque, commonly form as a result of excess cholesterol (fatty substances) in the blood, bringing on atherosclerosis, a blood vessel disorder sometimes referred to as hardening of the arteries.

Even without the formation of a thrombus, atherosclerosis is dangerous in that the plaque deposits can continue to grow, gradually narrowing the arterial passageway until it closes completely. The blood flow to the brain is then cut off just as it would be by a thrombus.

Sometimes, the blood clot forms elsewhere in the vascular (blood

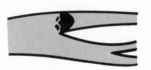

Thrombus or blood clot blocking the blood flow.

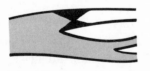

Buildup of plaque can reduce and eventually block blood flow.

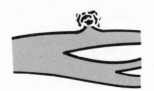

A rupture in the vessel walls (hemorrhage) disrupts blood flow beyond the point of rupture. The bleeding (hemorrhage) can also result in damage to the brain.

vessel) system. It can break off and be carried along in the bloodstream until it lodges in a brain artery or one of the neck arteries, impeding or completely cutting off blood flow to the brain. This wandering clot is called an embolism, and the condition is referred to as a cerebral embolism.

Another cause of stroke is the sudden bursting of blood from the ruptured wall of a weakened cerebral artery, known as a cerebral hemorrhage. The loss of blood to the neurons in the brain brings on the stroke. Additionally, the blood from the ruptured artery flows out into the surrounding brain tissues, then clots, and the clot exerts pressure on the tissues and on other blood vessels, causing further brain damage.

A cerebral hemorrhage also occurs when an aneurysm bursts. An aneurysm is a blood-swollen sac, or pouch, that forms on the artery wall. It can exist for some time, potentially dangerous but causing no discernible symptoms, until it distends enough to burst, flooding the brain with blood.

A brain tumor will also exert pressure on areas of the brain, and this can cause the same stroke effects as the other conditions just described.

Occasionally, a cerebral blood vessel may spasm, momentarily constricting enough to reduce or close off the blood supply. There's some question whether this is always a true "spasm" or perhaps a very small blood clot that temporarily blocks the flow of blood to the brain. Whatever the cause, these incidents are known as transient ischemic attacks (TIA) or, more commonly, as little strokes. The effects are temporary and can range from dizziness to weakness in an arm or leg to a momentary blackout, or even to the same symptoms as a full stroke.

TIAs have to be taken seriously, even though they may be only momentary and the individual recovers quickly and with no apparent ill effects. The appearance of a TIA can be the forerunner of a major stroke. Check with your physician and don't take any chances.

PREDISPOSING FACTORS

An examination by a physician, along with a thorough medical history, can disclose certain conditions that may indicate a risk of possible stroke. These predisposing factors, if present, do not mean you will have a stroke, but they can form the basis of a discussion with your physician of any treatment that may be required to help prevent a stroke.

Hypertension, or high blood pressure, is one of the primary predisposing factors to stroke. Hypertension is a "silent" disease in the sense that there can be an absence of observable symptoms. The one way to be sure is to have your blood pressure checked as part of a medical evaluation.

When the heart pumps blood through the vascular system, it creates pressure in the blood vessels, just as any pump uses pressure to move fluid along. Blood pressure (millimeters of mercury is the measurement standard used) is measured by an instrument called a sphygmomanometer, which indicates the pressure of the blood in the arteries at the beginning of a heart beat (systolic pressure) and between heart beats (diastolic pressure), when the heart is momentarily at rest.

Doctors and other health professionals take special notice of the pressure against the arterial wall during the diastolic phase of blood pressure measurement. When the pressure is higher than 90, they begin to treat the condition as borderline hypertension. If the diastolic pressure is consistently over 95 or 100, drug therapy may be started to control and lower the blood pressure. In addition, good eating habits, especially a reduced salt intake, and elimination of smoking will aid in controlling blood pressure.

Atherosclerosis is another significant predisposing factor to stroke. A well-balanced diet, regular exercise, and avoiding foods high in cholesterol will help prevent the development of atherosclerosis, or will substantially decrease its growth.

Heart disease of any kind is a potential stroke precursor. Anyone with heart disease should be under regular care of a physician or a cardiologist.

Diabetes, in addition to the other ravaging effects it can have on the body, increases the possibility of stroke. Again, the regular care of a physician is essential—and equally essential is the need for the patient to follow the physician's instructions and treatment plan faithfully.

The use of oral contraceptives by women, especially those who smoke heavily, increases the risk of stroke. Smoking, in general, is also considered a predisposing factor to stroke, as are obesity, undue stress, and a family history of hypertension, heart disease, or stroke.

One other important predisposing factor is race related. While different theories have been advanced to explain it, statistics show that black Americans, especially black males, are much more likely to develop hypertension than white Americans, which leads into another statistic: black Americans have more strokes, and at an earlier age.

WARNING SIGNS OF STROKE

Our bodies have ways of alerting us to trouble. Pain, for example, is the most obvious indication that something is wrong. There are indications of the possibility of an impending stroke that should be considered as warning signs from the body. The American Heart Association

has listed these warning signs, and if you experience any of them, don't ignore them. As mentioned before, play it safe and see your physician.
You may be at risk for a stroke if:

- You develop a sudden temporary weakness or numbness of your face, arm, or leg on one side of your body.
- You have some temporary difficulty with speech, or you find that you momentarily cannot speak at all, or you cannot seem to understand what others are saying.
- You have temporary visual difficulties such as dimness or loss of vision, especially in only one eye, or you start to see double.
- You have a temporary episode of dizziness or unsteadiness.
- You develop some unexplained headaches, or, if you usually do have headaches, the pattern of these headaches changes markedly.
- You seem to develop changes in your personality or your mental ability.

These warning signs can be momentary episodes, lasting for brief minutes, or they can extend for a few hours or almost a day. Whatever the length of time, the significant factor is that they have occurred. Don't ignore them. Let your doctor know what has happened—in detail.

You may have noted the similarity of the warning signs with the TIAs ("little strokes") described earlier. It's very possible that a TIA can take the form of one of these warning signs. Since TIAs lead to a stroke in about 50 percent of cases where they have occurred, this is still another reason not to ignore what has happened.

Prompt medical attention may result in being started on drug therapy, or possibly surgical intervention, as a preventive measure to avoid a stroke. Your physician will be better able to judge what treatment to recommend after he performs a thorough examination in conjunction with an exhaustive medical history.

TIAs and warning signs are a signal for you to make use of the medical expertise represented by your physician and other health care professionals. Doing so could save you from a major stroke.

REHABILITATION FOLLOWING A STROKE

Up to now, we've discussed what a stroke is, what it does to the mind and body, predisposing factors, and warning signs of a possible impending stroke. This information is intended as a guideline for the caregiver, as well as for the one receiving care at home, so that the nature of the patient's condition and what brought it about will be more readily understood. The more you know about stroke, the better you'll be able to provide the care needed at home for the stroke victim.

Also, since a second stroke is always a possibility, you have to know what to do to help prevent a second occurrence.

Proper care for the stroke victim involves not only a team of health care professionals but also coordination and cooperation between the hospital and the caregiver at home. In fact, it can be said that good home care for the stroke victim starts in the hospital. The role of the family (the caregiver is usually a spouse or family member) is of great importance in the recovery and rehabilitation of someone who has suffered a stroke.

The physical disabilities and personality changes that occur in the aftermath of a stroke indicate the part of the brain that has been damaged. Depending on which areas of the brain have been deprived of oxygen and the nourishing blood flow, or which areas may have become blood-soaked after a cerebral hemorrhage, the symptoms following a stroke may include: paralysis of one side of the body (hemiplegia) or of an arm or a leg; visual field disturbances; difficulties with speaking, writing, reading, or understanding language (aphasia); slurred speech (dysarthria); difficulty in performing voluntary movements (apraxia); personality changes.

The problems that are apparent during the first hours and days following a stroke do not necessarily reflect the long-term difficulties that will be faced by the patient and his family. Many of the early symptoms fade and abilities improve as the blood flow in the brain seeks and finds alternate vessels and pathways to neurons and swelling of the brain tissue goes down.

An all-out team effort is appropriate right from the start—to work with the patient and the family in an effort to preserve function and flexibility and prevent stiffness in the joints. The team players include the patient, his family, the family physician, and the rehabilitiation specialists: a physiatrist (a physician specializing in physical medicine and rehabilitation), a neurologist, physical and occupational therapists, a rehabilitation nurse, a speech pathologist, a social worker, and possibly a dietician and a vocational rehabilitation counselor.

Rehabilitation begins almost immediately, right in the hospital. It's not unusual for the patient to be partially or completely paralyzed on one side of the body. One side of the face may appear limp and flaccid, and one arm or leg may be motionless. If the right side of the body is affected, it usually means that the stroke occurred on the left side of the brain. Right-side brain damage will affect the left side of the body.

The nursing staff in the acute care hospital will take aggressive measures to assure that the patient will have as positive and speedy a recovery as possible. To prevent stiffness in the joints and relieve pressure on the affected side, the nurse will make sure that the patient is positioned correctly in the bed so as to maintain good body alignment. The nurse may use pillows and towels to prop up and position the patient to help prevent any deformities from occurring due to poor positioning during a long stay in bed. Since the arm or leg is without motion or sensation, it can slip into a position where it might become deformed or damaged—and the patient, of course, would not be aware of this since no sensory information is getting through from the damaged brain.

The nurse probably will also perform passive range-of-motion exercises on the patient several times each day. By lifting and carefully moving the limp arm or leg, she will work to prevent stiffness and any further deterioration of the muscles and nerves of the affected limb. Also, these exercises will stretch the soft tissues and aid in maintaining good circulation. Remember, the damage is in the brain and not the arm or leg, which are flaccid because messages that control movement are not coming through from the brain.

The nurse, or the physical therapist, if one has been requested, will want to teach members of the family to carry out these exercises on the patient during the hospital stay. Family participation has a two-fold purpose. First, it allows the family to do something to help the patient on the way to recovery. Watching someone you love lose functional ability is hard to take, and actively participating in the rehabilitation treatment works to keep family spirits and outlook positive and hopeful—which also has a good effect on the patient. Second, performing these exercises encourages family members to touch and stroke the patient, which becomes a soothing and caring exchange during a time of possible confusion and anxiety. This is especially true if the stroke has brought on communication and language difficulties (aphasia). The touching and stroking involved in the exercises will become, in effect, a means of communication and an expression of caring between the family and the patient.

The flexibility that passive range-of-motion exercises help maintain will be put to good use later when the physical therapist starts to work on more active exercises and, eventually, starts getting the patient to walk again. While it has been said that nine out of ten stroke victims regain the ability to walk, some of them will require the assistance of a brace, cane, or walker.

Physical therapy sessions may begin in the hospital "gym" and continue after the patient is discharged. At that time, the therapy sessions may take place during day visits to the outpatient department of the hospital, or at the patient's home, with the physical therapist making a series of house calls.

Depending on the type and extent of disability, the therapist will custom-tailor a therapy program to meet the particular needs of the patient. A leg brace may be recommended to help steady a weak or wobbly leg, and leg exercises may be prescribed to strengthen not only the muscles in the affected leg but also the muscles in the unaffected side.

If necessary, the therapist will help the patient to practice walking, often with the patient using a walker or a "quad cane" (a four-tipped cane) for added safety. At home, the therapist may have the patient practice walking up and down the stairs and getting in and out of the family car.

Together, the patient and the therapist will practice walking on smooth and rough ground as well as up and down ramps. Probably, they will also practice how to get up from the ground after a fall—in the event that the patient does trip and fall and there is no one around at the time to help him get up.

When weakness or paralysis affects the arm (often called the "upper extremity" by therapists and other health professionals), a sling may be used to help support the paralyzed arm. This is done to prevent the limp arm from possibly dislocating the shoulder because of the effect of its "dead weight" when the patient is sitting or standing.

Following a stroke, it may be necessary for the patient to be retrained in the activities of daily living if the paralysis affects the dominant side of the body. When a righthanded person has a stroke that weakens the left side of his body, minimal retraining will be necessary, since the paralysis (hemiplegia) does not affect the side of the body that is dominant in the physical activity of the patient. He has not lost the ability to use his right hand, although he may have perceptual disturbances that can create new problems. However, if the stroke has caused a weakness or paralysis on the right side of his body, some amount of retraining will be needed.

Since the right-handed person now cannot use his right hand, he will need retraining in how to dress and care for himself with the use of only his left hand. He will have to relearn how to write, this time with his left hand, and he will have to be taught how to feed himself with one hand. There are many devices for a one-handed person to use (see Chapter 5)—for example, a combination knife-fork—but the difficulty will be in switching from right-handedness to left-handedness. With patience and practice, it can be done.

This is where the skills and experience of an occupational therapist are needed. The therapist will evaluate the patient's self-care capabilities, often initiating this evaluation while the patient is still in the hospital. Once the person returns home, the assistance of an occupational therapist can be of great value.

As the person regains muscle function, other abilities may improve as well. The occupational therapist continually reevaluates the person's abilities. Moreover, the therapist works right in the location where those tasks will be performed—the person's home. The therapist can offer suggestions for improving function and independence right on the spot, at the particular moment these suggestions would be most helpful. Also, the therapist will be there to help the family cope with any problems that might arise as part of the home health care situation.

The goal of the occupational therapist will be to guide the patient and teach him the skills and techniques that will, if possible, permit complete independence. Also, the therapist will seek to identify the purposeful and recreational activities that will help add to the quality of life for the patient during his recuperation. Most people, with caring help and proper instruction and motivation, are able to relearn the self-help skills that foster independence.

APHASIA: A DEVASTATING CONSEQUENCE

Have you ever had the frustrating experience of trying to ask directions of a non-English-speaking person during a vacation trip—in a country where you do not speak or understand the language? You may speak slowly and clearly and use ample gestures and body language, but to no avail. You may find your listener speaks to you easily and fluently in his own tongue, or he may mumble something that probably means he doesn't speak English, and then will walk away.

Imagine, then, how the frustration and sense of anxiety and loneliness must be multiplied for the stroke victim when communication difficulties arise in his own family. The family faces are familiar—the patient usually does not lose the ability to recognize family members. Yet, depending on the location and extent of the damage to his brain, he may be unable to understand the words and phrases he hears his family saying (receptive aphasia). Or, he may be able to understand what he hears but unable to find the right words to express himself in response (expressive aphasia).

Aphasia is the loss of the ability to make sense of language, and is perhaps the most complex and disturbing symptom following a stroke. The loss may be total (global aphasia), but more often the loss is a partial one, affecting either the person's ability to understand what is spoken or written or his ability to speak or write what is in his mind.

The problem is not one of intelligence but rather one of communication. It's almost as though the switchboard in the brain's communication center had defective wiring. Sounds and words are heard, but the "connectors" to the part of the brain that gives meaning to language are faulty or dead.

Although any person who incurs brain damage may develop aphasia, it is most commonly seen in adults who have suffered a stroke. According to the National Institutes of Health, more than one million people suffer from aphasia in the United States, with strokes accounting for half the total. The balance are the result of head injury, infections, exposure to toxic materials, lead poisoning, and other causes.

In most people, the language function is governed by the left side of the brain, which accounts for the prevalence of aphasia victims with a right-side body weakness. While the exact locations in the brain of all the different language functions are not completely known, we do know that there are distinct areas of the brain responsible for speech comprehension, speech expression, and reading comprehension.

With expressive aphasia, the person knows what he wants to say but is unable to say what he wants. He may make unexplainable grammatical errors, or will have difficulty naming objects, or problems with using the telephone. However, this same person may be able to communicate through gestures, through writing, or by pointing to the object or to the printed word or phrase he has in mind.

The receptive asphasic has difficulty understanding spoken and sometimes written language. Many receptive asphasics may talk a great deal, but unfortunately they do not seem to make sense. They may become quite agitated when it becomes apparent their message is not getting through.

Two key concepts are critically important when you are trying to communicate with an aphasic person. First, the realization must be uppermost in your mind that this is an intelligent, feeling human being— and should be treated as such. Talking down to someone with aphasia can be disturbing—and talking over the aphasic's head to someone else is downright rude.

Second, you must also realize that through touch, gesture, body language, and other ways, you can have an exchange with this person. You can let him know you are there, ready to listen and communicate. This is where the speech pathologist can be of vital assistance. Through her evaluation of the various methods of communication, she may be able to identify the true extent of the difficulty and the best routes for optimal communication. Her counsel and guidance will help improve the interaction with the patient. In addition, by aggressively beginning a program of speech therapy, the patient will be actively working toward improvement in this most important capability.

Often, the speech therapist acts as an interpreter, helping the family or the doctors and nurses to understand what the patient is trying to communicate. The patient, for his part, feels that the speech therapist represents a vital and positive link that connects him to the outside world.

Although the outcome of aphasia cannot be determined in advance, patients with a better understanding of language seem to recover more than others. Many stroke victims show some spontaneous recovery from the symptoms of aphasia within a few days after the stroke occurrence, and they may continue to improve significantly for up to three months. After six months, though, further recovery will depend to a great extent on successful rehabilitation and speech therapy.

Although the results cannot be predicted, almost all patients will benefit from an early start of speech therapy. Whether the person recovers all language skills completely, or learns to rely on special cuing devices (pictures, words, or sounds) to assist him to communicate, the speech therapist does provide the positive therapeutic environment necessary for encouraging and motivating the patient.

When the patient has improved to the point of understanding most of what is being said to him, it is often helpful to seek a group experience. Group therapy helps to lessen feelings of isolation, and stroke victims will find support and encouragement as well as stimulation from the group. (A directory of Stroke Clubs is available from the American Heart Association. Refer to the Appendix for their address and other details.)

UNDERSTANDING THE BEHAVIOR OF
THE STROKE VICTIM

In the American Heart Association pamphlet, "Stroke: Why Do They Behave That Way?" (see the Appendix for their address) the following advice is offered for communicating and assisting stroke victims who have suffered left brain damage and thus have right-side paralysis (right hemiplegics):

Right hemiplegics will often have difficulties with speech and language. They also tend to be somewhat cautious, anxious, and disorganized when attempting a new task. Keep in mind the following suggestions:

1) Do not underestimate the patient's ability to learn and communicate even if he cannot use speech.

2) If he cannot use speech, try other forms of communication. Pantomime and demonstration are often useful.

3) Do not overestimate his understanding of speech and overload him with "static."

4) Do not shout. Keep messages simple and brief.

5) Do not use special voices.

6) Divide tasks into simple steps.

7) Give much feedback and many indications of progress.

On this last point, it's important to remember that the patient is depending on you for feedback as to how well he's doing. This doesn't mean he's expecting flattery. You must always realize that he has difficulty communicating or understanding what is happening. If you keep giving him feedback, no matter how trivial it may seem to you, you will not only encourage him but will also let him know that he's making progress. In this connection, don't lie to him. Don't try to encourage him by telling him he's doing better than he really is. You can be truthful without being harsh and without discouraging the individual. Patience and understanding will help both you and the individual struggling with the effects of stroke.

The left hemiplegic (right brain damage) may be able to talk better than he can actually perform. While the only speech problem may be sluggishness (dysarthria), there are likely to be problems with visual and spatial perception, resulting in impaired abilities because visual cues are affected. The left hemiplegic may be impulsive or careless and, to avoid the possibility of hurting himself, will need to demonstrate competence before being left completely on his own.

Tips from the American Heart Association include:

1) Do not overestimate his abilities. Spatial-perceptual deficits are easy to miss.

2) Use verbal cues if he has difficulty with demonstration.

3) Break tasks into small steps and give him much feedback.

4) Watch to see what he can do safely rather than taking his word for it.

5) Minimize clutter around him.

6) Avoid rapid movement around the patient.

7) Highlight visual reference points. (For example, outline a doorway in a bright color to aid the patient's spatial perception.)

VISUAL FIELD DEFICITS

Imagine what the world would look like to you if you wore goggles that restricted viewing to either side, allowing you to see only straight ahead—and then had the left half of each goggle covered with black tape. You would have a real problem seeing objects that were blocked by the tape. In time, you would learn to compensate for this visual deficit by turning your head from side to side.

Some stroke patients have this type of visual field problem and likewise compensate by turning their head. In some cases, people do forget about or neglect the impaired side. If the deficit is also a sensory deficit in which the impaired side lacks feeling, they may not even be aware, for example, that the arm and leg in bed with them is in fact their own.

This phenomenon is called one-sided neglect, and it can have a significant impact on the ability of the person to function. People with this problem may even ignore food on one side of the plate. If the plate is repositioned, the food will be noticed and eaten.

If the visual field is completely one-sided, a person may lose his way even if he is moving up and down the same corridor in, let's say, an airport. He will see one corridor with particular signs and arrows and perhaps windows as he walks along, and then, on the return trip, will see a completely different corridor because of his visual field deficit. (Pointing out landmarks to the right and left along the way will help orient the individual.)

The phenomenon of one-sided neglect can occur in both right and left hemiplegics, although it seems to be more prevalent in left hemiplegics. The American Heart Association suggests that you maximize the positive aspects of the person's viewing condition by keeping the unimpaired side toward the "action" and offering frequent cues to help orientation. Make sure the particular environment—bedroom, bathroom, etc.—has been arranged to maximize performance. Also, when conversing with the patient, make sure you sit on the unimpaired side.

MEMORY PROBLEMS

The stroke victim may have difficulty remembering things. For example, if you were to give him directions for performing a certain task and these directions involved several steps, he might remember only one or two steps out of the total you have given him. Yet, if you were to restate your directions one step at a time, as he performed them, you would probably see significantly improved functioning.

New information may be difficult for the person to retain. Repetition may help reinforce retention of the new information or task. For example, learning to slip on a brace or sling is awkward and represents "new information" for the patient. Many practice sessions, with much support, feedback, and repetition will help.

Don't be too surprised if certain skills that seem easy for the patient in one situation turn out to be impossible in another. The ability to apply learning from one situation to another is called generalization, and many poststroke individuals have quite a bit of difficulty applying new learning to another setting. For example, while the patient may be able to transfer from the hospital bed to his wheelchair, he may need to be retrained to transfer from his bed at home to the wheelchair.

For patients with this type of problem, creating some kind of structure in their lives by establishing a routine that is repeated daily will create a better sense of security and function. Wall calendars, notebooks, and other memory aids are helpful reminders.

EMOTIONAL INSTABILITY

One of the more perplexing symptoms following a stroke is the loss of emotional control. The stroke victim will laugh or cry for no apparent reason. While some of the crying can be attributed to the expected depression he may be experiencing in reaction to the profound changes that have happened to him, an individual will sometimes cry even though depression or sadness have not been the cause. It may help to interrupt this emotional behavior by distracting the patient with another activity.

This is a delicate matter, however, as you do not wish to supress or push aside feelings that the patient may want to express. Seek the advice of a social worker or other counselor if you question whether the emotional expressions are a reflection of true feelings or are a result of brain damage.

Each stroke patient is unique. The uniqueness of the individual prior to the stroke—in the way he lived, laughed, loved, and coped— becomes even more apparent after the stroke.

The purpose here in defining and describing the problems and symptoms that may be experienced by the stroke victim is to help you, the caregiver, to understand what is happening. Greater understanding will help you to provide a constructive environment that will maximize the abilities and the level of function for the brain damaged person.

Brain damage presents a frightening image and perhaps a grim view of the future. However, there is much that can be done to improve the quality of life for the stroke victim. With much patience and caring, you will be able to provide that desired quality of life.

18

Gastrointestinal Problems

Inflammatory Bowel Disease

ILEITIS OR Crohn's disease and ulcerative colitis are two debilitating diseases of the digestive tract that are collectively called inflammatory bowel disease (IBD). These are serious diseases of the small and large intestines. Estimates of their prevalence range from at least 500,000 chronic suffers to 1 or 2 million additional victims. The wide range here can be attributed to frequent delays in accurate diagnoses and the fact that many people are not hospitalized and therefore are not counted in the hospital census data on which these statistics are based. Younger people are afflicted with IBD more frequently than older people, with estimates that there may be as many as 200,000 children under the age of sixteen with these diseases.

Although both diseases cause similar symptoms—abdominal pain, diarrhea, fever, and weight loss—they reflect two dissimilar disease processes. Ulcerative colitis causes ulcerations or sores of the lining of the colon and rectum. In Crohn's disease, the layers of the wall of the intestine become inflamed and swollen. The lower part of the small intestine (the ileum) may be involved, or the inflammation may occur in the large intestine (colon). Other parts of the digestive tract may also be affected.

Young people and middle-aged people with symptoms of gastrointestinal distress generally undergo quite a bit of diagnostic testing before a definitive diagnosis is made. There is no single test that will unquestionably identify either Crohn's disease or ulcerative colitus. Barium X-rays of both the upper and lower GI tract and two additional tests that allow the doctor to look directly into the intestines through a lighted tube inserted through the anus (sigmoidoscopy and colonoscopy) can help to establish a diagnosis.

IBD is a disease that seems to occur more frequently in developed countries such as the United States, England, Scotland, and Scandinavia. Also, epidemiologists have established that the risk of developing either Crohn's disease or ulcerative colitis is about four to five times greater among Jewish people living in the United States and Europe. The reasons for this are unknown, as are the reasons why people of Oriental descent and black Africans develop IBD when these groups migrate to Western societies. No specific environmental factors or dietary differences have been found that would clearly explain these findings.

MANAGING IBD

Both Crohn's disease and ulcerative colitis are treated with drugs to reduce the inflammation. Most people with IBD take either sulfasalazine or prednisone (a corticosteroid) or both. Occasional immunosuppressive drugs are used to help control the disease. In addition, drugs to help control the diarrhea or reduce stomach pain may be prescribed.

Because the nutritional status of the individual may be adversely affected, nutritional supplements or vitamins may also be recommended. This is especially important for adolescents, as the teen years are important growing years and 15 to 20% of children with Crohn's disease and ulcerative colitis show signs of failure to grow. Scientists believe that the lack of growth in height and poor weight gain are due to an inadequate intake of calories and a level of undernutrition caused by diarrhea and the failure of the diseased bowel to absorb nutrients.

Physicians may recommend nutritionally complete liquid supplements, either alone or with regular food, to increase the caloric and nutritional intake. During a flareup of the disease, the individual may be too ill to eat normally (enterally). In such a case, total parenteral nutrition (TPN) or intravenous feeding will be used to improve the person's nutritional status and general health (see Chapter 6).

Active management of IBD can result in long periods that are symptom-free. Many people are able to live normal, active lives—completing school, competing in sports, pursuing professional careers—with only a brief period of acute illness, controlled by the use of medication. However, when medication is not able to control the symptoms, or if there is some other complication, such as an obstruction in the intestine, then surgery may become necessary.

In Crohn's disease, the diseased segment of the bowel often is removed and the two ends of the remaining healthy bowel are joined

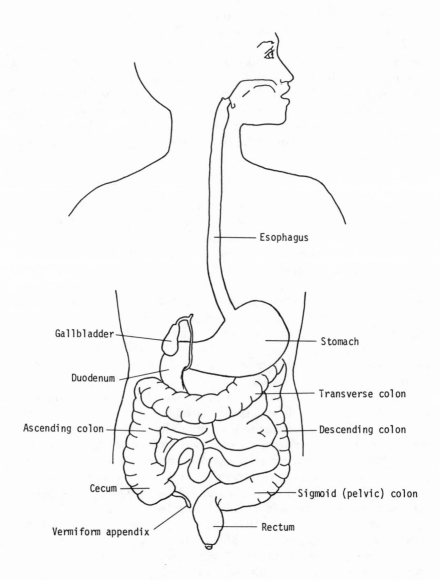

Esophagus

Gallbladder

Stomach

Duodenum

Transverse colon

Ascending colon

Descending colon

Cecum

Sigmoid (pelvic) colon

Vermiform appendix

Rectum

The GI tract.

together, resulting in many symptom-free years. This is not considered a "cure" since it is possible for the disease symptoms to recur with a concurrent inflammation in the same area as before.

A surgical cure for ulcerative colitis does exist. This entails removal of the entire colon and rectum, with the creation of an ileostomy (an artificial opening created in the abdominal wall through which liquid wastes are excreted). An appliance, sometimes called a bag or a pouch, is attached to the new opening (stoma) to collect the body wastes (see "Ostomy Care Techniques," p. 432).

Surgical alternatives have been designed to avoid the permanent ileostomy while still permitting the active lives sought by victims of ulcerative colitis. One procedure is called the Continent (Kock) ileostomy. In it the surgeon, after removing the colon and rectum, actually constructs an internal pouch out of the small intestine. The pouch is connected to the abdominal wall and to the "outside" by means of a flat ileostomy. Rather than emptying an external bag, the individual passes a catheter into the pouch and empties it regularly. Although this appliance-free alternative can have gratifying results, it carries with it an increased risk of infection and other complications.

Another procedure—highly experimental and presently under evaluation—retains the rectal sphincter while removing the upper rectum and colon. A collection reservoir is constructed in the ileum and connected to the remaining rectum. Many patients are then able to evacuate normally, or with the help of a catheter inserted through the anus to empty the pouch.

Understandably, victims of IBD, young and old alike, who have to deal with painful and sometimes embarrassing symptoms, need to work through the emotional adjustments that will lead them to as active a life as possible, despite the disease.

Some chapters of the National Foundation for Ileitis and Colitis have organized support groups in which afflicted people can give support to each other and learn from the experience of others. Professional counseling may also be helpful to come to terms with these debilitating and often interruptive chronic illnesses.

Managing with an Ostomy

Whatever the original disease that required creation of an ostomy, learning to live with the ostomy is another matter entirely.

For some, surgery may have cured severe bowel disease and offered a new lease on symptom-free living; for others, the ostomy may have resulted from lifesaving surgery for rectal cancer. Yet the major readjustment required with respect to body image and toileting habits can have a profound emotional impact on many patients.

There's now a part of their body that they may at first feel queasy about touching, a part that makes them different from everyone else. Also, previously there had been countless flights to the bathroom because of the severe bowel disease. It became almost commonplace. Now, however, there's an entirely new "bathroom" process to be learned.

Spouses and partners, too, will need to deal with their reactions and responses to the changes that have taken place. Along with the ostomate, they may worry about odor or the possibility of accidental leakage.

With information, guidance, support, and encouragement from others similarly afflicted, and with the help of specially trained nurses or enterostomal therapists, the new ostomate will learn how to take care of his ostomy. After a period of adjustment and acceptance, people living with a colostomy or an ileostomy can lead as full a life as anyone else.

COLOSTOMY VS. ILEOSTOMY

When the rectum and part of the colon are surgically removed, the normal channel for evacuation of body wastes can be replaced by a colostomy. The word "colostomy" in Greek means "cutting a (new) opening for the colon." The new opening (stoma) is usually located in the abdomen. Its exact location may depend on the amount of colon that has been surgically removed.

If the surgery removed only a small length of colon, the discharge through the stoma will closely resemble bowel movements prior to surgery. The higher up the colon the operation took place, the wetter, looser, and more liquid the discharge becomes. This happens because one of the most important jobs fulfilled by the large intestine is the reabsorption of water from the intestinal tract. The less colon present, the less water absorption that can take place, and the more liquid the discharge. Conversely, the more colon that remains, the more normal the discharge.

Many people with "low-placed" colostomies learn to regulate themselves and are able to discard the permanently placed collection pouch and use a simple piece of gauze over the stoma. By carefully controlling their diet and using irrigation techniques to evacuate body wastes, these colostomates feel secure with a simple stoma cap.

An ileostomy, in which the entire colon and part of the ileum or small intestine has been surgically removed, can redirect the small intestine to the surface at a stoma on the abdomen. Because minimal water absorption has occurred, the ileal discharge is liquid and continuous. While an appliance must be worn at all times, people living with an ileostomy can also lead full lives.

An enterostomal therapist (ET) or specially trained nurse will probably seek you out during your hospital stay. She will be the person who will visit your room, check the pouch that was placed during surgery, and talk with you about learning to manage your own ostomy care. The kind of training she will give you will depend on the type of ostomy that was performed during surgery.

Since an ileostomy requires that an appliance be worn at all times, the ET will teach you how to apply and remove the appliance, how to empty the pouch, special skin care techniques to protect the skin around the stoma, and how to manage odor control.

A low-placed sigmoid or descending colostomy will require that she not only teach you about appliances so you may feel more secure with them, but she will also discuss how to control the discharge through diet and irrigation techniques that will offer "pouch-free living" much of the time.

For colostomies that are higher on the colon, the information she will cover will be similar to ileostomy care.

Numerous products of various shapes, sizes, and materials are available for the management of an ostomy. The ET can select the proper appliances and skin care products that meet the person's needs. The specific appliance that is initially recommended will depend on the type of surgery, the type of discharge, skin sensitivity, and the shape of the stoma and the abdomen.

Disposable or reusable appliances can be selected, depending upon the individual's needs and wishes. At first, there may be a bit of experimentation in order to select the appliance that is easier to change and offers the best fit. During the weeks following surgery, as the swelling goes down and the real shape of the stoma becomes apparent, some changes may need to be made.

Even after the final decision has been made and the type of appliance has been selected, many ostomates have made further changes as they learn about newer appliances that are easier to use. Through interaction with other ostomates or through their ostomy product supplier, they learn about specially designed pouches for special situations. The United Ostomy Association supplies many additional contacts for ostomates (see the Appendix).

You and your ET will ultimately decide on the basic appliance you use. Choosing the right appliance can assure a better quality of life.

As their name implies, disposable appliances for ileostomates are

OSTOMY CARE TECHNIQUES

HOW TO EMPTY YOUR OSTOMY POUCH

Here are some guidelines to help you empty your ostomy pouch in your bathroom at home.

You'll need to empty it when it's about one-third full. If you have a colostomy, the pouch will usually need to be emptied once or twice daily. If you have an ileostomy, the pouch will have to be emptied five or six times daily.

To prepare for this procedure, place a cup of warm water within reach. Then, sit on the toilet with the pouch hanging between your legs.

Or, if you prefer, sit on a chair next to the toilet. Be sure the pouch's opening is inside the toilet bowl.

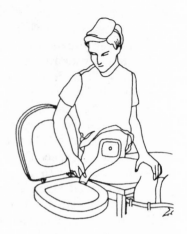

To empty your pouch, turn up the bottom of it and remove the closure clamp.

To prevent splashing, place some toilet paper on the surface of the water or flush the toilet as you point the pouch's unclamped opening into the bowl.

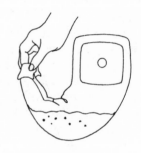

Slide your thumb and index finger down the outside of the pouch, squeezing all the contents into the toilet.

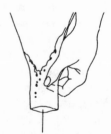

Next, use tissue or a disposable wipe to clean any remaining drainage from outside and inside the pouch opening.

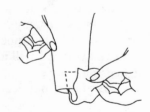

Hold the pouch opening upright and pour the cup of water into the pouch, as shown here. Swish the water around to remove any remaining drainage. As you work, avoid wetting your stoma or the pouch adhesive. A little water won't do any harm, but too much could break the seal.

Now, direct the pouch opening into the toilet. Let the pouch drain thoroughly.

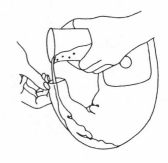

If you use a pouch deodorant, place it in the pouch, following the manufacturer's directions. Then, using a clean disposable wipe or toilet tissue, clean and dry the outside of the pouch. Finally, close the pouch with a clamp or rubber band. Then wash your hands well.

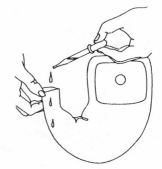

HOW TO CLEAN A REUSABLE POUCH

To increase the life of your reusable pouch and help prevent odor, clean your pouch thoroughly every time you change it. Having at least two pouches is advisable. This way you can clean one while you're wearing the other.

Here's how to clean your pouch:

Remove the double adhesive disk from the faceplate. If you can't remove all of the adhesive, try rolling the rest of it off with your fingertips.

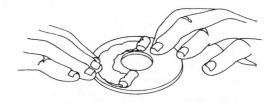

Or try loosening the adhesive with a gauze pad moistened in adhesive solvent. But remember, always use solvent sparingly. Too much may erode the faceplate.

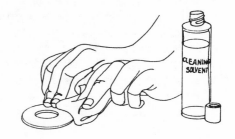

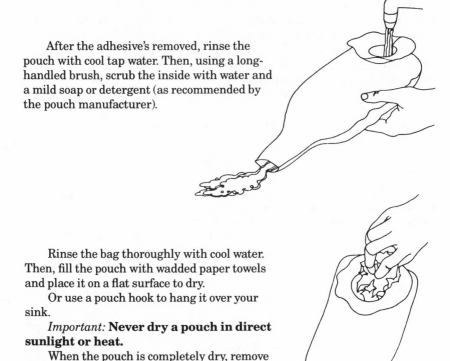

After the adhesive's removed, rinse the pouch with cool tap water. Then, using a long-handled brush, scrub the inside with water and a mild soap or detergent (as recommended by the pouch manufacturer).

Rinse the bag thoroughly with cool water. Then, fill the pouch with wadded paper towels and place it on a flat surface to dry.

Or use a pouch hook to hang it over your sink.

Important: **Never dry a pouch in direct sunlight or heat.**

When the pouch is completely dry, remove the paper towels, if you've used any. Store the pouch in a cool, dry place.

usually changed daily; "permanent" appliances are often left in place for three to seven days before changing. These long-term appliances can be cleaned, deodorized, dried, and reused. Often, the ostomate has two or three permanent appliances and rotates their use to allow time for drying and airing an appliance after it has been removed.

Many colostomates choose from a wide variety of lightweight, disposable appliances. Some are two-piece combinations, with a reusable mounting ring on a belt that encircles the stoma. Others have a square of adhesive that surrounds the stoma opening and is simply pressed against the skin and worn without a belt.

Careful skin care is of great importance for the successful management of an ostomy. The discharge from an ileostomy or colostomy is rich with skin-irritating enzymes, and special care must be taken to keep the discharge away from the skin. Numerous skin products—washes, creams, skin protectors, and adhesives—are available. (Stomahesive is a skin barrier in wafer form.)

Karaya gum (a compound that comes from the sap of an Asian tree) is another effective skin barrier. It's available in gum powder form and also as part of the protective covering of a one-piece appliance.

Through careful selection of the right size and shape of appliance for your stoma, and by keeping the skin under the appliance clean and dry at all times, you can prevent development of annoying and uncomfortable skin problems.

DIET

The person who previously suffered through years of gastrointestinal discomfort because of IBD will find that the presence of an ostomy can open up dietary doors that previously had been closed. The greater freedom of food selection and enjoyment usually evokes much appreciation in ostomates.

Not all foods can be consumed, of course. For example, eating high-cellulose foods such as corn, nuts, celery, or coconuts should be minimized. At least a quart of water should be drunk every day, especially by the ileostomate who is losing fluids. Odor-producing foods such as beans, onions, asparagus, cabbage, and cheese should be limited—or a deodorant product can be used to help absorb the potentially embarrassing odor. Also, a correctly fitted appliance will confine the odor.

EMBARRASSING SITUATIONS

Patience with yourself (or with your spouse) and a sense of humor can work wonders to carry you through those embarrassing and frustrating situations. There may be times when it seems things just aren't working as they should—an appliance loosens and a leak threatens to stain a new formal, or a sudden flow of excrement occurs after careful showering and cleansing, and you have to start all over again. It happens, and it's disappointing. Try to put the isolated incident into perspective and not let it get you down.

While living with an ostomy does require extra personal care, it need not be the excuse for avoiding the pleasures of a normal and active sex life. Certainly, there are understandable feelings about lost attractiveness and a new body image to sort out. If you are in an ongoing relationship, your partner has been there every step of the way. There should be few surprises.

Most partners readily accept the new plumbing, especially when compared to the alternatives that a refusal of surgery presented. By carefully emptying the bag, folding it neatly, and taping it against itself to create a smaller bulge, you can prevent its flopping around during lovemaking.

For the ostomate who dates, there comes a time when it's necessary to tell. With luck, the partner will be receptive and sensitive and not offended by the presence of an ostomy. Young people with ostomies do require emotional and psychological support to learn to manage their own care as well as to deal with the periodic feelings of rejection that may be experienced. The support of peers—perhaps through the United Ostomy Association—can help tremendously.

Today, more and more people are talking about their ostomies. For years, a cloud of secrecy and embarrassment had kept the postsurgical presence of an ostomy literally "under wraps." With improvements in products and procedures made by innovative manufacturers, ostomates can and do participate in all types of activities. They travel extensively, have babies, enjoy active sex lives, swim, ski, and enjoy all that life has to offer.

19

Circulatory and Cardiovascular Problems

THE HEART is an essential organ that starts pulsing before birth and continues for many decades to sustain life by pumping blood and nutrients throughout the body. The figures are awesome: the average heart beats 100,000 times a day, each and every day; 4,300 gallons of nourishing blood are sent daily through 60,000 miles of blood vessels into all the body tissues. Nothing man-made can match this performance.

Because of the complexity of the heart and the extent of its function, much can happen to disrupt or damage its operation. Volumes have been written on the heart and the care it requires when injured. In this section, we'll cover the two major heart problems that relate to home health care: heart attack and angina.

Heart Attack: Sudden Onset and Step-by-Step Recovery

Not too long ago, if you managed to survive a heart attack, it marked the end of the good life for you. Weeks and sometimes months were spent convalescing. Long days and nights were spent in bed, and then, when you were finally allowed out of bed during the day, you had to sit in a chair and do nothing except read a little, or have someone read to you.

Tennis racquets were stored away, as were golf clubs and other sports equipment, because exercise was considered taboo. You could not be allowed to exert yourself. Travel plans had to be curtailed, or perhaps even completely prohibited, since it might be too "stressful."

Two decades ago, research findings were instrumental in bringing about changes in these ingrained patterns and practices concerning recuperation from heart attack. Researchers found that, contrary to what had been the prevailing medical opinion, "total rest" was not all that beneficial, and, in fact, inactivity could bring about even more incapacitation.

This fact was dramatically shown in a study in which normal, healthy college students were confined to bed for twenty days. Examination of the students disclosed that this enforced rest actually reduced the heart's ability to deliver oxygen to the body tissues and increased the heart's oxygen requirements. Also, the inactivity significantly weakened all other muscles. It took time and much exercise to enable these students to return to their prior levels of health and strength.

The implications of these and other findings to the postcoronary patient were clear. Today, health professionals seek to minimize any deterioration in strength or endurance that can be brought about through excessive bed rest. A carefully supervised program of gradually increasing activity is set up as soon as possible, depending on the particular needs and health problems of the individual patient. In some hospitals, qualified patients are placed in such a program within a few days of being transferred out of the CCU (coronary care unit).

As much activity as the patient can reasonably tolerate has replaced the total bed rest approach of twenty years ago. The heart attack victim is now encouraged to return to a normal life at a reasonable and responsible pace. The health care team, through education and counseling, works with the patient and the family to control the risk factors that originally led to the heart attack and to modify the patient's life style and habits to prevent a recurrence.

THE WARNING SIGNS OF A HEART ATTACK

If you've had a heart attack, or have witnessed the heart attack of someone close to you, the sequence of events will undoubtedly remain forever in your memory. Most likely, nothing out of the ordinary was happening immediately prior to the heart attack. Heart attacks can happen at work, at home, during leisure activities, at exciting moments, when calm, when under stress—anywhere and anytime.

Often, the first feeling of tightness in the chest is brushed off as being due to indigestion. Ignoring this warning sign, especially when combined with the others listed below, can be hazardous. The American Heart Association estimates that each year 350,000 people die of a heart attack before they reach the hospital—many because they refused to consider the possibility that they could be having a heart attack.

Warning signals of a heart attack are:

- Pain in the center of the chest, sometimes starting as a feeling of pressure or fullness, that lasts more than two minutes.
- A spreading of the pain to the shoulders, neck, arms (especially the left arm), or the lower jaw.
- An increase in the severity of the pain, accompanied by dizziness, nausea, sweating, fainting, or shortness of breath.

Many people do not have symptoms. These are known as silent coronaries. The heart muscle is damaged by the attack, despite the lack of symptoms.

Short, sharp, stabbing twinges of pain are generally not an indication of a heart attack. If you experience any of the above symptoms for more than a few minutes, get medical attention immediately. Call your doctor or get to the emergency room of a hospital. It could save your life.

WHAT HAPPENS IN A HEART ATTACK?

The common medical term for what most people call a heart attack is myocardial infarction (MI). This occurs when there is a complete blockage in one of the arteries that carry blood to the heart muscle, the blockage usually being due to a clot formed in an artery narrowed by the accumulation of fatty deposits over the years (atherosclerosis). The area of the heart muscle beyond the point of blockage dies from lack of oxygen and nutrients that are carried in the blood. A heart attack may damage a small, focused area of heart muscle or, in the case of a major attack, may cause extensive heart muscle injury.

The first few touch-and-go hours after a heart attack are usually spent in a hospital's coronary care unit (CCU). The patient, if conscious, will undoubtedly be frightened and apprehensive. However, it is here in the CCU that the trained staff vigilantly cares for heart attack patients, constantly on guard for signs of irregularity in heart function and ready to take appropriate action at any moment. It is only after the patient has stabilized and the doctors and staff are sure that he's out of immediate danger and on the way to recovery that the patient is moved out of the CCU to a more restful and conventional hospital room.

In time, a tough scar usually will form as the heart muscle heals. New circulation may form blood vessels near the blocked artery to help bring blood to the deprived muscle tissue. This is called collateral circulation, which is the body's way of helping the heart to mend after a heart attack.

The first days and weeks after a heart attack require the maximum amount of rest to give the heart a chance to heal (but not the complete inactivity of total bed rest). At first, activity may be limited to getting out of bed to use the toilet or to sit in a chair. Soon, short walks around the room or down the hall are encouraged. By this time, plans are usually being made for the discharge of the patient from hospital, to continue recuperation at home.

Today, people are being discharged from hospitals sooner and sicker, and—especially for the post-MI patient—going home is often greeted with mixed feelings. Once survival from the heart attack has been assured, the person begins to take stock of the emotional as well as the physical impact of what has happened to him.

The weeks and months following a heart attack offer ample opportunity for reflection. A heart attack that has usually come on with no prior warning has disrupted the normal flow of daily events and has threatened the individual's very existence. Life outside the protective security of the hospital with its trained staff often becomes filled with fear and apprehension. Will I have another attack? Will I die because I cannot get the swift help of an on-call hospital staff? Will the pain return? Have I really recovered enough to be at home?

Attention is paid to every twinge, to every strange sensation. Instant mental flashbacks to the scene in the CCU with its beeping monitors and frightening realization that death may be hovering nearby are not uncommon. Most experts agree that these fears usually lessen with time.

Once the reality of what has happened sets in, it is not uncommon for a case of the "blues" to take hold. A sense of being struck down overwhelms the patient, and there is the fear that the active life style the person enjoyed before the heart attack will never again be possible. Questions hammer away at the mind. Will I be able to work again? Will I be as competent at my job as I was before? Will I be able to function at home as I once did? Will I ever be able to enjoy sex again?

The "blues" may take many forms, including changes in sleep patterns, memory problems, loss of interest in sex, and even recurring thoughts of death. Persons not forewarned and prepared for the onset of these frequently experienced reactions during the initial weeks following a heart attack may become unduly concerned and emotionally upset. In a sense, these are the mental and physical aftershocks of the upheaval of a heart attack; they usually lessen and are gone within three months.

The husband or wife and other family members of a heart attack victim are also subject to emotional and physical upsets. They, too, have suffered through the heart attack. They will feel concern for the loved one, resentment for what the heart attack has done to all their lives, and possibly even personal guilt for somehow having caused the heart attack.

Everyone involved—heart attack victim and family alike—has to face the reality of what has happened. The victim has been weakened by the heart attack, and time now becomes an all-important factor. Although the amount of time will vary with the individual, it usually will take about four to six weeks for recuperation to take hold, and perhaps another month before returning to work will be feasible. Patience and understanding will be needed by all concerned.

Recuperation at home has many hills and valleys and bumps and ruts, with good days and bad to be expected. Here's where the positive emotions that come from taking an active part in the recovery process can work magic. Fears, anxieties, and depression have to be made to evolve into a determination for making the recovery work. Regaining health is the goal that both victim and family must work at diligently.

Since, for the time being, the daily demands of a job and the workplace are not pressing, there's time for the person recovering from a heart attack to rethink living patterns and actively work at changing the behavior and habits that previously contributed to the potential for a heart attack. Now is the time to start making changes that will bring about regained strength, increased endurance, restored heart health, and the resumption of normal living patterns. The accomplishment of these goals depends upon adhering strictly to the diet, exercise, and medication plan that has been prescribed to prevent a second heart attack.

DIET

The prudent diet—the heart-healthy diet—has received quite a bit of attention in the press and in a number of cookbooks and other publications. Many people are now quite familiar with the list of no-no's that have come to be associated with a high-fat, high-cholesterol diet. A more complete discussion of good eating guidelines appears in Chapter 6; however, it is worthwhile here to highlight what you can do to maintain good heart health through diet:

1) Get to your ideal weight. It makes little sense (especially if you've already had a heart attack) to make your heart work harder carrying around all those extra pounds. With your doctor's help, you can develop a calorie-controlled eating plan that will help you lose unwanted pounds safely and at a reasonable rate.

2) Eat small meals more often. Many of us have little more than juice and coffee for breakfast, eat lunch on the run, and overeat at dinnertime. This, too, is asking your heart to work harder than neces-

sary. By eating smaller meals more often, you allow your body to digest the food more easily.

3) Control the type and amount of fat in your diet. It has been demonstrated that high-fat, high-cholesterol diets can add to the risk of heart attack. Learn to eat the low-fat way by substituting chicken and fish for the high-fat content of meats such as beef and organ meat. Use the no-cholesterol alternative to butter, namely, margarines made with liquid vegetable oils. Sensible substitutions are readily available. It's just a matter of selecting the low-fat alternatives that food stores now offer—skim milk or 1 percent milk instead of whole milk, for example, or low-fat cheese instead of regular cheese.

4) Modify cooking methods. Broil or bake food instead of frying it, and prefer roasts to heavy cream-filled casseroles.

5) Add complex carbohydrates to your diet. Vegetables, fruits, and enriched cereal and grain products are nutritious alternatives to the high-fat and high-cholesterol foods you are trying to avoid.

6) Use lemon or freshly ground pepper and other spices instead of adding salt to your food. Although the relationship between high sodium levels and high blood pressure (a definite heart risk factor) has not been firmly established, limiting the added salt in your food is easy to accomplish, and it can help maintain good health.

There's ample guidance available from the American Heart Association (contact your local chapter) and in almost every bookstore. The AHA publishes its own cookbook filled with simple and delicious recipies. Also, Jane E. Brody has prepared a sequel to her best-selling *Jane Brody's Nutrition Book.* Called *Jane Brody's Good Food Book,* it offers easy-to-follow guidelines and recipes for sensible and delicious meals.

Some final notes. Periodic blood tests can document the level of cholesterol and triglycerides (fatty acids) in your blood and will indicate to you and your doctor just how effective your eating habits now are. Also, although your doctor may okay the use of moderate amounts of alcohol, keep in mind that there are many calories in liquor, beer, and wine—and very little nutritional value. So if you are watching your weight, be sure to count the calories in any alcoholic drinks you may consume.

EXERCISE

Exercise plays a vital part in the rehabilitation program following a heart attack. Heart attack victims who were dangerously out of condition before the incident will need to establish an exercise program to help them get into shape and maintain good physical condition. Others, who may have exercised before the heart attack, will have to work back slowly to their previous activity levels.

Some hospitals now offer outpatient cardiac rehabilitation programs to provide the guidance and motivation necessary for many post-MI individuals. These programs fill an important need. A progressive exercise program for the cardiac patient has to be as carefully planned and implemented as a medication prescription. Without a planned exercise program, there is danger of a potential "overdose" that can bring on unwanted and hazardous "side effects." Contraindications for exercise have to be reviewed carefully by your physician and other members of the health care team.

In the supervised environment, blood pressure, heart rate, and electrocardiogram (ECG) readings can be monitored before, during, and after exercise. These readings help the exercise therapist modify the program to mesh with the responses of the individual to the various exercises. Also, continual tracking of the individual's condition may help disclose and identify any previously unseen problems that may have existed.

The progressive exercise program begun in the hospital usually is geared to increasing the energy expenditure of the patient to a level of three "mets" (a measure of three times the body's metabolic rate at rest). Simple stretches and arm, leg, and trunk movements are performed under the guidance of a health professional. Heart rate, blood pressure, and ECG readings can be monitored. Often the individual can be taught to take his own pulse and monitor his pulse rate following exercise. Walking up and down stairs may be practiced with supervision, and short walks around the hospital unit may be undertaken as the patient's exercise tolerance increases.

At the time of discharge from the hospital, written instructions may be given to the patient to serve as guidelines for continuing the exercise program at home. The progressive exercise program can provide objective and concrete documentation that the heart is healing and endurance is building. In time, the individual will note that his walking distance has increased while his need for frequent rest periods has declined.

Participation as an outpatient in a cardiac rehabilitation unit adds the further support of many other people similarly working to regain strength and endurance. The support and camaraderie of the group and the ongoing supervision and instruction of the health professionals can spark the less motivated individual to participate in the exercise program. Ultimately, the motivation and perseverance to continue the program must come from the individual, but the support, supervision, and encouragement of others can provide the initial incentive.

Cardiac rehabilitation programs will vary, but all will include a sequence of warm-up exercises, followed by aerobic or dynamic exercises to increase the heart rate to the target level, and concluding with cool-down movements to allow the return of the heartbeat to its normal slower rhythm.

Walking, jogging, bicycling, rowing, jumping rope, and swimming are some of the dynamic exercises that may be included in a cardiac rehabilitation program. People on a home exercise program, working under the supervision of their physician and other health professionals, will probably work on building walking distance over a period of time before adding other forms of dynamic exercise. In some cases, the individual may learn how to take his own pulse and blood pressure readings before and after exercise and to plot the readings on a chart. The chart will give graphic indication of progress being made. The slower pulse rate charted for walking a previously difficult distance will serve as much needed concrete evidence of progress toward recovery and better health. The individual will then have a sense of control over his body and the destiny of his life.

SMOKING

In a word—don't! According to the American Heart Association, smokers who continue to smoke after a heart attack double their risk of a recurrence. Moreover, smoking increases the heart rate, raises the blood pressure, and narrows the blood vessels—all of which are dangerous even to someone who has not had a heart attack, and doubly dangerous to someone who has. Your family physician, the local cancer association, and the American Heart Association all can be of assistance in setting up a "stop smoking" program.

SEX

Unfortunately, commonplace myths and misconceptions about sexual activity after a heart attack are often not discussed at all, or, if they are, the subject is glossed over or even ignored. The impact of abstention from any sexual activity after a heart attack for fear that it is too strenuous can have a harmful effect on both patient and partner. The partner may not wish to "impose" on the patient under the mistaken impression that it may be hazardous, and the patient may be concerned about a lost interest in sexual activity, or be overly conscious and apprehensive about the normal changes in heart rate, breathing, and blood pressure that occur during sex.

A well-written pamphlet entitled "Sex and Heart Disease," available by contacting your local chapter of the American Heart Association, dispels the myths surrounding this subject and provides guidelines for resuming sexual activity.

First and foremost, it is simply *not* true that sex after a heart attack can cause another attack, or even death. Sexual activity, including intercourse, is appropriate as soon as the individuals involved feel ready. Readiness for sexual expression may evolve in stages. The couple may first seek only the pleasure of being close to each other, touching, holding, stroking, caressing. These emotions and actions impose little strain and are life-affirming.

Feelings of depression following a heart attack and anxiety about the ability to perform can have a deleterious effect. By keeping the recovery process in perspective and maintaining a high degree of flexibility in accepting the emotional ups and downs, the couple can find many ways to enjoy closeness and approach lovemaking with patience and understanding.

Here are some suggestions about how to enhance sexual expression:

- Let your exercise program work for you. The program designed to maintain and improve physical conditioning can also help the post-MI individual become better prepared for sexual activity. Exercise builds a sense of vitality, and vitality can work as a strong antidepressant.
- Wait at least one hour after a meal before lovemaking to allow the food to be digested.
- Choose a time and place where both you and your partner will feel rested and free from day-to-day responsibilities and interruptions.
- Be sure to take any medications prescribed by your doctor before lovemaking.
- Talk to each other about feelings, fears, and desires. With communication comes understanding, and understanding leads to greater closeness.

If, with time and exploration, you find that there are problems in sexual function or that, unhappily, things just aren't the same, talk with your doctor, either individually or together. This may help you find answers to lingering questions and doubts. Further counseling by a trained therapist may aid in the resumption of an interrupted sex life.

Because sexual expression and enjoyment adds to all dimensions of life, the return to a normal sex relationship is a critical part of the recuperation process following a heart attack.

LIFE STYLE AND WORK

A life-threatening experience such as a heart attack can lead to a reexamination of priorities and values held prior to the incident. Career goals, job opportunities, and self-imposed life style stresses that had been so all-consuming before the heart attack now become less critically important. Alternatives to the fourteen-hour day may be explored and new career paths and goals may evolve.

The exercise program may become a new high-priority task, to be done each day, and the need to work harder and longer hours than anyone else at the office may well decline in urgency.

About 80 to 90 percent of heart attack victims do return to work within two to three months following the attack, and usually to their old jobs. Some modification of old work habits may have to be made to accommodate the exercise and rest schedule that has now become a part of daily living for the heart attack victim. More effective methods of delegating work will have to be instituted for the busy executive, and less demanding and exhausting travel schedules will have to be worked out. Easing back to work in this manner helps both the heart attack victim and his co-workers and associates to adjust.

For many people, the experience of having a heart attack and spending weeks in recovery serves as a needed incentive to make positive changes in life-style and working and recreational activities— something that could not have been easily accomplished previously. The new habits and patterns may, in fact, lead to a happier and better adjusted person, as well as a healthier one.

It has been said, somewhat ironically, that in some ways a heart attack can become one of the more positive experiences for an individual. It can make you determined to enjoy the rest of your life in the best health possible.

Angina: The Pain that Warns

For some, it happens while shoveling a path through newly fallen snow, or when carrying the groceries from the car to the kitchen. For others, it can happen almost each time they climb a flight of stairs or hurry across a street. Chest pain, tightness, shortness of breath . . . it's scary and it hurts. It's called angina pectoris, and it sounds a body alarm each time it happens.

Angina is not a heart attack. The pain may be similar in nature to that of a heart attack, but it is much less severe and does not last long. Angina occurs when the blood flow to some part of the heart muscle is less than it should be. Discomfort, chest pain, and tightness can be felt when there is an oxygen insufficiency in the coronary arteries that bring oxygen and nourishment to the heart.

The build-up of atherosclerotic plaque over the years narrows the inside of coronary arteries, reducing the normal blood flow. During periods of emotional stress or physical exertion, when the demands of the heart are greater, the narrowed blood vessels are not able to supply the needed oxygen. Oxygen deprivation of the muscle brings on the pain of angina or the typical sensation of tightness in the chest. It is usually short in duration, disappearing after the person calms down and rests a bit. Nitroglycerin, a prescription medication, is the mainstay of treatment for angina and should be taken before pain develops. (If your doctor prescribes nitroglycerin, remember that air, light, heat, moisture, and the passage of time inactivate nitroglycerin. Carry it with you at all times in its original dark glass bottle. Do not carry nitroglycerin in a metal or plastic pill box.)

In time, the development of collateral circulation, with other blood vessels increasing in size to assist in bringing blood to the heart muscle, will help alleviate the discomfort of angina. This extra circulation can help prevent a total blockage (a heart attack) or lessen the potential damage to the heart muscle should a heart attack occur.

PREVENTION—AN IMPORTANT PART OF
TREATMENT

Since the underlying cause for development of angina is usually atherosclerosis—a condition that can also cause a heart attack—your doctor will probably treat your angina by prescribing a diet, an exercise program, and life-style modifications that will help prevent further restriction of coronary artery blood flow. A weight control plan should be set up if overweight is a problem, along with the standard low-fat, low-cholesterol diet and exercise program your doctor advises. By making these critical changes after the initial angina incident, you can reduce the risk of a future heart attack.

As already mentioned, nitroglycerin tablets are generally prescribed for angina. This is a safe, non-habit-forming drug that is usually very effective in relieving the pain and discomfort of angina. It can also be used to prevent an angina incident if taken prior to anticipated physical exertion or a very stressful situation.

Nitroglycerin works by reducing the heart's demand for oxygen, thus better equalizing the supply and demand of blood flow to the heart muscle. Nitroglycerin comes in several forms: tablets that are placed under the tongue; another kind of tablet that is swallowed; capsules, and ointments (disc, patch, or paste) that are absorbed through the skin. If your doctor has prescribed nitroglycerin, keep a fresh supply on hand at all times. As mentioned, do not transfer the tablets from their original dark glass bottle to your pocket or purse. These tablets are sensitive to light and can lose their effectiveness if exposed to light, heat, or air. Fresh nitroglycerin tablets will cause a little stinging under

Table 23 ■ A<small>NTIANGINAL</small> D<small>RUGS</small>*

Generic names	Brand names[a]	Usage information / precautions[b]	Possible side effects[c]
Verapamil	Calan, Isoptin	Take at same time each day 1 hour before or 2 hours after eating • Works 1 to 2 hours after taken • Avoid driving if you feel dizzy • Learn to take your pulse rate; if it drops to 50 beats per minute or lower, do not take medication until you consult your doctor • Avoid taking with alcohol; may cause severe low blood pressure *Overdose symptoms:* unusually fast or slow heartbeat, loss of consciousness, cardiac arrest	*Common:* tiredness *Infrequent:* dizziness, nausea, constipation, unusually fast or slow pulse, cough, shortness of breath, numbness, tingling in hands and feet, difficult urination
Isosorbide dinitrate	Iso-Bid, Isordil, Sorbitrate	Take at same time each day, 1 or 2 hours after meals • Sublingual or chewable tablets work 3 to 5 minutes after taken and swallowed; pills 30 minutes after taken • Periodic lab blood tests may be recommended • Drug relaxes blood vessels, increasing blood flow to heart muscle *Overdose symptoms:* vomiting, sweating, shortness of breath, loss of consciousness	*Common:* headache, flushed face, nausea, vomiting, rapid heartbeat *Infrequent:* fainting *Rare:* skin rash

| Nitroglycerin (glyceryl trinitrate) | Nitro-Bid, Nitro-Dor, Nitrodisc, Nitroglyn, Nitrol, Nitrostat, Transderm-Nitro | Tablet or capsule—swallow whole with liquid; don't chew • Ointment—apply as directed • Sublingual tablets—place under tongue every 3 to 5 minutes at earliest sign of angina; if you don't have complete relief with 3 or 4 tablets, call your doctor. Sublingual tablets work in 1 to 3 minutes. Other forms work 15 to 30 minutes after taken • Will not stop an attack, but may prevent attacks • Avoid taking with alcohol • May cause headache and fainting • Keep sublingual tablets in original container; always carry with you

Overdose symptoms: flushed face, vomiting, weakness, sweating, fainting, shortness of breath, coma | *Common:* faintness, dizziness, headache, flushed face, nausea, vomiting, rapid heartbeat
Infrequent: skin rash
Rare: severe skin irritation, peeling |

* Some of these medications may be prescribed by the doctor for other uses.
a These brand names are only a sampling. Several generics reviewed are available under additional names not listed here.
b Check with your doctor for specific directions and precautions when taking these and any other medications.
c This does not list all of the possible side effects. Check with your doctor regarding the safety and possible side effects when taking these and or any other medications.

Source: H. Winter Griffith, M.D., *Complete Guide to Prescription Drugs* (Tucson: HP Books, 1983).

the tongue, which is one way to make sure they haven't lost their effectiveness.

In addition to nitroglycerin, your doctor may also prescribe other medications called beta blockers that lower the heart rate and blood pressure. These drugs reduce the workload of the heart during exercise, thus helping prevent the development of anginal discomfort. Other drugs called calcium blockers are also used. They work by reducing the blood pressure and, like nitroglycerin, dilate the arteries supplying the heart muscle. Table 23 lists frequently used angina medications.

CORONARY BYPASS SURGERY, THE NEW LEASE ON LIFE

When medications are not sufficiently effective in reducing the occurrence of angina, or when, through diagnostic tests such as coronary arteriography, it is learned that one or more of the coronary arteries is severely clogged, your doctor may recommend coronary bypass surgery. This surgery, developed fifteen years ago, replaces the clogged coronary arteries by grafting blood vessels (usually taken from the leg) as detours around the clogged arteries. If two of these bypass vessels are grafted onto the blocked artery, the operation is known as double bypass surgery; three bypass grafts make it a triple bypass operation.

More than one million Americans have had this surgery, and for many it has offered a new lease on life. With more than 170,000 procedures done each year, there is some question as to whether this surgery is needed in all instances. Yet, for individuals whose arteries have become so clogged that merely walking across the street leaves them panting for breath and in pain, the surgery works like a heavenly gift. Its ability to increase the blood flow to the heart muscle reduces the symptoms of angina and improves the individual's endurance and exercise tolerance.

Coronary artery bypass surgery is major surgery, lasting from three to six hours. Following surgery, the patient is usually taken to an intensive coronary care unit, where fluids, heart function, and breathing can be monitored. Nurses or respiratory therapists usually assist the patient with breathing and coughing exercises to clear the lungs and prevent development of infection.

As with any major surgery, there has to be a period of rest and recuperation to aid the healing process. Like the post-MI patient, the individual recovering from coronary bypass surgery will need time to restore strength and build endurance. A program of progressively more active exercises will be initiated as part of the rehabilitation and recuperation effort.

Time will be needed also—just as with recovering heart attack patients—for the individual and the family members to come to terms with what has happened and to sort through the emotional and physical adjustments that have to be made.

Although surgery does offer significant relief from the discomfort, pain, and debilitation of angina, it does not cure the disease process that led to its development. The new lease on life that the surgery provides will be short-lived unless changes in the individual's behavior, diet, exercise patterns, and life style are made so as to reduce the possibility of a recurrence. In other words, we're back again to the low-fat, low-cholesterol, planned-exercise regimen prescribed by the doctor for heart attack victims. The home recovery process for the postsurgical coronary bypass patient is similar to that of the post-MI patient, with the additional discomfort of a healing surgical wound for the patient to contend with.

In time, the postsurgical coronary bypass patient may find he experiences little or no angina after physical exertion and can now return to living a more active life. Although there is still some controversy over the benefits of bypass surgery for patients with mild angina, and also over whether or not patients who have had bypass surgery actually live longer than those who have not had it, there is little question that the benefits in improved quality of life are appreciated by the thousands of former angina victims now living active, pain-free lives following surgery.

ANGIOPLASTY

Although it is not applicable to all cases of coronary occlusion, the procedure known as coronary angioplasty can be used for a small percentage of angina victims. In this procedure, an inflatable balloon is inserted into the coronary artery on the tip of a flexible tube called a heart catheter. When the clogged portion of the artery is reached, the balloon is inflated, dilating and stretching open the blockage in the artery.

The procedure is significantly less invasive than bypass surgery, and it can successfully open blocked vessels without the weeks and months of recovery needed following surgery. Once again, though, this procedure does not reverse or cure the underlying cause of angina—atherosclerotic disease. As before, life style and dietary changes are needed.

With heart attack and angina, there is no substitute for following good health practices. It's the best way of helping to prevent future attacks.

Hypertension

It's a scene that TV viewers have seen over and over again in hospital dramas, paramedic adventures, or "family doctor" stories. The patient, conscious or unconscious as the case may be, has a blood pressure cuff wrapped around his arm, the bulb is pumped, the stethoscope is placed above the crook of the elbow, and the frowning, very concerned intern, paramedic, or family doctor studies the blood pressure gauge intently, and then . . .

There's no need to go on with the scenario. We all know it pretty much by heart. The above example has been used not to poke fun at television but to point up how familiar almost everyone is with at least the basic motions involved in taking someone's blood pressure. It's a common procedure, and television programs are not leading us astray by showing it to us so often. In every doctor's office, for example, taking a patient's blood pressure is a regular aspect of routine physical examinations. During every operation, a constant check is kept on the blood pressure of the patient and the surgeon is informed of any significant deviations. In other situations—an accident in the streets with paramedics working to save a life, or a hospital emergency room where a stricken patient has just been rushed in by ambulance—blood pressure is monitored as a vital part of the emergency procedure.

Why is blood pressure so important? What, exactly, is being measured?

In checking blood pressure, a measurement is taken of the pressure of the blood against the walls of the arteries as the blood is being pumped through the vascular system by the heart. As long as a person's heart continues to beat, there will be pressure in the arteries. There will be a higher pressure as the heart muscles contract and push the blood out into the arteries and a lower pressure as the heart pauses between contractions to fill up with more blood to pump out on the next beat.

Two measurements are needed to give a full picture of the blood pressure, and they are written one above the other with a line in between, similar to a common fraction (Blood pressure, however, is not derived mathematically, that is, the top figure is not divided by the bottom figure. The two figures are written this way for ease of notation.) The figures represent pressure recorded in millimeters of mercury. The first figure indicates the pressure when the heart contracts and pumps blood into the arteries. This is known as the systolic pressure and is the top figure in the reading. The bottom figure represents the measurement of the pressure when the heart pauses between beats and is known as the diastolic pressure.

The two readings tell the doctor with what force the heart is pumping blood through the body. This gives an indication of how hard the heart is working. A sudden very low blood pressure reading during an operation, for example, or during emergency treatment of an accident victim, indicates serious trouble (the patient is going into shock) requiring immediate medical action. If, on the other hand, a blood pressure measurement is abnormally high, this shows that the heart is straining to pump the blood—and a continued strain of this nature can eventually damage the heart, leading to cardiac disease and heart failure. Additionally, hypertension—the term for persistently high blood pressure—can, in time, bring on a stroke or severely damage the kidneys.

It's in these three areas—heart disease, stroke, and renal (kidney) disease—that hypertension works its greatest havoc by damaging blood vessels in the heart, brain, and kidneys. The walls of blood vessels are fairly elastic, being able to expand to accommodate an increased blood flow under high pressure. However, this elasticity can be lost if the pressure against the vessel walls remains persistently high over a long period of time. This loss of elasticity of the blood vessels in the brain, for example, can weaken them and lead to the bursting of a vessel—a cerebral hemorrhage.

A consistently elevated blood pressure also contributes to the formation of fatty deposits in the lining of blood vessels (atherosclerosis), possibly as a result of the added stress on the inside of the blood vessels. When atherosclerosis develops, the inner diameter of the blood vessels narrow as more and more deposits are accumulated, and this restricts the flow of blood.

A reduction of blood flow to the brain, to the muscles of the heart, and to the kidneys causes damage to these organs. Heart muscles can weaken; brain cells can be deprived of nourishing blood; and kidneys can be kept from functioning properly.

The kidneys have a special relationship to blood pressure. Under normal circumstances, the kidneys help to regulate the blood pressure. For example, if blood pressure drops and less blood flows to the kidneys, they secrete two substances, renin and aldosterone. Through a complex biochemical process, renin causes constriction of blood vessels in the body, which increases the pressure of the blood flowing through these vessels. At the same time, the aldosterone causes sodium and water—the excess of which is normally eliminated by the kidneys in the urine—to be retained in greater quantities in the vascular system. This acts to increase the blood volume, which also raises the blood pressure. Once a normal blood flow to the kidneys is reestablished, renin and aldosterone are no longer secreted.

Damage to blood vessels in the kidneys caused by hypertension can affect the various functions of the kidneys, such as eliminating wastes, regulating blood pressure, and balancing the amount of sodium and water in the system—and can also lead to kidney disease and eventual kidney failure.

The insidious nature of hypertension lies in the fact that no symptoms of it are apparent while it's doing its damage. This is why it is known as the silent killer. Often, it isn't until heart, brain, or kidney damage is severe enough to produce symptoms that the individual will become aware that something is wrong. However, this can be avoided by the simple action of having regular blood pressure checks, which will detect an elevated blood pressure and allow the physician to start treating it—and there are treatments (see below) that can help.

TYPES OF HYPERTENSION AND CAUSES

There are two major types of hypertension: essential (primary) hypertension; and secondary hypertension. About 90 to 95 percent of all known cases are essential hypertension. The exact causes of essential hypertension are not known. Many researchers and physicians believe that a combination of factors contribute to essential hypertension—obesity, a diet high in sodium, heredity, stress, age, and atherosclerosis, for example.

To the average person, stress seems to lead the list. It's quite common to caution someone to "watch your blood pressure" when that individual gets unduly excited. Anger, tension, and excitability—especially when accompanied by a red face and sputtering speech—are the hallmarks of a raised blood pressure to most people. There's truth in this, of course, since persistent and excessive stress can, and often does, lead to an elevated blood pressure. However, hypertension does not necessarily denote that a person is under "hyper" tension. There can be both outward and inner calmness and still the blood pressure will be high, perhaps due to some of the other factors already mentioned.

The causes of secondary hypertension are usually easier to determine. This type of hypertension is a secondary symptom of a primary disorder, such as kidney disease, brain injury, circulatory system disease, or cardiac damage. Once the primary causes have been accurately diagnosed and, if possible, corrected, the secondary hypertension will be eliminated.

DISCOVERING HYPERTENSION

Over 60 million American adults have high blood pressure, which includes about 50 percent of all those over sixty-five. Many are not even aware of its presence. Almost twice as many blacks as whites have hypertension (the reasons for this are still unknown), and hypertension strikes equally at all social and economic levels of society. However, whether it's essential hypertension or secondary hypertension, it's vital that it be detected as early as possible before it can do extensive damage.

Finding out if you have hypertension is a simple matter. The first step is to have your blood pressure checked. You can do this yourself; you can have it done during special drives when blood pressure is checked free in shopping malls and similar places; or you can have your doctor do it.

No matter which method you choose, you should eventually see your doctor. Only a trained medical professional, such as the family physician or a cardiologist, can correctly interpret blood pressure readings. Blood pressure can vary from hour to hour, changing as you walk or sit or stand or move about. Your pressure will be different when you wake up than it is during sleep, and it will also be different at various times during the day. What you eat, what you drink, how you feel at the moment, what kind of stress you may be experiencing—all these and other factors contribute to your blood pressure.

A careful physician will take more than one blood pressure reading on more than one occasion before he makes a diagnosis of hypertension. The record of your blood pressure measurements will be considered along with your general physical condition, your previous medical history, your hereditary background insofar as it relates to hypertension, your present emotional state, and all the other varied factors that your doctor knows have an effect on your blood pressure.

He'll even examine inside your eyes with an ophthalmoscope (that hand-held device the doctor uses to shine a narrow beam of light into your eye while he stands nose to nose with you) to determine the condition of your retina. A retinal examination will disclose whether the small blood vessels in the retina have been affected by high blood pressure, which will give the physician a good general indication of what has happened to the blood vessels in the rest of your body.

How high does high blood pressure have to be before it becomes hypertension? There have been many answers to this. A popular standard used to be that "normal" blood pressure consisted of a systolic pressure (the top figure) of 100 plus your age, and a diastolic pressure (the bottom figure) of 80. Thus, if you were fifty years old, your pressure should be 150 over 80 to be considered normal.

As with most popular conceptions, this one had some truth in it. A diastolic reading of 80 is neither high nor low, and it's a known fact that pressure tends to rise to some degree as we age. However, the 100-plus-your-age-over-80 standard was never really endorsed by knowledgeable physicians.

It also used to be said that the diastolic reading was more important than the systolic reading, since the diastolic reading indicated the blood pressure when the heart was at rest, and if this were high, then it meant the heart was working even harder than the systolic pressure would indicate. Once again, there was a kernel of truth in this, but it didn't tell the full story, nor was it an acceptable standard.

Today, physicians and other health professionals generally agree that a systolic pressure that persistently rises above 140, with a diastolic pressure that remains higher than 90–95, can be diagnosed as hypertension. For individuals over sixty, a systolic pressure of 150–155 would not be considered hypertension. However, it's up to a physician to interpret blood pressure readings, and this physician must know the individual—not necessarily personally, but most certainly medically—in order to assess correctly the series of blood pressure readings and other information that has been gathered about the patient. Also, if necessary, the physician will order tests, not only to add to the medical knowledge about the patient but also to determine whether some disorder other than hypertension is causing the high blood pressure readings.

The patient has to work very closely with the doctor on this. He has to give the doctor all the information he needs, and he has to cooperate with the doctor in all respects. In turn, the doctor has to discuss his findings in detail with the patient, and the two of them should reach a determination together as to the nature of the problem and the various courses of action and treatments available to them.

As part of his examination, a knowledgeable physician will be aware that often a patient's blood pressure responds to the inner tension created merely by the approach of the doctor (or the nurse) to take a blood pressure measurement. It has been demonstrated that a patient's blood pressure can rise in anticipation of the taking of a blood pressure reading. Moreover, it begins to rise not when the arm cuff is being inflated, which to some individuals is a tense moment, but well before the blood pressure measurement is even started.

A patient who had been diagnosed at various times as: (1) "mildly hypertensive," (2) "at the stroke level," (3) "fairly normal," and (4) "having a labile blood pressure that responds to the slightest excitement" was asked when he felt the most tense during a blood pressure measurement. His answer was that his inner tension seemed to rise slowly as he anticipated the coming procedure, then rose swiftly as the cuff was inflated, and peaked when the doctor opened the bulb's release valve and started to take the pressure reading. If the patient was watching the descending column of mercury or the movement of the needle on the gauge (depending on which measuring device the doctor was using), then his tension was most apparent each time the mercury column seemed to "blip" or the gauge needle momentarily wavered. Looking away didn't help much.

This patient may or may not have been typical. However, it has been determined in various tests that both systolic and diastolic pressure readings of some patients varied during the time the doctor was in the room to take a series of blood pressure measurements. Pressure readings were higher during the early part of the doctor's visit, diminishing somewhat as time went by.

Some medical researchers have cautioned that patients can be given medication and a course of treatment started for mild hypertension on the basis of the somewhat elevated readings brought on by the approach of the doctor and the knowledge of the patient that a blood pressure reading was about to be taken.

To counteract this phenomenon, some doctors will place the cuff on a patient's arm and leave it there with the tubing and the bulb dangling while conducting another aspect of the examination or merely talking to the patient. The theory here is that the patient will become accustomed to the cuff, and the tension brought on by his anticipation of the coming blood pressure measurement will thereby be reduced. This technique sometimes works, but on a truly tension-ridden patient it will have little effect.

The reason for all these precautions and qualifications concerning blood pressure readings is that hypertension, in itself, is not so much a disease as it is an indicator of future medical problems. If a misdiagnosis of essential hypertension is made, then there's always the possibility that a primary cause of the hypertension has been overlooked (kidney disease, for example, or brain damage), and treating the hypertension will not attack the main problem. Also, since hypertension often requires a lifetime adherence to the treatment plan and the medications prescribed, the physician (and the patient, too!) must be certain that it is, indeed, hypertension and not some momentary disruption of the patient's blood pressure.

TREATMENT

Once a correct diagnosis of essential hypertension has been made, the matter of treatment has to be considered. Let it be said at the start that, except for extremely severe cases (there is such a disease as malignant hypertension), treatment for hypertension is carried out at home.

It isn't likely that an individual will require home health care solely for hypertension. It is generally not the kind of disorder that requires a person to stay at home. Hypertension, however, can accompany other diseases (diabetes, for example, or renal disease) and so will have to be dealt with at home along with the primary disease.

Hypertension can be successfully treated with drugs. There are many drugs available for this purpose, enough to provide the physician with an arsenal of medications with which to combat hypertension. However, all medications have side effects, and most physicians prefer to try other methods before resorting to drugs. It should be noted, though, that there are physicians and other health specialists who insist that aggressive drug therapy be the treatment of choice. The controversy is still not settled.

What does nondrug therapy involve in the treatment of hypertension? Basically, the problem is attacked on several fronts: weight reduction; limited salt (sodium) intake; a well-balanced, nutritious diet that is low in fat; eliminating smoking (if the patient is a smoker); regular exercise; and learning to cope effectively with stress.

Losing Weight • Obesity is the bane of the hypertensive individual. Excessive fat in the body requires increased blood flow to nourish the fatty tissue, and this puts an additional strain on the heart, forcing it to pump harder. Also, a diet high in fat and cholesterol can lead to the formation of fatty deposits on the walls of the arteries (atherosclerosis), which will narrow the arteries and force an increase in blood pressure in order to maintain the necessary blood flow to the various body organs.

Although many hypertensive individuals are thin, obesity and high blood pressure often go hand in hand. It is not at all unusual for a physician to tell a patient who has mild hypertension, or a blood pressure that is borderline high, that each pound lost will bring the patient that much closer to the complete elimination of the blood pressure problem. In other words, sometimes a significant weight loss will be all that's needed to bring blood pressure down to safe levels.

It's not easy to lose weight, especially if the excess fat represents the accumulation of years of overeating. It must be done, however, if hypertension is to be brought under control. No matter what other treatment methods are tried, including drugs, the presence of excessive fat and a body overburdened with excess weight will reduce the effectiveness of the hypertension treatment.

The family physician can be consulted regarding a diet plan, or he may refer the patient to a trained nutritionist or reputable weight loss clinic. There are more than enough sensible diets (forget the fads!) to give the patient many avenues to weight loss while still maintaining enjoyment of food. Diets do not have to be deadly.

Watch That Salt Intake! • For many years, scientists and medical researchers have been exploring the effect of sodium on blood pressure. Sodium is part of ordinary salt, and there is general agreement that excessive use of salt—at the table, in cooking, and in processed foods—has a direct bearing on the development of hypertension. Conversely, and of great significance, it has been shown that many hypertensive individuals can reduce their blood pressure by cutting down on salt intake.

Does this mean everyone with hypertension has to go on a salt-free diet? Not necessarily. Not everyone who uses salt excessively will develop high blood pressure, and not every hypertensive person will succeed in reducing his blood pressure merely by cutting down on salt. There have been studies that have determined that salt is not as great a contributing factor to high blood pressure as was believed in the past. However, these studies are not conclusive, and some of the methods used in conducting the studies have been questioned.

All of the answers aren't in yet, but what is presently known, based on many years of previous research, indicates that the intake of sodium, mostly through the consumption of ordinary salt, does have a direct effect on the blood pressure.

It's easy enough to use less salt in cooking and to cut down, or even eliminate, the use of salt at the table. It takes a bit more effort, though, to reduce your intake of salt from the consumption of processed foods, which generally make heavy use of salt in their preparation. Product labels can help—if the food manufacturer has listed the sodium content on the label. (If the manufacturer claims his product is "salt-free" or has a "low-sodium" content, or uses similar wording, the actual sodium content must be listed by law.) As a general guide, if salt or sodium is near the top of the list of ingredients on the label, you can be sure the food product is high in sodium.

It's not too difficult to arrange a diet that will significantly restrict the amount of sodium consumed and, at the same time, allow a person some freedom of choice in food selection. Common sense will tell you that you should not attempt to set up a diet of this type on your own. A knowledgeable physician should be your guide. Also, there is much information available in various books on the subjects of hypertension and nutrition, and organizations such as the American Heart Association (see the Appendix) can provide useful literature.

Drug Therapy • One of the first medications a physician may prescribe when starting a drug therapy treatment program for hypertension is a diuretic. A diuretic increases the excretion of urine and decreases the amount of sodium and water retained in the body. Less sodium, as has already been explained, will work to reduce hypertension. In addition, the diuretic action removes excess water from body tissues, reducing fluid volume and helping to bring down blood pressure.

The most commonly prescribed diuretics are the various thiazides, for example, chlorothiazide (Diuril) and hydrochlorothiazide (Esidrix). These drugs generally act within an hour after being taken. In addition to their beneficial action, some diuretics may cause a loss of potassium from the body, which can lead to muscle pains or cramps, excessive tiredness, or nausea and vomiting. To avoid these side effects, be sure to add foods high in potassium to your diet—for example, bananas, raisins, oranges, melons, and avocados. In some cases, your doctor may want to prescribe a potassium supplement.

Prolonged use of a diuretic can sometimes lead to an attack of gout (see Chapter 20 on arthritis). This is a highly painful disorder, and there are drugs available (colchicine is the most common) to relieve the pain of the attack.

Patients who have diabetes have to be careful when taking diuretics, as these drugs may increase blood sugar levels. A blood test will tell the physician whether this has happened, and he can compensate for it by changing the insulin dosage (if the patient is an insulin-dependent diabetic) or by suggesting dietary changes for the patient.

Other medications are used to increase the effectiveness of the treatment program. Usually, the next drug tried is what is known as a beta blocker, which acts to relax and expand blood vessel walls, thus bringing about a decrease in blood pressure. One of the most common beta blockers usually prescribed is propranolol (Inderal). Side effects of this drug can include fatigue, insomnia, and asthmalike symptoms. It may also increase the effects of oral antidiabetic drugs and insulin, which means that diabetics taking Inderal or other beta blockers should be extra careful and check with their physicians.

Many other drugs are available to the physician in setting up the treatment program for hypertension. Each of these drugs has a specific purpose and possible side effects. Table 24 lists frequently used hypertension medications. The patient and the doctor should discuss the suggested medications, the dosage required, the possible side effects, and anything else that will add to the patient's knowledge and understanding of the treatment program and how it will work to help him.

MONITORING YOUR BLOOD PRESSURE AT HOME

It wasn't too long ago that you could get your blood pressure checked only in your doctor's office or in a hospital. Moreover, most of the time

Table 24 ■ ANTIHYPERTENSIVE DRUGS*

Generic names	Brand names[a]	Usage information/precautions[b]	Possible side effects[c]
Atenolol Metoprolol Nadolol Propranolol Timolol	Tenormin Lopressor Corgard Inderal Blocadren	Prescription required • Take as prescribed • Drug starts working 1 to 4 hours after taken • Don't drive until you learn how drug affects you • Take with meals or immediately after • Do not discontinue without consulting your doctor • Dose may need gradual reduction if you have taken medication for a long time *Overdose symptoms:* weakness, slow or weak pulse, blood pressure drop, fainting, convulsions, cold and sweaty skin	*Common:* drowsiness, numbness or tingling of fingers or toes, dizziness, diarrhea, nausea, pulse slower than 50 beats per minute, cold hands and feet, fatigue, weakness, dry mouth *Infrequent:* hallucinations, insomnia, headache, confusion, depression, nightmares, reduced alertness *Rare:* skin rash, sore throat, fever, unusual bleeding and bruising
Prazosin	Minipress	Prescription required • Drug starts working 30 minutes after taken • Do not drive until you learn how drug affects you • First dose likely to cause fainting • If over 60 do not stand while taking • Sit or lie down if you feel dizzy *Overdose symptoms:* extreme weakness, loss of consciousness, cold-sweaty skin, weak-rapid pulse, coma	*Common:* vivid dreams, drowsiness, dizziness, rapid heartbeat *Infrequent:* headache, irritability, depression, rash, blurred vision, dry mouth, appetite loss, constipation, diarrhea, nausea, vomiting, chest pain, shortness of breath, increased urine *Rare:* decreased sexual functions

(Table 24 continued)

Generic names	Brand names[a]	Usage information / precautions[b]	Possible side effects[c]
Captopril	Capoten	Prescription required • Take as prescribed • Works 60–90 minutes after taken • Avoid driving if you become dizzy • Do not stop using without consulting your doctor • May need periodic lab blood counts and urine tests • Take on empty stomach (1 hour before or 2 hours after eating) • First dose, if taken with a diuretic, may cause severe blood pressure drop *Overdose symptoms:* fever, chills, sore throat, fainting convulsions, coma	*Common:* skin rash, loss of taste *Infrequent:* dizziness, fainting, chest pain, irregular heartbeat, swelling of face, hands, and feet *Rare:* sore throat, nausea, vomiting, indigestion, abdominal pain, cloudy urine, fever, chills
Chlorothiazide (diuretic) Chlorthalidone Hydrochloro- thiazide	Diuril Hygroton Hydrodiuril	Works 4–6 hours after taken • May take several weeks to lower blood pressure • Hot weather and fever may cause dehydration and drop in blood pressure • In people over 60, may cause severe dizziness and excessive potassium loss *Overdose symptoms:* cramps, weakness, drowsiness, weak pulse, coma	*Infrequent:* dizziness, mood changes, headaches, blurred vision, dry mouth, nausea, vomiting weak pulse, weakness, tiredness, weight changes *Rare:* rash, sore throat, fever, jaundice

| Triamterene and hydrochloro-thiazide (diuretic) | Dyazide | Works 2 hours after taken • May take 2–3 days for maximum benefit • If 1 dose per day, take after breakfast; if more than 1 dose per day, take last dose no later than 6 PM • In people over 60, long use may increase blood clots • May cause rash or sunburn in areas exposed to sun

Overdose symptoms: lethargy, irregular heartbeat, coma | *Infrequent:* anxiety, drowsiness, confusion, dry mouth, thirst, diarrhea, irregular heartbeat, unusual tiredness, weakness
Rare: headache, sore throat, fever, red-inflamed tongue, unusual bleeding or bruising |

*These drugs may be prescribed by the doctor for other uses.

ᵃThese brand names are only a sampling. Several generics reviewed are available under additional names not listed here.

ᵇCheck with your doctor for specific directions and precautions when taking these and any other medications.

ᶜThis does not list all of the possible side effects. Check with your doctor regarding the safety and possible side effects when taking these and or any other medications.

Source: H. Winter Griffith, M.D., *Complete Guide to Prescription and Non-Prescription Drugs* (Tucson: HP Books, 1983).

you were never told what your pressure was, just that it was "all right" or "normal," or perhaps that it was "high" or "slightly elevated" or maybe "a bit low." Even if you were given the figures, you probably wouldn't know what they meant. And certainly the technical name for the device used to measure blood pressure—a sphygmomanometer—was foreign to most people, who wouldn't even attempt to pronounce it.

As in so many other aspects of our lives, time has wrought changes. Today, not only are many people knowledgeable about the meanings of blood pressure readings, but they take their own pressure at home. The old standby of the doctor's office—the upright gauge with the column of mercury riding up and down in a glass tube between a double line of figures—is still around. However, you can now purchase, at fairly reasonable prices, just about any type of home blood pressure monitor to fit your individual needs.

The selection of home monitors available include manual, electronic, and digital monitors, each of which has special features that will allow an individual to pick the one best suited to him.

Manual monitors often have the stethoscope attached to the edge of the cuff to facilitate one-handed operation. To use such a monitor, wrap the cuff around your upper arm, following the directions supplied by the manufacturer and making sure that the stethoscope is properly positioned over the upper arm artery. Pump the bulb attached by tubing to the arm cuff, inflating the cuff and putting pressure on the artery until the flow of blood is stopped.

Next, open the release valve on the bulb and slowly let the air out of the cuff, listening through the stethoscope for the tapping sounds that indicate blood is once again flowing through the artery. The pressure indication on the gauge at this point is the systolic pressure.

You continue to release the air from the cuff while still listening through the stethoscope. The tapping sounds you first heard have now become louder and more pronounced. Then, as more air is released and the pressure of the cuff on the artery is reduced, the sounds become muffled and finally disappear. The point at which there is a distinct change in sound or the sounds can no longer be heard is the diastolic pressure.

It takes a bit of practice, but in a short time it will no longer be a strange procedure to you. It's not something that you can sluff off or perform carelessly, however. As the manufacturer's instruction booklet will no doubt explain, you have to be careful to get the cuff properly positioned over the upper arm artery and also have the stethoscope set up so that you hear the sounds without difficulty. If the cuff has been placed wrong, it may take more pressure than it should to shut off the artery, and you'll then get an erroneous blood pressure measurement.

The same holds true if the stethoscope is not positioned above the artery. The sounds may not appear when they should, which will also give a false reading.

To make certain you are using the device correctly, you may want to take it with you when you visit your doctor and have him watch as you take your own blood pressure. He can then compare your reading with the one he gets on his sphygmomanometer and will be able to advise you if you are doing it correctly and, if not, tell you how to correct your errors.

Physicians today realize the importance of making the patient a full partner in his own health care, and this includes home monitoring of blood pressure. At one time, many doctors and other health professionals thought it would be counterproductive to encourage patients to monitor their own blood pressure at home. There were dire predictions of patients panicking and running to the doctor or the emergency room of the hospital if they obtained unexpectedly high readings when taking their blood pressure. At the very least, it was reasoned, the ordinary patient would not know what to do with the blood pressure reading once it was obtained, and this would bring about a flood of phone calls to the doctor asking for an interpretation of the reading.

None of these things happened, and home monitoring of blood pressure is now firmly entrenched, both as a part of home health care and also for people who wish to check the status of their health between visits to the doctor.

The electronic and digital home monitors now being offered to the general public represent state-of-the-art devices. Using microphones to pick up artery sounds, flashing lights, microprocessors, and computer displays, these devices make it easy to check your blood pressure with almost foolproof accuracy. Prices vary almost as much as special features of the monitors. Your local pharmacy will often have a display of monitors or, at the very least, a catalog from which you can make your selections.

COPING WITH STRESS AND HYPERTENSION

One of the uses of a home blood pressure monitor is to learn how to cope with stress to reduce your blood pressure. It's a simplified form of biofeedback for those who do not have the money or the time to visit a laboratory and get hooked up to the machines that tell the patient how his body is reacting to the influence of his thoughts. People can reduce their blood pressure in this way, and it has proven to be an effective technique.

In its own way, home monitoring of blood pressure has also proven effective. By taking your blood pressure at various times of day and under different circumstances, you can obtain a better understanding of how your body is reacting to various types of stress. With better understanding will come relaxation and a lessening of inner tensions, and in time a lowering of the blood pressure.

Relaxation and reduction of inner tensions is the key to blood pressure control. There are many techniques for obtaining relaxation. One of the most common methods is to sit quietly in a dim room, close your eyes, and think of each part of your body as you command it to relax. You can start with your toes and work your way up to your head, or do it in reverse. Practice is needed, of course, but this technique can be made to work. Once again, books are available. Check with your local library or browse around the bookstore, if possible, or consult your doctor or a therapist. Help is there if you wish to avail yourself of it.

The hypertensive person is not necessarily unduly nervous. However, stress can build in many ways, and too much stress will have an effect on your blood pressure. If you learn to live with stress and control its effects on you (see the section on dealing with stress in Chapter 4), you will be able to prevent stress from increasing your hypertension—or perhaps from bringing it on if you are presently free of it.

COMPLIANCE PROBLEMS

This is a term doctors use when referring to the problem of getting patients to follow a treatment program. Compliance represents a special problem with hypertension, and it's one the patient should be knowledgeable about.

Because hypertension often has no symptoms and the individual feels good, it's difficult to get that individual to follow a strict regimen of taking medication, eating properly, and cutting down on salt intake. It becomes even more difficult if the medications produce unwanted side effects. Many a patient has stopped following the doctor's treatment program because of this.

Researchers have found that compliance depends on a number of factors, mostly having to do with the patient's knowledge of hypertension and his perception of its seriousness. If the patient perceives his hypertension as something that's not bothering him and that may disappear if he just watches his weight and what he eats, then that patient will not be at all likely to keep taking the medications prescribed by his doctor.

If the patient does not perceive any immediate benefits from the treatment, or if he feels that the treatment will cause more difficulties and problems than the hypertension itself, then he will not be at all inclined to stick with the treatment program.

Control of hypertension often means a complete change of life style, and the patient will find many reasons to resist this change—especially if his hypertension is at the stage where no symptoms have appeared. The patient may balk at taking prescribed medications if it doesn't make him feel any better and usually makes him feel a bit worse in some respect.

If you have hypertension you should be aware of the pitfalls represented by this compliance problem. Knowledge of what hypertension is and what damage it can do is a good starting point for encouraging compliance in yourself. It's difficult enough to fight hypertension without bringing in the additional difficulty of fighting your natural inclination not to comply with a treatment program that limits and changes the way you want to live.

Think through all of your perceptions of hypertension and the requirements of the treatment program you and your doctor have worked out. You may find that many of these perceptions are a form of self-deception about the seriousness of the disease, the efficacy of the medication, and the severity of the consequences if you do not control the hypertension.

Hypertension may have no symptoms at the start. But if you let it get out of control, you're likely to have more unpleasant and possibly life-threatening symptoms than you care to deal with.

Hypertension can be controlled. How well it is controlled is up to each individual.

20

Arthritis

IF YOU HAVE arthritis, you are in considerable company. It is presently estimated that 15 percent of Americans have to contend with more than 100 different arthritis-related diseases. That's more than 31 million people, at an annual cost (including treatment and lost productivity) of almost $17 *billion*.

Among the 100-plus kinds of arthritis and related diseases, there are some familiar names such as rheumatoid arthritis, osteoarthritis, and gout, and also many less familiar—systemic lupus erythematosus, for example. Each of these rheumatic diseases is distinct, with its own causes, treatment, and therapies. The effects on people coping with these diseases can range from a mild stiffness and infrequent pain to severe disabling pain and loss of certain functional abilities.

Research laboratories, both government and private, have spent hundreds of millions of dollars seeking causes and cures. Theories abound, but there is not as yet any identified cause, or causes. However, because of these research efforts, medical scientists have gained considerable insight into these diseases and have been able to devise, test, and make available a variety of methods and therapies for treating and coping with the effects (symptoms) of these diseases.

We now have a wide variety of drugs available to treat the pain and inflammation associated with arthritis. For severely deformed hips or knees, replacement joints have been developed and used with exciting results. These symptomatic treatments help arthritis sufferers live a fuller and more functional life.

Unfortunately, many people with arthritis believe its presence is an unavoidable part of growing older for which nothing can be done. They delay obtaining proper medical treatment and seek to treat themselves with a variety of unproven therapies. Self-treatment, in itself, is not wrong. Taking responsibility for your own health and actively managing and participating in your health care regimen is an excellent approach to maintaining good health. You cannot do it alone, however—and this is especially true when arthritis is concerned. You need to include, as a vital part of your health care team, a trained physician.

Together, you and your doctor will be able to evaluate the effects and benefits of the various therapies and arthritis medications available that are designed to help avoid or reduce the possibility of a crippling disability. Often, the treatment for stiffness or pain is only part of the story. There should also be an ongoing effort to prevent any permanent damage or further loss of function.

In this section, we will be discussing the major arthritis-related diseases, with an overview of some of the arthritis management techniques you and your doctor can evaluate to maximize function and limit disability.

The word "arthritis" actually means inflammation of the joint. The joint itself consists of a number of different types of tissues working synergistically (producing a combined effect greater than the sum of the individual effects) to allow for movement of the two bones that meet at the joint. In the normal joint, each of the bones has a protective pad of cartilage at each end. This rubbery covering acts as a shock absorber and prevents the bones from rubbing against each other as they move.

The joint is surrounded by a synovial sac that protects the entire joint. The synovial fluid that is released here helps lubricate the joint for easy movement. The bones themselves are encased by muscles, connected to the bones by the fibrous tissue of the tendons. When you bend your knee, for example, certain muscles become shorter (contract), and others become longer (relax). This push-pull action on the tendons attached to the bones in the knee joint causes the knee to bend. The knee cartilage and the synovial fluid within the knee joint work to make this motion smooth, easy, and pain-free.

Rheumatoid Arthritis

The main symptoms of rheumatoid arthritis are hot, stiff, and inflamed joints. For reasons that are still unclear, the synovial membrane in the joint becomes inflamed, and the joint becomes swollen and feels puffy to the touch. The inflammation causes an increase of blood flow to the joint, which makes the area feel warm. Enzymes are released into the joint space, and this can cause additional irritation. Over the course of years, enzymes can irreversibly damage the cartilage and bone.

This chronic inflammatory disease affects both large and small joints. The wrists and knuckles are almost always involved. Rheumatoid arthritis can cause pain, weakness, fatigue, and immobility. It can have an erratic course, with periods of inflammation and disease activity followed by periods of remission. Of great concern to doctors and therapists during periods of activity is the protection of the tissues of the joint to prevent deformity and help preserve function during periods of remission.

Rheumatoid arthritis is more than a joint disease. Many doctors refer to it as rheumatoid *disease* so as to include the entire body or "systemic" impact of this condition. In addition to the tired and weak feeling generally associated with infections in the body, rheumatoid arthritis may involve other tissues and organs of the body, including the heart, lungs, and eyes.

According to Kate Lorig, R.N., Dr. P.H., and James J. Fries, M.D. in *The Arthritis Helpbook* (Reading, Mass.: Addison-Wesley, 1980), "Even the worst cases of rheumatoid arthritis tend to get better with time. The arthritis usually becomes less aggressive." This finding provides even more reason to treat and protect the joints during the early stages to help preserve function when disease activity lessens.

Once an accurate diagnosis of rheumatoid arthritis is made—after a physical examination and a series of tests—the physician will recommend an individualized and comprehensive treatment plan. This treatment plan will probably include rest and exercise because the appropriate balance of each is important in maintaining flexibility while preventing deformity.

Varying regimens of anti-inflammatory and pain-relieving drugs may be tested in order to select the approach that offers the most benefits with minimal side effects. Quick-fix treatments are not necessarily the approach doctors prefer. They know that although it is difficult to predict, it is possible that rheumatoid arthritis may be present on and off for quite some time. This is one of the reasons why potent painkillers are not prescribed too readily. Some medications could completely eliminate any sensation of pain; however, doctors usually prefer to focus their drug treatment on reducing inflammation, which is the cause of the pain. If pain were to be completely eliminated with little or no reduction of the pain-causing inflammation, joint damage would most likely result. The warning cue of pain causes the individual to limit the stresses that additional activity would place on the joints during a period of inflammation.

Since the cause of rheumatoid arthritis (and, therefore, the cure) has not yet been determined, the treatment plan has to focus on relief of symptoms. However, an entire new generation of modern drugs now makes it possible to help most people lead productive and comfortable lives and avoid the potentially crippling effects of the disease.

Osteoarthritis

Of the 100-plus varieties of arthritis, by far the most common is osteoarthritis, which is not an inflammation of the joints but rather a degenerative disease. Osteoarthritis is a deterioration of the cartilage that supports the bone connection at a joint. It is often considered a "universal" problem associated with the aging process, for virtually everyone over the age of sixty will show some deterioration on an X-ray. Fortunately, few of these people actually experience the symptoms that can accompany osteoarthritic changes.

As the cartilage wears, it becomes thinner. For some as yet unexplained reason, the bony surface next to the cartilage becomes thicker. Little spurs of bony bumps also form. This combination of worn cartilage and thicker bone surfaces, along with the presence of spurs, can cause pain when the joint is flexed. Bone can move against bone—much like a creaking unoiled door or gate—resulting in stiffness and pain.

Lorig and Fries, in *The Arthritis Helpbook,* describe three kinds of osteoarthritis. The mildest form affects the joints of the fingers, resulting in the knobby bumps usually associated with the aging process.

Another form of osteoarthritis affects the discs of the spine. Bony growths appear when the spaces between the vertebrae narrow. Here, the discs rather than the cartilage become frayed. Once again, symptoms of stiffness and pain can occur, although the changes in the spine can begin relatively early in life, and the individual may be completely symptom-free.

The third form of osteoarthritis, more common than the other two and often more painful, affects the weight-bearing joints of the hips and knees. An X-ray of an affected joint will show a lessening of the apparent space between the bones as the cartilage occupying this space thins and frays and bony spurs appear.

Pain in the joint may come and go, accompanying walking or other movement of the joint. In addition, the muscles attached to the bone will need to work harder to accomplish a simple task, with the result that these muscles may tire and show signs of fatigue not normally to be expected for such a simple task. Yet movement of these joints and their associated muscles is vitally important to maintain range of motion and flexibility and to retard or reduce the stiffness that can result from lack of use.

The additional bulk of an overweight person can add further stress to the vulnerable joints. Loss of extra pounds will significantly reduce the wear and tear on the joints.

Research is providing more and more information about osteoarthritis, but it is still not known exactly why some people experience mild symptoms and others more severe discomfort. Some people can have osteoarthritis in many of their joints, yet they may feel stiffness or discomfort in only one area. The pain can be present each day for weeks on end and then disappear for weeks or months at a time. Moreover, it is difficult to predict how the illness will progress over time, or even which treatment plan will be most helpful.

People with osteoarthritis can learn the techniques that help to manage and control the stiffness and pain of the disease. A regular routine of exercise to maintain flexibility and function, plus rest to reduce or prevent disability, can help to ensure an independent and active life style for the osteoarthritis victim.

Joint Replacement Surgery

Surgery for arthritis problems of pain and stiffness was once considered the treatment of last resort: when all else failed, surgical intervention was tried. In the past twenty years, however, the development of replacement joints and the surgical techniques for implanting them has been an exciting advance in the treatment of arthritis.

In hip replacement surgery, for example, the worn and stiffened ball and socket of the hip is replaced with plastic and metal parts. The new joint is constructed by replacing the top of the thigh bone with a metal ball on a stem. The socket, or cup, of the pelvis is replaced with a plastic cup.

Using a fast-hardening glue, orthopedic surgeons can equip a person with a new joint that can eventually permit pain-free movement of the previously diseased joint. With exercise, physical therapy, and a commitment to rehabilitation, the previously disabled person will find that the replacement joint will allow him to walk free of pain—and only someone who has been through this pain can appreciate what this means to the arthritic patient.

This remarkable achievement in hip replacement has served as a model for replacement of joints in other parts of the body. Knee joint replacements are becoming increasingly more common, and shoulder and elbow joint replacements are beginning to emerge.

Usually, the decision to perform a joint replacement can be made without the pressures of an emergency situation. This gives the patient—

the replacement candidate—and the surgeon a chance to evaluate the risks and benefits of such a procedure. All surgery carries with it an element of risk. Moreover, the recuperation and rehabilitation process can be quite demanding and will require a long period of time.

The nonemergency nature of this type of surgery gives a gift of time to the arthritis sufferer, allowing her to obtain answers to all questions she may have—and the opportunity to get a second (or even a third) opinion. Once these preliminaries have been attended to and the patient has developed confidence in the surgeon, the operation can proceed.

Gout

Gout was once considered a disease of the wealthy, since they were the only ones who could afford to gorge themselves on the rich food and fine wines that were supposed to bring on an attack of gout. Today, we know that food and drink are not that much to blame, and gout is more economically democratic (it strikes both rich and poor), although it can be called sexist since nine out of ten people with gout are male.

Gout is a painful, serious, and potentially crippling form of arthritis. Fortunately, for most of the close to 1 million Americans with gout, use of proper medication makes it a controllable disease.

During the last thirty years, research scientists have been able to identify the key factors responsible for this painful disorder. It has been found that gout occurs when the body has too much of a substance called uric acid. Uric acid is one of the by-products of another substance—purine. Purines can be found in organ meats and in anchovies and sardines. Also, the body manufactures purines from other substances.

When the uric acid level in the blood is too high, the body usually excretes it to maintain a more normal level. However, if the healthy balance of uric acid production and excretion goes awry, the excess of uric acid in the blood can precipitate out as tiny crystals of sodium urate. These crystals seem to seek out and settle in the joints—usually the big toe, but also in the knees, elbows, and wrists.

These crystals are "foreign" substances in the joints, and their presence causes the body's protective white blood cells to invade the joints and remove the offending crystals—which then allows additional crystals to settle in. This cycle creates an extremely painful inflammation, a swelling and reddening of the affected joint area. In some cases, there is a slower buildup of these crystals into puffy, disfiguring skin lumps called tophi at or near the joints.

Gout attacks may occur for no apparent reason, or they may follow a minor injury, surgery, or overindulgence in food or drink. During a gout attack, there can be extreme pain; between attacks, the person can be completely symptom-free. Untreated attacks can last about a week.

DIAGNOSIS AND TREATMENT

The unique symptoms of gout help doctors in making a diagnosis. A blood test can reveal an abnormally high level of uric acid, which is an important clue for the doctor. Also, since the drug colchicine offers definitive relief during an inflammation, its effective use usually affirms gout as the diagnosis.

Although the causes of gout are now clear, there continues to be no known cure. However, a number of medications have been found to be quite effective in treating an attack in progress, and even preventing future attacks. These drugs help by increasing the excretion of uric acid (probenecid) or by decreasing the body's production of uric acid (allopurinol). A drug used to fight inflammation (phenylbutazone) is also used.

Gout sufferers need not eat special diets, although avoiding foods high in purines may be recommended. During a painful attack, adequate rest and protection of the affected joint can be helpful in recovery.

Managing with Arthritis

Exercise, rest, proper medication, avoidance of fatigue, and the "right" attitude help the arthritis sufferer to live as independently and as pain-free as possible. This approach may require a reevaluation of an individual's current life style and the adoption of new habits and new commitments. Let's take a logical look at what is involved if you have to manage with arthritis and the potential benefits that you can enjoy.

It's helpful to remember that the changes in your functional abilities—and even the endurance of discomfort—have usually taken place over quite a long period of time. Even if you make drastic changes in your life style, it will take a certain amount of time for the effects to become apparent.

EXERCISE: KEEP MOVING TO KEEP MOVING!

Living with arthritis can mean that pain will be the result of many movements you may make; nonetheless, movement and exercise are important parts of arthritis treatments. Although on the surface this may sound contradictory, it makes good sense.

When you make any kind of bodily movement, you have to use the muscles, ligaments, and tendons that surround and attach to the bones in the joints to accomplish that movement. Stiffness in a joint has an impact on the muscles and tendons that move the articulating bones. By keeping these muscles as strong and as flexible as possible, you are increasing the probability of maintaining the highest possible level of function.

This not only makes sense—it's a must. Without working to maintain flexibility and to build strength in the muscles, you may be multiplying the functional impact of the arthritis-affected joint. Weakened muscles will have an all but impossible task of trying to move a stiffened joint.

Exercise has numerous other benefits. Regular exercise helps to control weight. Swimming, walking, cycling—all of these burn calories. No matter what your age or condition, when you burn more calories than you consume, the result will be a loss of weight. Trimming down and losing extra pounds reduces stress on the weight-bearing joints. Moving about can be easier if you are moving less of a load.

The extra energy that you expend during exercise can add energy to the rest of the day. The increase in blood flow during and immediately after exercise helps bring nourishment to the synovial fluid and the joint cartilage and helps remove the waste products present.

Assuming that the exercise program is begun slowly and increased gradually and you are not exercising too strenuously during a period of inflammation, you can actually increase your stamina and reduce fatigue. Best of all, exercise can make you feel better about yourself and your appearance and will add confidence to the way you carry yourself and move about.

You should plan your exercise program with the advice and guidance of your doctor or physical therapist. With this type of professional help, you can schedule a daily regimen of warm-up exercises or activities. Simple stretches or small movements in the "pain-free" range can help get the blood flowing.

Sometimes the application of heat prior to exercise—a hot bath or shower, hot packs, paraffin wax, a heating pad, or a hot water bottle—will help relax the joints and muscles and relieve pain. "Taking the waters" at a spa can have a similar effect.

In other instances, applying cold may also be effective. The application of cold can relax the muscles and will have a numbing effect. This may help with a "hot joint."

Your exercise program should include exercises to maintain range of motion and to gently stretch the muscles and tendons of the joints. These range-of-motion exercises can be done daily to ensure the continued motion of joints and can be performed actively (by yourself) or passively (by someone else moving the affected body part). Each of the numerous joints in your body has its own range of motion. With daily movement and exercise, function and flexibility will be maintained. (See the section on "Keeping Fit" in Chapter 8 for some simple range-of-motion exercises.)

A second form of exercise consists of strengthening exercises. By building up the strength of your muscles, you will add support and stability to stiff or weakened joints. A word of caution here: lifting heavy weights and placing this burden on vulnerable joints is *not* the way to build muscle strength. The added stress of too much weight can hurt more than it helps. You and your therapist or your doctor will have to develop a plan that works to strengthen the appropriate muscles without adding an extra burden to the joints. The combination of a carefully planned program of strengthening exercises and range-of-motion and flexibility exercises will help maintain and improve function.

A third form of exercise, designed to add to your endurance level, is aptly called endurance exercise. "Fun" activities such as swimming, walking, cycling, and dancing promote better heart health and improve the way you feel. Over a period of time, there can be an improvement in blood circulation and breathing capacity and an overall increase in your feelings of fitness and well-being, despite the impact of arthritis.

After exercising, a cool-down period helps return your heart rate to a normal level. As you cool down, be careful not to get chilled. At all times, as you progress through your exercise regimen, be sure to listen to your body. It will help prevent exercise-induced injuries. The idea is to maintain the stretch and motion of your muscles and slowly work to increase range, strength, and endurance. If there is considerable long-lasting pain after exercising, you may be overdoing it. Listen to your body. Cut back on the exercise a bit until you can build it up once again.

REST AND ENERGY CONSERVATION

As important as exercise is to maintaining joint movement, resting an inflamed joint is equally important to helping reduce the inflamation. However, too much rest—or just plain inactivity—can lead to stiffened joints and eventually more painful joints.

The challenge here is achieving a balance. You have to learn your own body signals in order to work out the appropriate balance for yourself. There may be times when a particular joint has to be splinted to permit it to rest safely in a healthy position. However, you will not want too much time to elapse before you begin using the joint again—albeit gently at first—to ensure flexibility and build good muscle tone.

With rheumatoid arthritis, for example, you have to be particularly careful to rest when needed and to increase your exercise regimen gradually during periods when there is no inflammation.

In general, people with arthritis should learn the techniques of energy conservation. It's not difficult to accomplish. If you think about it, you'll realize that we do often "spend" more energy during the day than is necessary. All those trips up and down the stairs in your home may include many unnecessary trips. Preparing extra snacks or performing additional household chores or trying to squeeze in one more hour of work on some special project often serves only to deplete your energy reserves.

Each of us wakes up each morning with a "cupful of energy." If we spend it wisely, we will find that we have adequate energy to complete all the necessary tasks of the day, with a bonus amount left over to spend on hobbies and social activities.

If, however, we deplete our energy reserves too early in the day, we are left too tired and fatigued to continue during the day. Short naps or rest periods at intervals during the day will help to restore some of the lost energy level.

Learning the two guidelines of energy conservation—organization and efficiency—can be of great help in guarding that cupful of energy. Spend some time thinking about the activities you wish to complete,

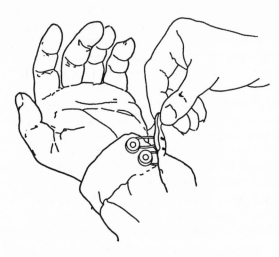

Button extenders can ease the morning routine when arthritis limits dexterity.

ARTHRITIS

either on a daily or a weekly basis, whichever is most convenient for your situation. Plan to accomplish these activities in such a way as to take advantage of your periods of higher energy. Do this by setting priorities and clustering chores.

By planning ahead, you will find that you do, indeed, have more time and energy to finish tasks without becoming rushed or exhausted. In addition, by sprinkling periods of rest among periods of exertion, you will help to recharge your "batteries" for continuation of your activities. Added help comes from planning your work areas to avoid unnecessary steps—by sitting at work rather than standing, for example, and by prioritizing your activities and eliminating tasks that are unnecessary.

Further suggestions on getting the most out of your day can be found in Tables 9–15, "Tips for Daily Living," which contain practical suggestions for efficiently performing activities we engage in each day. Dressing, cooking, housekeeping, self-care, and other essential tasks can often be made easier and less taxing by planning ahead and modifying your approach, where necessary, to conserve energy.

MEDICATION: HELPS AND HAZARDS

There's quite a variety of prescription and nonprescription drugs available today to treat the assortment of symptoms associated with arthritis. Flare-ups of rheumatoid arthritis can be treated with anti-inflammatory medications that have been developed for this purpose. Antipain medication (analgesics) works to reduce or even eliminate the pain associated with osteoarthritis or rheumatoid arthritis. Antigout drugs are also quite effective in preventing an attack or in relieving the symptoms of the attack once it has begun.

The therapeutic effects and the accompanying side effects of the available drugs can vary from person to person. Although increased dosages of aspirin may relieve the pain associated with osteoarthritis for some, or reduce the inflammation of rheumatoid arthritis for others, it may also cause unwanted side effects in many people.

You and your doctor will probably have to work together for a period of time to devise the drug regimen that will work best for you. Although the overall goals of treatment may be clear and simple—reduce inflammation, preserve function, control pain, and restore any lost function—the paths to reaching these goals can differ for each individual. For example, tolerable pain for one person may be intolerable for another.

Here's where your partnership with your doctor is critically important. You will want to learn as much as you can about the drugs that may help you and the schedule for taking these medications. Know what your dosage is, what side effects to watch out for, and which side effects, if they do occur, should be brought to the immediate attention of your doctor. Keep a record of the effects of the drugs on you and bring this record with you when you visit your doctor. Don't experiment on your own with changing your medication schedule or the dosage or, because of impatience, stopping the medication on your own because no immediate relief seems apparent to you. It may take a while before you begin to see and feel results. Give the medication your doctor has prescribed for you a chance to do its work.

Aside from aspirin in its many forms and dosages (time-released aspirin, buffered aspirin, etc.), which is available without a prescription at your local pharmacy and at a host of other stores, including supermarkets, there are a considerable number of prescription drugs for your doctor to choose from in treating your arthritis. Table 25, pages 480–485, summarizes some frequently used arthritis drugs, listing the primary purpose of each drug and the more common side effects.

Be sure to ask your doctor or pharmacist for more complete information about the specific drugs you are taking.

Good Eating and Arthritis

It would indeed be wonderful if these pages could list the ten foods that would treat or even cure your arthritis. Unfortunately, it cannot be done.

Although many have made claims for special foods or special drugs, proclaiming their special benefits for arthritis sufferers, there is no accepted scientific justification for modifying the basic, well-balanced, nutritious diet recommended by most physicians and nutritionists. The guidelines to good eating for all of us are applicable to arthritis sufferers.

Observing good eating habits—including in your diet all of the basic nutrients—maintains your health and helps you to feel more energetic. A balanced diet consisting of low-calorie, high-nutrient foods will help you lose extra pounds. A trimmer person is usually healthier and easier on the weight-bearing joints.

Vitamins are important (see Chapter 6), but megadoses of specific vitamins may not be effective and, as in the case of drugs and other medications, may have dangerous side effects.

To date, the special "miracle cures" claimed for some diets are felt to be unfounded. The research was based on case histories (the benefits derived by a few people) rather than on scientifically constructed experiments (allowing comparisons with a control group on a standard diet).

Table 25 ■ ARTHRITIS DRUGS FREQUENTLY USED

Generic names	Brand names[a]	Usage information / precautions[b]	Possible side effects[c]
Acetaminophen	Tylenol, Datril	Drug starts working 15–30 minutes after taken • Take as needed, no more than every 3 hours. *Overdose symptoms:* stomach upset, irritability, convulsions, coma	*Rare:* extreme fatigue, skin rash, sore throat, fever, unusual bleeding or bruising
Phenylbutazone	Butagesic	Prescription required • Take as prescribed • Drug starts working 4–24 hours after taken • Maximum benefit: may require 3 weeks	*Common:* dizziness, headache, stomach upset *Infrequent:* depression, drowsiness, ringing in ears, constipation or diarrhea, vomiting, swollen feet or legs *Rare:* convulsions, confusion, skin rash, blurred vision, sore throat, fever, mouth ulcers, black stools, vomiting blood, difficult or painful urination
Oxyphenbutazone	Tandearil	Prescription required • Drug starts working 4 to 24 hours after taken • Maximum benefit: may require 3 weeks • Don't drive until you learn how drug affects you • Do not discontinue without consulting doctor • Dose may demand gradual reduction if you have taken medication for a long time.	*Common:* dizziness, headache, stomach upset *Infrequent:* depression, drowsiness, ringing in ears, constipation or diarrhea, vomiting, swollen feet or legs *Rare:* convulsions, confusion, skin rash, blurred vision, black stools, vomiting blood, unusual bleeding or bruising, bloody urine

Overdose symptoms: confusion, agitation, incoherence, convulsions, possible hemorrhage from stomach or intestine, coma

Common: dizziness, headache, nausea, pain
Infrequent: depression, drowsiness, ringing in ears, constipation or diarrhea, vomiting, swollen feet or legs
Rare: convulsions, confusion, skin rash, blurred vision, black or bloody stools, breathing difficulty, unusual bleeding or bruising, bloody urine, painful urination

Sulindac

Clinoril

Prescription required • Drug starts working 4 to 24 hours after taken • Maximum benefit: may require 3 weeks • Don't drive until you learn how drug affects you • Do not discontinue without consulting doctor • Dose may demand gradual reduction if you have taken medication for a long time.

Overdose symptoms: confusion, agitation, incoherence, convulsions, possible hemorrhage from stomach or intestine, coma

Common: flushed face, difficult urination, less urine, unusual tiredness
Infrequent: depression, confusion, hallucinations, severe constipation, abdominal pain, vomiting
Rare: skin rash, blurred vision, slow heartbeat, irregular breathing

Meperidine

Demerol

Prescription required • Drug starts working 30 minutes after taken • Don't drive until you learn how drug affects you • People over 60 should avoid prolonged use.

Overdose symptoms: deep sleep, slow breathing, slow pulse, flushed and warm skin, constricted pupils

(Table 25 continued)

Generic names	Brand names[a]	Usage information / precautions[b]	Possible side effects[c]
Propoxyphene	Darvon	Prescription required • Drug starts working 30 minutes after taken • Don't drive until you learn how medication affects you *Overdose symptoms:* deep sleep, slow breathing, slow pulse, flushed and warm skin, constricted pupil	*Common:* flushed face, difficult urination, less urine *Infrequent:* depression, confusion, hallucinations, severe constipation, abdominal pain, vomiting *Rare:* skin rash, blurred vision, slow heartbeat, irregular breathing
Indomethacin	Indocin	Prescription required • Drug starts working in 4 to 24 hours • Maximum benefit: may require 3 weeks • Don't drive until you know how drug affects you • Do not discontinue without consulting doctor *Overdose symptoms:* confusion, agitation, incoherence, convulsions, possible hemorrhage from stomach or intestine, coma	*Common:* dizziness, headache, nausea, pain *Infrequent:* depression, drowsiness, ringing in ears, constipation or diarrhea, vomiting, swollen feet or legs *Rare:* convulsions, confusion, skin rash, blurred vision, bloody or black stools, breathing difficulty, unusual bleeding or bruising, bloody urine, painful urination, fatigue
Meclofenamale	Meclomen	Prescription required • Drug starts working 4 to 24 hours after taken • Don't drive until you know how drug affects you • Do not discontinue without consulting doctor	*Common:* dizziness, headache, nausea, pain *Infrequent:* depression, drowsiness, ringing in ears, constipation or diarrhea, vomiting, swollen feet or legs

Drug	Instructions / Overdose	Side Effects
	Overdose symptoms: confusion, agitation, incoherence, convulsions, possible hemorrhage from stomach or intestine, coma	*Rare:* convulsions, confusion, skin rash, blurred vision, bloody or black stools, breathing difficulty, unusual bleeding or bruising, bloody urine, painful urination
Ibuprufen Mofrin, Rufin	Prescription required • Drug starts working 3 to 24 hours after taken • Maximum benefit: may require 3 weeks • Don't drive until you know how drug affects you • Do not discontinue without consulting doctor *Overdose symptoms:* confusion, agitation, incoherence, convulsions, possible hemorrhage from stomach or intestine, coma	*Common:* dizziness, headache, nausea, pain *Infrequent:* depression, drowsiness, ringing in ears, constipation or diarrhea, vomiting, swollen feet or legs *Rare:* convulsions, confusion, skin rash, blurred vision, bloody or black stools, breathing difficulty, unusual bleeding or bruising
Fenoprufen Nalfon	Prescription required • Drug starts working 4 to 24 hours after taken • Do not drive until you know how drug affects you • Don't discontinue without consulting doctor • Dose may demand gradual reduction if you have taken medication for a long time *Overdose symptoms:* confusion, agitation, incoherence, convulsions, possible hemorrhage from stomach or intestine, coma	*Common:* dizziness, headache, nausea, pain *Infrequent:* depression, drowsiness, ringing in ears, constipation or diarrhea, vomiting, swollen feet or legs *Rare:* convulsions, confusion, skin rash, blurred vision, bloody or black stools, breathing difficulty, unusual bleeding or bruising, bloody urine, painful urination

(Table 25 continued)

Generic names	Brand names[a]	Usage information / precautions[b]	Possible side effects[c]
Penicillamine	Cuprimine	Prescription required • Drug starts working in 2 to 3 months *Overdose symptoms:* ulcers, sores, convulsions, coughing up blood, coma	*Common:* skin rash, joint pain, fever, swollen lymph glands *Infrequent:* sore throat, fever, appetite loss, nausea, diarrhea, vomiting, unusual bleeding, swollen feet or legs, bloody or cloudy urine *Rare:* double or blurred vision, ringing in ears, mouth ulcers, breathing difficulty
Prednisone	Colisone	Prescription required • Drug starts working in 2 to 4 days • Do not discontinue without consulting doctor • For 2 years after discontinuing, the drug influences your response to surgery, illness, injury or stress • Make doctor aware of this *Overdose symptoms:* convulsions, heart failure	*Common:* acne, poor wound-healing, thirst, indigestion, nausea, vomiting *Infrequent:* mood changes, insomnia, blurred vision, sore throat, fever, black or bloody stools, muscle cramps, frequent urination, irregular menstrual periods *Rare:* irregular heartbeat, rash

Tolmelin Sodium	Tolectin	Prescription required • Drug starts working 4 to 24 hours after taken • Do not drive until you learn how drug affects you • Do not discontinue without consulting doctor • Dose may demand gradual reduction if you have taken medication for a long time *Overdose symptoms:* confusion, agitation, incoherence, convulsions, possible hemorrhage from stomach or intestine, coma	*Common:* dizziness, headache, nausea, pain *Infrequent:* depression, drowsiness, ringing in ears, constipation or diarrhea, vomiting, swollen feet or legs *Rare:* convulsions, confusion, skin rash, blurred vision, bloody or black stools, breathing difficulty, unusual bleeding or bruising, bloody urine, painful urination
Piroxicam	Feldene	Prescription required • Inform your doctor: if you have a history of stomach problems; If itching, fever, fatigue or a rash occur after taking medication, consult the doctor	*Infrequent:* diarrhea, vomiting *Rare:* dizziness, abdominal pain, skin rash

[a]These brand names are only a sampling. Several generics reviewed are available under additional names not listed here.
[b]Check with your doctor for specific directions and precautions when taking these and any other medications.
[c]This does not list all of the possible side effects. Check with your doctor regarding the safety and possible side effects when taking these and or any other medications.
Source: H. Winter Griffith, M.D., *Complete Guide to Prescription Drugs* (Tucson: HP Books, 1983).

The "Right" Attitude

It is inappropriate and even dangerous to ignore the fact that arthritis and its discomforts and pains exist (some people attempt this form of "denial"); however, it is unfortunate and unnecessary to abandon other healthy, life-supporting activities because of the presence of arthritis. Chapter 5 offers tips on managing the tasks of daily living and also suggests devices and aids that will be of help to arthritics.

The person with arthritis will do well by focusing on the positive actions and goals that are of importance in his or her life. This changes the person's inner outlook and attitude from focusing solely on the pain and other symptoms of arthritis to thinking in terms of managing to make the goal despite the arthritis and its accompanying stiffness and pain. The sense of well-being and accomplishment when the goal is reached and new goals are established can be the best treatment around.

Take a moment to think about the goals and pleasures that are important to you. State them positively and in the present tense. Write them down.

For example, if planting tomatoes is important to you, or if you want to give a dinner party for family and friends, let that be your goal. Think through the techniques you can use to reach the goal. The methods may have to differ from what you would have done in earlier days— you may have to sit on a chair in the garden rather than kneel on the ground as you used to, or you may have to work a little each day in the kitchen to prepare the food for the dinner party. However it happens, though, the tomatoes will grow, the guests will enjoy the dinner in your home. You will have accomplished your goal and you will feel better for the accomplishment.

Old friends, as well as new friends who are in a situation similar to yours, can work wonders to help you. The Arthritis Foundation chapter in your area may offer the opportunity to join one of their self-help groups or to attend various activities. Building friendships and learning from others can provide incentive or rekindle the determination to become an active participant in life rather than a victim of one of life's most frequently encountered diseases.

It's up to you.

21

Renal Disease

PLAN NOW FOR Your Vacation in Florida."
"Vacation in Bavaria."
Advertisements in the travel section of the Sunday papers?
Perhaps. But how about this one?
"Dialysis at Sea."

Actually, these ad headlines were mixed in among the advertisements for surgical supplies and hemodialysis home delivery services in a recent issue of the *NAPHT News* (National Association for Patients on Hemodialysis and Transplantation). These travel ads represent the many opportunities now being offered to patients with end-stage renal disease, who are being kept alive with kidney dialysis treatment, to pursue alternatives to staying at home as they enjoy their second chance at life.

Today, the innovations of modern medical technology and the financial support of the U.S. government give over 60,000 people in the United States another turn at living a normal, active life. With hemodialysis centers located all over the world, it takes just a little extra planning for people on dialysis to be able to work or play in many different locations of their choice.

Fifteen to twenty years ago, end-stage renal disease meant certain death. This harsh reality was inescapable because of the vital life-sustaining tasks performed by the kidneys. These two bean-shaped organs work as the body's purification and control system. The five to six quarts of the body's blood supply pass through the kidneys twenty-five times a day. With each pass through the kidney—with its 140 miles of tubes and its millions of filters—waste products and toxins are filtered out of the blood for excretion in the urine. The frequency of urination and the relative concentration of these toxins in the urine are regulated by the kidneys as a means of controlling water balance in the body.

The kidneys also work to regulate the balance of salts and acids in the body. In addition, the kidneys help to control the blood pressure and produce the hormone erythropoietin, which stimulates the development of red blood cells in the bone marrow. Further, the kidneys aid in the body's maintenance of proper levels of calcium, phosphorous, and vitamin D.

Clearly, properly functioning kidneys are essential to life. Improperly functioning kidneys compromise health, causing high blood pressure, anemia, and the uremic syndrome—a constellation of symptoms resulting from the effects of the accumulated toxins and metabolic wastes occurring because of loss of kidney function.

Kidney problems can also be brought on by other diseases. In diabetes mellitus, a disease in which the body has difficulty using glucose, one of the unfortunate complications can be progressive injury to the kidneys. About one in four of the newly diagnosed kidney failure patients in the United States is a diabetic.

Kidney failure can result in an excess retention of fluids, an impairment of myocardial function, and congestive heart failure. The uremic syndrome can also affect the neurologic system, causing lethargy, irritability, confusion, or an altered personality. Additionally, the syndrome will take its toll on the skin and the gastrointestinal systems. A combination of chronic anemia and a buildup of uremic pigments causes the grayish-yellow appearance nurses call the uremic look. The sweat of someone with uremic syndrome if left on the skin can cause a severe itch and, if untreated, can lead to further skin irritations. Gastrointestinal upsets and a loss of appetite can cause debilitating weight loss, although this may be masked by the swelling caused by fluid retention and edema.

A New Life with Dialysis

Today, when both kidneys can no longer do an adequate job, there are three alternatives from which to choose. The oldest option is hemodialysis, the process by which the blood is channeled through an artificial kidney, removing the impurities and excess fluids. The prototype for the modern artificial kidney was developed during World War II. However, until 1960, when Dr. Belding Scribner developed the means to permit repeated dialysis treatments, the original artificial kidney was reserved for use only in acute reversible kidney failure.

Once the "shunt" was devised (a connection between an artery and a neighboring vein, in the arm or leg, allowing a connection to be made between the patient's blood supply and the artificial kidney), people with nonreversible kidney failure, who needed ongoing and repeated dialysis, could now be treated.

During dialysis, the blood flows from the patient to the artificial kidney, where it is cleansed and returned to the patient. Inside the artificial kidney, the blood flows across one side of a membranous sheet or inside specially constructed tubes. On the other side of the membrane is a dialysate, a cleaning bath solution. Impurities in the blood flow through pores in the membrane, which are not large enough to pass the blood cells. The blood and the dialysate never mingle, and the impurities that have passed through the membrane are carried away by the dialysate.

Schedules vary, but patients can undergo two to three dialysis treatments a week, with each treatment lasting four to eight hours.

The first dialysis program, which began in Seattle in 1960, grew in size, and soon other programs were launched. By 1972, there were 18,000 patients on dialysis nationally at an annual cost of $229 million. In 1972, landmark legislation was passed that resulted in the virtually total financial support of all persons with chronic renal failure by the Health Care Financing Administration.

On July 1, 1973, almost all kidney patients, regardless of age or income, became eligible for Medicare coverage. The coverage begins the third month after a person starts hemodialysis and pays approximately 80 percent of the annual costs, which average $15,000–30,000 per year per patient.

During the next ten years, hundreds more dialysis centers opened, some of them hospital based and others outpatient treatment centers. The refinements of the dialysis unit itself encouraged its use by certain patients in the comfort of their own homes.

By 1982, the government was paying for the treatment of over 55,000 patients at an annual cost of $1.8 billion. Approximately 42 percent of these patients were dialyzed at a hospital-based center; 41 percent were treated at an independent or free-standing dialysis center; and the remaining 17 percent were routinely dialyzed at home, often with the supervision and involvement of one of the home dialysis service companies that grew in response to the increased demand.

The second method for treatment of end-stage renal disease is another form of dialysis: peritoneal dialysis. This method evolved as a result of greater understanding by researchers of the body and the dialysis process. Here, rather than using an external artificial kidney machine, the dialysate solution is introduced by tube directly into the peritoneal cavity (the abdominal and pelvic areas) of the body. Using the mechanism of osmosis, the patient's own venous system and the peritoneal membrane work as the filtering mechanism. Toxic wastes and excess fluids are filtered into the dialysate solution, which is then removed from the body and discarded.

A refinement of this approach, called continuous ambulatory peritoneal dialysis (CAPD), can be done by the patient himself without the need for machinery, trained nurses, or technicians. In CAPD, the patient introduces the dialysate solution into his own body through a surgically created catheter. The solution is packaged in a plastic bag, which connects to the catheter through a plastic tube. When the bag is raised above the waist, the solution responds to gravity and flows down into the patient's body. Approximately two liters of special dialyzing solution is used. Once the plastic bag has emptied, the person can roll up the bag and place it under his clothing. He is then free to resume his normal daily activities.

While the patient is engaged in everyday activities, the solution is at work, drawing in and retaining the toxic wastes and excess fluids from his body. Approximately four to six hours later, the patient, by holding the plastic bag below his waist, can once again use gravity to aid him. The toxin-filled dialysate drains from his system into the plastic bag. After the bag has filled, it is disconnected from the tubing and discarded. A new bag filled with solution is connected, and the process is repeated.

With approximately four exchanges every twenty-four hours, the patient more closely replicates the natural filtering process of the kidneys. Also, the individual is freed from spending any time hooked up to special machinery or equipment.

CAPD, however, is a complicated process and is not for everyone. There are many risks involved. The process requires careful, meticulous attention to the sterile procedure that must be used to prevent the possibility of dangerous infection to the peritoneal lining. Peritonitis can be fatal.

Transplants

Kidney transplanatation offers the promise of complete freedom from artificially accomplished dialysis. By replacing individuals' diseased and nonfunctioning kidneys, surgeons have successfully helped thousands of people to begin life again.

Renal transplantations cannot be done for everyone. Much depends on the patient's age and medical condition and, most important, the availability of an "acceptable" kidney. Because the newly transplanted kidney is a foreign organ, careful matching of donor and recipient is needed to reduce the incidence of rejection once the kidney is surgically attached in the new host's body.

One kidney is sufficient to do the job. However, because of the problem of rejection, the "batting averages" of the surgeons are less than perfect. Ideally, the transplanted kidney comes from a donor who is related to the patient, with blood type and other tests demonstrating that there is a close match of blood type and tissue type, reducing the chances of rejection.

Transplanted kidneys from a donor who is a living relative have an overall success rate of approximately 80 percent after two years. However, most patients do not have a relative who is a suitable donor, in which case they are placed on a waiting list for a kidney from a person who has died and has donated his or her kidneys for transplantation.

Although tissue types are carefully matched, the success rate is lower for transplants from nonrelated donors—approximately 55 percent after two years. If the new kidney is rejected, the patient must then return to dialysis and await the call that another matching kidney has been found. Today, there are virtually thousands of kidney patients waiting for the call so they can have one of the 4,000 kidney transplants that are performed annually.

Most of the costs for transplantation are covered by the special renal Medicare program. The National Kidney Foundation, through its affiliates, works to assist patients to locate the appropriate resources and assistance. The foundation's nationwide donor program, education of professionals, and public information service all help kidney patients in their quest for a better quality of life. The NKF recommends that patients under the age of fifty-five should seriously consider renal transplantation because of the improved survival rate and rehabilitation success rate when compared to dialysis.

Today, dialysis can be considered a temporary alternative for some patients as they wait for the "cure" that comes when a new, functioning kidney is transplanted. More than 10,000 people are now living with someone else's kidney.

Living with Dialysis

People living on dialysis—whatever the method or mode—usually find that it changes their lives, mostly for the better. Often, the knowledge that dialysis looms as the eventual treatment has been in the minds of patients long before it actually occurs. With ample opportunity to reflect on its impact, many patients now on dialysis report that they had anticipated a perpetual nightmare of restrictions and complications, only to find that dialysis, when it did happen to them, was "no big deal."

How an individual copes with the scheduling and the planning that come after the start of a dialysis treatment program, and how this will affect his life, depends on his own outlook and inner strengths and the support and information that comes from the medical team with whom he is working.

Learning how to operate a hemodialysis machine is not difficult. Many patients can do this and, to allow themselves freedom during the daytime, hook themselves up to the machine in the late evening and even sleep while the machine is doing its work (there are automatic alarms if something goes wrong).

More serious problems can arise concerning the emotional impact of dialysis and the knowledge it brings to a patient. Realistically, the patient knows that end-stage renal disease can mean a greatly shortened life because of all the possible complications.

Those individuals who get a kidney transplant can look forward with some hope to the possibility of many years of being able to function normally. The dialysis patient, however, has to contend with a different outlook. Dialysis can go on indefinitely—but the human body undergoing dialysis cannot. Many complications can develop: cardiovascular disease, congestive heart failure, stroke, infection, hepatitis, anemia, hypertension, loss of energy. Knowledge of all this takes its toll on the patient and on the caregiver.

Depression in the patient is to be expected, and with depression comes a host of other ills—apathy, loss of sexual function, fear of dying, and feelings of deprivation, to name the most common effects.

In addition to depression, there can be emotional distress over being dependent on a machine for a lifetime. Also, anxiety concerning health can develop, and the patient may become suicidal. Symptoms of denial are also not uncommon, with the patient refusing to acknowledge his disease or the seriousness of his state of health.

All of this can affect the family and the caregiver. Feelings of resentment against the patient can build, along with the constant worry about the future. Family conflicts can erupt and intensify, bringing on recriminations and a lack of understanding and communication. The outlook admittedly can be bleak, but many patients and their families have learned to cope with dialysis and what it signifies.

At the University Hospital in Ann Arbor, Michigan, a program utilizing patient-to-patient contact has been formalized to help patients newly diagnosed with end-stage renal disease. The program trains its participants to counsel new patients and their families in clinics, in dialysis centers, in intensive care units—wherever these new patients are found.

The program participants, who are patients on dialysis themselves, function as role models for the newly diagnosed patients. They share feelings, information, and resources with the new patients and work to alleviate the anxiety that is always present and to lessen the sense of isolation and loneliness experienced when coping with this disease. Professionals at the University Hospital give high marks to the positive impact that the peer counseling sessions have had.

The National Association for Patients on Hemodialysis and Transplantation (NAPHT) is a national organization that helps patients and their families by providing information about kidney disease, treatments, and rehabilitation. The association's newsletter, the *NAPHT News,* is filled with articles and stories geared to the interests and information needs of this unique group.

In cooperation with the National Kidney Foundation, NAPHT has published a helpful pamphlet entitled "Working with Kidney Failure: Rehabilitation and Employment." It addresses the issues concerning rehabilitation for the dialysis patient. It also identifies resources such as the vocational rehabilitation services available in each state that will assist people in learning new job skills if they are unable to return to previous employment. Some practical advice is offered on how to handle the job hunt, the job interview, and any questions from potential employers concerning the health care and scheduling needs of the person on dialysis.

For individuals considered by their physicians to be unable to return to work, the pamphlet reviews the guidelines for qualification for Social Security disability benefits. (See the Appendix for addresses of NAPHT and the National Kidney Foundation.)

Peter Madden, a psychologist living in Richmond, Virginia, was on dialysis for about four years when he wrote his four tips to others coping with dialysis:

I live a better life on dialysis than I ever did before. I have continued working with very little time lost to dialysis-related problems. The regularity of the dialysis program has forced me to organize my life and plan more efficiently. My family life has improved since all of us have had to pull together to deal with the impact of a chronic disease. Finally, I appreciate each day and activity a little more.

His four tips:

1) *Be positive.* Approach dialysis with a positive frame of mind. Seek out ways to alter your thinking and your life style to compensate for your weaknesses and build up your strengths.

2) *Be independent.* Madden is a firm believer in home dialysis and the active involvement which it entails. He does not endorse the passivity that may occur when health professionals at a dialysis do it for you. He states: "I am certain that it is no coincidence that very few center-based patients continue a normal working life, while most home patients of working age apparently do continue supporting themselves."

3) *Be useful.* Madden's words again: "I believe we have a moral obligation to make our lives count by continuing to contribute back to society as much as we can by working to support ourselves or by volunteer work. I am hopeful that the day will soon end when every dialysis patient is automatically considered totally disabled and that we will have to face the same tests as everyone else."

4) *Be happy.* Every day you live is a bonus gift from God. Focus on activities you enjoy and maintain as normal a life as you can. Take vacations, start new activities, and maintain your zest for life.*

---

*For more information about living with dialysis, Edith T. Oberley and Terry D. Oberley have published a practical guide for patients, *Understanding Your New Life with Dialysis: A Patient Guide for Physical and Psychological Adjustment* (Springfield, Ill.: Charles C. Thomas, 1983). The book covers kidney failure, human and artificial kidney function, diet and medications, psychological adjustments, finances, and much more.

22

Respiratory Disease

SHORTNESS OF BREATH, the inability to get enough air into the body, can not only limit the physical activities a person can perform, but can also be desperately frightening. Walking across the street may be almost impossible, and the simple, everyday acts of taking a shower and getting dressed may require exertion at the limit of the individual's capacity.

Respiratory difficulty may be related to chronic obstructive pulmonary disease (COPD), lung cancer, cystic fibrosis, or occupational lung diseases such as silicosis, black lung disease, and asbestosis. Also, respiratory problems may be brought on by neuromuscular disease. The symptoms of amyotrophic lateral sclerosis (ALS, See Chapter 17) or muscular dystrophy can include respiratory difficulty. In the frail, elderly patient, respiratory problems may be related to infections such as pneumonia.

COPD: A Major Disabler

With an estimated 9 million Americans fighting the impact of COPD, the experience of "not getting enough air" is, unfortunately, an all too common problem. COPD encompasses the two major disabling respiratory diseases—emphysema and chronic bronchitis. According to Social Security disability records, COPD is second only to heart disease as a cause of disability, and as with heart disease, the discovery of COPD often occurs after damage has already been done—in this case, to the respiratory tract.

Most cases of COPD probably are preventable, since their origin can often be traced to smoking. Fortunately, treatment can, if begun early enough, successfully improve the quality of life and maximize function in the individual. Of course, the treatment regimen has to be followed carefully and strictly if it is to be at all effective. Patients and the health professionals assisting them can choose from a variety of treatments, including medication, physical therapy, respiratory therapy, oxygen therapy, and even something as simple as plain exercise.

Treatments are available—but the cure has yet to be found.

WHAT IS BREATHING?

To better understand the respiratory impact of emphysema and chronic bronchitis, it will be helpful to have a basic knowledge of what is involved in the normal breathing process.

When you breathe, you use the muscles of your stomach and your chest. The stomach muscles raise and lower the diaphragm, the membrane that separates the chest and the abdominal cavities in your body, and the chest muscles expand and contract as needed. When you inhale, the movement of the diaphragm and the action of the chest muscles expand the area of the chest cavity, thereby allowing air to be drawn into the lungs through the nose and mouth.

The path followed by the inhaled air involves a descent through the windpipe (the trachea) to a fork where the two bronchi (one for each lung) branch off. Each bronchi then divides and subdivides into a tree-branch configuration, finally terminating in clusters of tiny air sacs, or alveoli. These elastic sacs are surrounded by a web of tiny blood vessels (capillaries). It is here that the exchange of gases (incoming oxygen for outgoing carbon dioxide) takes place. When you breathe out, your chest muscles and your diaphragm contract, and the carbon dioxide is expelled out of the air sacs and back up the bronchiole branches to the bronchial tubes, then up through the windpipe and out through the nose or mouth.

THE EFFECT OF COPD

COPD can involve a blockage in the air pathway or a limitation of the amount of air that can be taken in or expelled by the lungs. This results in less oxygen being available for absorption into the bloodstream.

In chronic bronchitis, the obstruction is caused by a thickening of the bronchial walls and a hypersecretion of mucus. This limits the volume of air drawn into the lungs. In emphysema, the reduced amount of oxygen available is caused by changes in the normal structure of the lungs. The tiny capillaries that surround the air sacs become reduced in number and lose their elasticity, and the air sacs become varied in size. These changes reduce the total area available for the important exchange of gases in the lungs.

The disruption and diminution of airflow to the lungs may be intermittent, occurring only with strenuous activity, or it can be continuous, depending on the extent of the disease. Whether the respiratory problem is bronchitis-related or emphysema-related, the COPD patient needs to be treated and carefully followed by trained medical professionals. Without treatment, the health of COPD patient may deteriorate to the point of heart failure and death because the heart muscles do not receive an adequate amount of oxygen to function.

COPD is thought to develop early in life and progress over a long period of time (sometimes twenty or thirty years). Its earliest signs and symptoms usually do not attract any attention until their impact is quite pronounced—and at that point there will probably be significant damage to the lungs and respiratory tract.

Smoking is known to play a major role in the development of chronic bronchitis and emphysema. A "smoker's cough" and "running out of wind" upon exertion may be subtle and not very noticeable symptoms at first. Many smokers feel their morning cough is just part of the waking up routine each morning and so pay it little heed. Also, shortness of breath upon exertion may not become apparent until the person experiences an unusual loss of "wind" after just some routine physical exertion. By that time, there is undoubtedly a significant reduction in lung capacity.

As the disease progresses, a greater number of respiratory infections may occur, and, in addition, an increasing experience of shortness of breath may impede the individual's ability to continue with his or her usual activities. At first, recreational activities may be reduced or eliminated because of the discomfort experienced upon attempting physical exertion. A more sedentary life style will be adopted. And then, as the disease takes stronger hold on the person, shortness of breath may interfere with and impair the person's ability to work. This can lead to a loss of job or forced early retirement.

All of this can put a strain on family relationships, and it will take its toll of the person's emotional as well as his physical health. The potential for clinical depression will always be present because of the less than satisfying life style now being forced upon the individual, plus increasing anxiety about finances and the ability to function as time goes by.

TREATMENT

Because prevention of the complications of COPD is the treatment goal, early detection is most important. Subsequent damage to the lungs can then be avoided, and if COPD is caught early enough, the disease can be arrested and, in some cases, reversed.

The administration of oxygen may become necessary to ensure an adequate level of oxygen in the system. Physical therapy to promote and build endurance will be helpful. Various medications may be prescribed to fight off infection or to help thin and loosen secretions, and postural drainage will help to keep the lungs clear.

There are two major goals throughout the treatment program: to maximize breathing function while improving the quality of life for the individual coping with the disease. Home health care can work wonders in helping to achieve both these goals. Many people with respiratory disease find themselves bouncing in and out of hospitals to treat infections or to clear breathing passages. A well-designed and carefully controlled home care program can ensure the person's continuing ability to function at home while, at the same time, working to prevent repeated hospitalizations. The home health care staff, the physician, the pharmacist, the oxygen supplier (if oxygen is required), the family, and, of course, the patient all have to work together to plan for and to cope with the many physical and emotional needs that will warrant attention.

A home care program for respiratory problems will consist of at least three basic components: breathing control; bronchial hygiene; and rehabilitative exercise. Depending on the needs of the individual, additional therapies such as special aerosol medication, the occasional or full-time use of oxygen, or special exercises may also be employed. Also, any other health conditions and the medications and therapy they require will be reevaluated and integrated into the home care respiratory program.

An important first step in setting up a home care respiratory program is the sharing of information among the patient, the caregiver, the patient's family, the physician, and the other members of the professional health care team. The physician, the nurse, and the respiratory therapist will want to know all about the patient—his life style, the nature and duration of his breathing difficulties, and his mental attitude toward his disease. Goals of the treatment program will be discussed and a course of action planned to accommodate the individual's needs, life style, and illness pattern.

A test of breathing function will be performed. The physician may use a number of different devices, but the focus here is to quantify both the amount of air that can be inhaled and exhaled and the force and duration of the exhalation.

Needless to say, avoid smoking—a point that will be stressed by all the health care professionals. They will also probably discuss the nature of the particular respiratory problem with the patient and will give specific information about lung function and the rationale for each aspect of the treatment program. This is the preferred way for the all-important treatment partnership to begin.

STEPS TO BETTER BREATHING FUNCTION

Whether the respiratory problem is mild or severe—and whether or not special medications such as bronchodilators are used—there are certain basics that work to maximize breathing function for all patients. The first basic is to breathe correctly. With the possible exception of athletes and singers, most of us have never been trained in how to breathe. We begin life with a reflexive cry when we are born and probably never give breathing more than a passing thought until there is a noticeable loss of function.

It's best to breathe in through the nose (not the mouth). This filters, humidifies, and warms the air being taken into the lungs. The home health nurse or the therapist can observe and advise the patient as he or she practices breathing in several positions. Air distribution in the lungs changes as the position of the chest changes, and it is important that the patient breathes correctly in all positions.

Most people with emphysema or chronic bronchitis work hard at breathing—but do so in an ineffective manner. Shallow, "shoulder breathing" is far less efficient than deep, abdominal breathing. By breathing in a slow, relaxed manner, allowing the belly to protrude with each breath, you will be increasing the area in which the lungs can expand.

Take your time breathing out. One way to slow down breathing is to purse your lips as if to whistle, then breathe out slowly. This approach is far more efficient than the rapid in-and-out panting that can occur with shortness of breath.

Place your hands on your belly as you breathe in and out and feel the movement of your stomach. Practice this technique until the habit of slow, relaxed deep breathing becomes second nature to you.

This more efficient method of breathing can help improve function in emphysema patients, including an increase in their tolerance of exercise.

The additional secretions of mucus due to the stimulation of the respiratory tract by an inflammation make productive coughing a necessity. All of us cough reflexively when there is an irritant in our respiratory tract. This helps to clear the airway and encourages free breathing. Nonproductive coughing is exhausting and of little help in clearing the airway. Your home care nurse or physical therapist can teach the patient how to cough productively without exhausting himself in the process. By using a combination of deep breathing exercises and stomach contraction, the therapist can help promote a more efficient cough. Sputum is always discarded in a tissue, never swallowed, and a period of rest may be helpful following a coughing session.

When the mucus or lung secretions are difficult to mobilize, the therapist may use a technique called postural drainage. By changing the patient's position, the therapist can use gravity to help drainage and percussion to mobilize the mucus. The therapist may use cupping of the hands or vibration on the patient to loosen secretions and, with the patient cooperating with breathing and productive coughing techniques, succeed in clearing the airway.

There are medical considerations and contraindications to this procedure, so do not attempt your own postural drainage program unless you first check with your physician. Your therapist can instruct a home health aide or family member in how to assist in the coughing technique, if this is determined to be an appropriate treatment.

Respiratory ability can be greatly improved by drinking plenty of water and other liquids. Normal breathing uses up moisture. The air we breathe in is humidified by the moisture of the respiratory tract. The effects of low humidity (as in heated rooms or a desert environment) and of certain medications can create a potential for dehydration. Without adequate moisture in the respiratory tract, all secretions become thickened. It is difficult to clear these thick secretions from the lungs, and if the secretions stagnate too long, bacteria may multiply, bringing on the hazard of respiratory infection.

Water intake helps to thin these secretions and ensures a proper level of body hydration. In addition, a humidifier can help to provide much-needed moisture to the respiratory tract. Humidification of the respiratory tract can be accomplished with a humidifier or a nebulizer (a device that humidifies in the form of an aerosol).

Any use of direct humidification requires absolutely clean equipment. Special care must be taken with the mask that directs humidity into the airway. Keeping equipment clean helps to reduce the risk of infection resulting from bacterial contamination of the devices being used.

The importance of bronchial hygiene cannot be overstressed. Because the nose and the mouth are gateways to the respiratory tract, they must be kept particularly clean to protect the airway from irritants and unwanted bacteria. This means the patient will have to make proper use of a toothbrush and dental floss, as well as antiseptic mouthwashes and denture cleansers. Unclean teeth and gums provide a medium for bacteria that can bring on infections of the respiratory tract. Also, keeping the nasal passageway clean and clear will help to promote free breathing.

The purpose of these measures is to avoid any possible source of infection, to prevent congestion, and to maintain a clear airway for free breathing.

Making the environment for the COPD patient as dust-free as possible is a major requirement. It's not as simple as deciding to dust regularly and vacuum once a week. Dust has to be banished as much as is humanly possible from the home—and that's more than just a mere housekeeping job.

The first general rule to observe is that if it's washable, it's all right to use. This holds true for drapes, curtains, and bedding (wool is out!). Foam pillows should be used, but remember to replace them before the foam disintegrates. Mattresses should be encased in plastic or vinyl casings, fastened with zippers. For comfort, a mattress pad can be used, as long as it's washable.

Generally, water keeps down dust. There are some things, however, on which water cannot be used—books, for example. Keep shelves full of books out of the bedroom and any other room the COPD patient will be using on a regular basis. Go over everything in the rooms being used with an eagle eye. This does not mean you have to strip the rooms bare of furniture and accessories, but you should eliminate any obvious dust catchers and plan to clean what remains regularly and thoroughly.

Why all this fuss about dust? Household dust is usually composed of particles of dirt, animal hair, pollen, parts of insects, and any other contaminants and irritants that can find their way into your home. For the person with respiratory disease, this particle-laden dust can be both a source of irritation and annoyance and a real danger to free breathing, as well as a potential source of respiratory infection.

Bear in mind, too, that no matter how dust-free you make your home (especially those rooms the patient will use on a regular basis), the whole effort will be for naught if the patient or a family member decides to go out gardening. It doesn't take much imagination to see what can happen to a dust-free room when someone comes into it after a session in the garden, where dirt and pollen and insects can run rampant. So gardening and all other dirt- and dust-producing activities have to be approached with caution.

Asthma

In addition to COPD, which encompasses emphysema and chronic bronchitis, asthma is another major respiratory disease that affects large numbers of people, many of them children. It has been estimated that 9 million Americans have asthma and that almost 3 million of these are children.

Asthma is a chronic disease characterized by repeated attacks of wheezing, labored breathing, tightness in the chest, and coughing. In a severe attack, the victim appears to be suffocating as he struggles for breath. His face can have a bluish pallor, and he will perspire heavily. Such an attack is frightening to all who witness it, although in all but the most extreme cases, asthmatics can eventually catch their breath.

Fortunately, most asthma attacks are mild. Some people are completely free of all symptoms between attacks, which vary in frequency, length, and severity for different people. Other victims may continue to have mild coughing episodes most of the time, with more severe attacks from time to time. The attacks can occur at any time and often occur at night. They can start slowly or strike abruptly, and sometimes the wheezing is so loud it can be heard across a room.

During an asthma attack, the airways into the lungs are blocked by three different actions. The smooth muscles around the small bronchial tubes (bronchioles) constrict and narrow the air passageways; the mucous membranes inside the bronchioles swell, further narrowing the passageways; and the membranes begin to produce thick secretions, still further cutting down on the space inside the bronchial tubes. The victim of an asthma attack cannot get enough air into his lungs, nor can he expel sufficient air to leave room for air being inhaled, thus precipitating the struggle to breathe and the feeling of suffocation.

There is no cure for asthma. The symptoms can be treated, but the disease, at the present time, cannot be cured.

There are two types of asthma—extrinsic and intrinsic. Extrinsic asthma is basically an allergic reaction, and it can be triggered by a variety of substances: pollen, house dust, car exhaust fumes, smoke, animal hair, feathers, certain foods (dairy products, nuts, and chocolate, for example), paint fumes, fish, and many more.

Allergy tests and the slow and careful elimination of suspected allergens can help pinpoint what may be bringing on the attacks. If the person is found to be allergic to a certain substance, then every effort must be made to avoid that substance.

About 25 to 35 percent of asthmatics suffer from the extrinsic type, which usually strikes before the age of thirty.

Intrinsic asthma has no known cause. Medical researchers have so far been unable to determine what happens to bring it on, although it would appear that a viral infection such as flu can trigger the attack. Also, there is the possibility that the autonomic nervous system, which controls breathing and other automatic bodily functions, somehow malfunctions and the nerve controlling the muscles around the bronchioles is stimulated, causing the muscles to contract and bringing on the asthma attack.

An intrinsic asthma attack can also be brought on by strenuous physical exercise, the stress of emotional turmoil (including excessive laughing or crying), and sometimes even common medications such as aspirin.

For those who develop asthma in childhood, there is some hope in the statistics that show a good percentage of them (as high as 70 percent in one study) "outgrow" the disease, at least to the extent that attacks do not continue to occur. About 20 to 30 percent of those who get asthma as adults will outgrow it in time.

Although these statistics may seem to offer hope, the total number of asthmatics represents a serious health problem in this country, and except for the most extreme case, where hospitalization is required, the disease is essentially treated at home.

Treatment of asthma usually involves inhalation of medications, although drugs are also available in sustained-release preparations and injections. Inhalation of bronchodilators (drugs that open up the airways by relaxing the constricting muscles) can be accomplished with a metered-dose device that the patient holds in his mouth, forming an airtight seal. The medication canister is pressed down while the patient inhales, and the dose of medication is delivered to the lungs in aerosol form. Medication can also be taken with a nebulizer, a device that releases the medication in a mist that the patient inhales.

Families and caregivers of asthmatics can help by knowing what to do when an attack strikes. Here are some basic guidelines:

- Make sure all medications and inhalation devices are clean, ready, and on hand when an attack begins.
- Note the time the first dose of medication is taken so the next dose can be timed according to the schedule prescribed by the doctor.
- Help the asthmatic to get into a position that will help minimize breathing difficulties—usually sitting up and leaning forward.
- Make sure that the room is well ventilated and that fresh air is available.
- Remain calm even though the asthmatic may be struggling mightily to breathe. If you panic it will only add to the stress of the situation and may make the attack worse.
- Know where and how to reach the doctor or hospital emergency facilities if the attack should become severe enough to require immediate medical attention.

An asthma attack can be frightening and dangerous. Asthmatics, with the help of families and caregivers, have to learn to adjust their life styles to the ever-present problem of coping with this disease.

Engaging in Activity to Tolerance

"Activity to tolerance" is the amount of energy a person can expend without becoming unusually tired. It is a measure of endurance and productivity. Usually, the level of tolerance for an activity will increase with repetition of that activity over a period of time. For example, an individual with severe respiratory disease may, at first, be able to get out of bed and sit upright in a chair for only ten minutes; repetition of this activity will significantly increase the time out of bed and in the chair. Working to increase this level of activity helps improve the rate and depth of respiration.

It is far more healthy for the COPD patient to sit or stand than to lie down, and, of course, it's even better to move around. The lungs will expand more fully and coughing can be even more productive. Walking—even if only a few steps—helps to promote deep breathing and speeds up the heart rate. By promoting regular exercise designed to build tolerance, you can strengthen the cardiac and respiratory systems. Muscle tone will improve, and the joints will maintain their flexibility and move with less effort. Equally important, regular exercise helps to promote a sense of fitness and well-being and fosters a higher level of independence.

Lifelong habits do take their toll. It is more difficult for a smoker who seldom exercises to increase his activity than it is for a nonsmoker who exercises regularly. By working with a trained exercise physiologist or a physical therapist, the individual with respiratory disease can learn how to exercise to the limit of tolerance rather than to the point of exhaustion. The benefits of this type of exercising are far-reaching and health-restoring, producing an increased ability to tolerate activity and function more productively.

All of this activity—deep breathing, productive coughing, and increased activity—requires energy. Also, additional energy is needed to combat any infection that may develop with respiratory disease. The basic source of energy is the diet. Adequate calories and nutrients must be a part of the daily diet for any person—and especially the compromised patient—in order to provide the energy fuel necessary to function. Often, small frequent meals are better tolerated than large meals. A nurse or dietician can be of much help in working with the patient to set up a well-balanced and nourishing diet.

The improved nutritional status and physical tone resulting from a good diet will aid in efforts to improve breathing, coughing, and level of activity.

Medications

When breathing function is compromised, the physician will consider alternative courses of action. One of these is the use of medications.

Medications such as bronchodilators may be prescribed to bring about relaxation of the smooth muscles of the bronchial airways, thus promoting easier breathing. These medications may be administered in an aerosol form, which will require special equipment to assist in placing the medication deep into the bronchial tubes.

The equipment can vary from a metered-dose inhaler—offering a self-contained system of a measured amount of medication in an "applicator device"—to a special and rather complex piece of equipment called an intermittent positive-pressure breathing (IPPB) apparatus, which helps to push the medication into the lungs. This IPPB device, once commonly used, is now usually reserved for people with compromised breathing capability who require this type of assistance in inhaling.

Hand-held nebulizers can be used to break up the prescribed medication into a fine mist. The individual then squeezes a bulb, while inhaling, to direct the medication-impregnated mist into the lungs. Another model of nebulizer works in tandem with an air compressor to help place the medication deep into the lungs. The mouthpiece and nebulizer of these respiratory therapy devices must be rinsed after each treatment and thoroughly cleaned every few days to prevent the equipment itself from becoming a source of respiratory infection. (This holds true for any and all equipment used for respiratory therapy.)

Oxygen

There are many circumstances in which the addition of oxygen helps to relieve shortness of breath, increases the level of oxygen in the system, and aids in improving the quality of life for the patient. Usually a blood gas analysis—measuring, among other things, the levels of oxygen and carbon dioxide in the blood—is performed to document the need for supplemental oxygen. (This can be of help when applying later for insurance reimbursement.)

Various choices of oxygen systems are available. The individual's life style, interests, and oxygen needs will determine the type of oxygen system selected. Liquid oxygen systems have been developed that combine a reservoir for in-home use with a lightweight, portable, refillable tank for use outside the home. Some units have an oxygen flow rate that permits up to eight hours of portable oxygen supply, providing ample time for local visits away from home, holding down a part-time job, or visits to the doctor's office.

For individuals who remain in their homes and who seek to be free of the need for regular oxygen tank deliveries, an oxygen concentrator may be the answer. The oxygen concentrator is a device that takes in room air and, through a process involving filters and compressors, chemically removes most of the nitrogen from the air, leaving a mixture containing 90 to 98 percent oxygen to be inhaled by the patient.

When supplemental oxygen is required, the patient and the physician or other health professionals involved should evaluate the monthly oxygen costs, patterns of oxygen use (part-time or full-time), the level of planned activity, personal preferences, and the type of home environment. All of these factors should be taken into consideration when making the decision on which oxygen system to use.

Whatever the choice, there is a vital need for information and instruction on the correct use of the equipment, its maintenance, and the role of relaxation and energy conservation in avoiding unnecessary shortness of breath and its accompanying discomfort. (See Chapter 5 for energy-saving tips in daily living.) All of this should be coupled with an exercise program that will help maximize function and increase independence, activity level, and endurance.

WARNING

Oxygen supports combustion. There is always the danger of fire when oxygen is in use. Follow these rules for the safe use of oxygen:

- *No smoking.* Put up a sign on the door of the room to this effect, and alert all family members, visitors, and anyone else who may enter the room.
- Do not use grease or oil on any of the oxygen connections.
- Do not keep alcohol or ether next to the oxygen.
- If an oxygen tent is being used, do not place an electrical device in the tent.
- Keep oxygen cylinders away from heat.
- Keep a charged and functioning fire extinguisher available—and know how to use it.

CHOOSING YOUR OXYGEN SUPPLIER

Your physician or therapist may identify a few suppliers in your area who will provide the particular equipment you will need. Your home health nurse or the hospital discharge planner may offer additional choices. As an educated consumer, you may want to confirm and clarify the kind of equipment and service that is being offered to make sure it meets your needs.

By obtaining answers to the following questions, you will be better able to compare your options and make a knowledgeable choice:

- Does the company rent, lease, or sell the equipment that has been recommended for you? Or are they offering an alternative, which should be double-checked with your physician?
- Are they open twenty-four hours a day, seven days a week, including holidays? Is there a knowledgeable person on call around the clock (not just a phone answering machine)?
- What kind of training program do they have for new patients? Who provides the training? Are the instructors registered respiratory therapists?
- What happens when the equipment needs repair? Do they repair their own, or is the "service department" really just another nonrelated company?
- What are the charges and costs for the equipment, accessories, servicing, and deliveries? Are there any extras not covered by their basic estimate?
- How is insurance reimbursement handled? Do they obtain the proper substantiation and complete the necessary paperwork?

By checking with a number of companies in your area, you will get a sense of whether they are simply equipment suppliers or people-oriented professionals working as part of your home health care team. If you can, talk to other people who are using home-delivered oxygen from the various companies you are researching. Ask them what their experience has been with these companies.

Although in some areas your choice of suppliers may be limited, asking these questions will let you know what to expect. With knowledge, you will be able to plan for emergencies and lessen your anxiety of the unknown by making sure you are completely informed. Moreover, by letting each company know your level of need and what questions you want answered, you are conveying a strong message. The oxygen supply business is becoming more competitive; your questions and interest may help to improve the services being offered in your area.

Living Each Day

Walking long distances may be difficult for an individual coping with respiratory disease—yet driving a car may be possible. Portable oxygen can be used while driving the car, and the use of a car (or even pulling oxygen along in a cart while walking) can increase mobility without undue energy expenditure.

Supportive counseling is often helpful for any person coping with a chronic illness, but it becomes virtually essential for a person with respiratory problems. Anxiety, depression, guilt, anger, and frustration are common reactions to the multiple stresses created by chronic respiratory disease. Difficult breathing brings on increased anxiety, which in turn further compromises breathing ability.

Learning techniques for relaxation and stress control can help in achieving optimal functioning. Groups of individuals sharing common experiences, such as Emphysema Anonymous, Inc. (see the Appendix) provide friendship, support, and understanding that cannot be experienced any other way. Support groups also guide the families in reaching a better understanding of the disease, the sense of loneliness it engenders, and its impact on the patient's personality and self-image.

The COPD patient may not need a great deal of direct personal home health care; however, he or she may—if living alone—require housekeeping assistance. Cleaning, laundry, shopping, and cooking may require a level of energy and activity that places too great a demand on the compromised patient. The help of a support person, such as a housekeeping aide, reduces the anxieties and fears that ill health can bring to the person living alone. Even if the household chores are performed by a family member who stops by every day, a housekeeping aide can be of value in providing respite for the family member.

Setting priorities are of utmost importance. The limited energy reserve of the COPD patient has to be expended with great care and selectivity. One individual, writing in *Batting the Breeze,* a newsletter of Emphysema Anonymous, Inc., notes:

Since we can't do everything we want to, each must set his own priorities. If I want to go to lunch, I have two choices: First, the conventional one of taking a shower, dressing, leaving the apartment in apple pie order, arriving just in time, too exhausted to thoroughly enjoy the lunch. Then there is *my* way—take a shower the night before, concentrate on getting ready early so that I can relax with the paper while recuperating from the activity of dressing; plan to get to the restaurant in time to rest before others arrive, and enjoy my lunch.

This person learned her limits and was clear about her priorities. Her energy was geared to planning for her own enjoyment and giving herself what she needed, while letting go of things she was unable to do.

Each of us can profit from this example, regardless of the state of our health. The respiratory-impaired person, however, *must* follow this example or else live with the unhappiness of unfulfilled expectations.

Appendix

A Resource Directory

T HIS APPENDIX is organized by problem area and is designed to provide you with suggestions of places to contact for information and assistance. The resources listed cover a wide variety of social organizations, community groups, health associations, and government agencies. Be prepared when you call. *Have your questions ready.* If the operator answering the telephone cannot answer your questions, ask to speak with the public relations department. People working as public information specialists may be more knowledgeable about the scope of services offered by their organization. They may know about groups and organizations not mentioned here (especially local or community-based resources). Use the Home Health Care Resource Record on the next page to keep track of your inquiries and the suggestions that are offered. I've tried to make this section as complete as possible. Please write to me % W. W. Norton & Company if you know of an organization which should be included in future editions.

Contents

Aging	513	Miscellaneous	550
Arthritis	519	Neurological and Neuro-	
Blindness	520	muscular Diseases	551
Cancer	524	Alzheimer's Disease	551
Community Services (Social		Amyotrophic Lateral	
and Legal)	528	Sclerosis	551
Death and Dying	531	Huntington's Disease	552
Dentistry	536	Multiple Sclerosis	553
Diabetes	536	Muscular Dystrophy	553
Digestive Disorders	537	Myasthenia Gravis	554
Equipment and Supplies	538	Parkinson's Disease	554
Hearing Disorders	539	Nutrition	556
Heart Disease and Stroke	541	Pain	557
Home Care Services	542	Physical Disability	558
Information Services	545	Recreation	560
Institutionalized Patient		Respiratory Problems	564
Services	547	Sexuality	564
Kidney Diseases	548	Skin	564
Mental Health	549	Speech	566

HOME HEALTH CARE RESOURCE RECORD

Date _____

Organization and / or person contacted _____

Position or title _____

Address _____

_____ Phone no. _____

Questions asked   Answers

_____   _____

_____   _____

_____   _____

_____   _____

_____   _____

_____   _____

_____   _____

ADDITIONAL RESOURCES

Organization	Contact Person	Telephone

Next steps _____

_____

AGING

■ AMERICAN ASSOCIATION OF RETIRED PERSONS (AARP)
The AARP is an organization dedicated to improving the lives of the nation's elderly population. Local AARP groups across the country combine to deliver a variety of programs and services. Among them are:

> *Consumer programs* • consumer rights, financial planning, insurance purchasing
>
> *Driver improvement* • designed to meet the needs of motorists fifty-five and over
>
> *Health advocacy* • provides the elderly with information on nutrition, preventive health care, chronic disease, Medicare, etc.
>
> *Second career opportunities* • for those in need of advice on continuing to work beyond age sixty-five; finding a part- or full-time job; doing volunteer work
>
> *Widowed persons service* • to give emotional support to one who has lost a spouse

In addition, AARP publishes booklets covering a wide range of topics. Of interest may be:

> *How to Write a Wrong: Complain Effectively and Get Results*
>
> *More Health for Your Dollar:* an older person's guide to health maintenance organizations (HMOs)
>
> *The Prudent Patient: How to Get the Most for Your Health Care $*

For your free copy of AARP booklets, please write

AARP Fulfillment
P.O. Box 2400
Long Beach, CA 90801

Membership in AARP is $5 a year or $12.50 for three years. Membership includes a subscription to the bimonthly magazine *Modern Maturity* and the *AARP Newsletter.*

To request program / service / membership information, please contact AARP and specify the type of information you seek.

American Association of Retired Persons
1909 K Street, N.W.
Washington, DC 20049
(202) 872-4700

■ GRAY PANTHERS PROJECT FUND
The Gray Panthers work to change laws and attitudes that discriminate against people on the basis of their age. They lobby, testify before Congress, organize letter-writing and telephone campaigns—all concrete steps toward effecting social change. In the area of health advocacy, they have brought many issues

to public attention: pensions, nursing homes, special problems of older women and of the aged minorities, Medicare and Medicaid funding.

The Panthers publish a flyer, "Be Careful, Older Americans: Know Your Rights and Responsibilities About Medicare, Part B," free on request (include a stamped self-addressed envelope).

To learn about the location of a group near you, contact

Gray Panthers Project Fund
311 S. Juniper Street
Philadelphia, PA 19107
(215) 545-6555

■ NATIONAL ALLIANCE OF SENIOR CITIZENS (NASC)
NASC is based in Virginia and is forming chapters in New York and Florida. A chapter has already been established in Arizona. This organization acts as an advocate for senior citizens in Washington and in state legislatures. They charge a $1 membership fee, which entitles you to receive *"The Senior Guardian,"* a monthly newsletter, and a bimonthly newspaper, *Our Age.*

In addition, members can participate in a discount program offering savings on such items as prescriptions, hotel and auto rental rates, and tours. If you would like to know more, contact

National Alliance of Senior Citizens
2525 Wilson Boulevard
Arlington, VA 22201
(703) 528-4380

■ THE NATIONAL ASSOCIATION OF AREA AGENCIES ON AGING (N4A)
The N4A is a private, nonprofit, national organization based in Washington, D.C., representing over 600 area agencies across the country. The focus of the association is to promote a national policy that would permit older Americans to remain independent in their homes and communities for as long as possible. Each member agency identifies and attempts to respond to local needs and conditions in both the short and long term. Individuals can become members of both their local area agency as well as the national association. Check with both for membership fees.

Area agencies' range of services vary, but can include:

Home health aid	Counseling
Personal care	Telephone reassurance
Nutritional counseling	Shopping assistance
Housekeeping	Transportation
Home visiting	Information and referral
Chores	Recreation
Home repairs	

In addition to providing the aforementioned services, the organization welcomes volunteer participation in a number of interesting areas, such as advisory council, political advocacy, home visiting, telephone reassurance, and much, much more. For further information regarding services, participation, membership, or the location of the area agency nearest you, contact

National Association of Area Agencies on Aging
600 Maryland Avenue, S.W., Suite 208
Washington, DC 20024
(202) 484-7520

■ NATIONAL CLEARINGHOUSE ON AGING
The Administration on Aging of the National Clearinghouse on Aging collects, analyzes, and disseminates information on the problems of the aging. It responds to inquiries by sending fact sheets, bibliographies, and other publications or by making referrals to other information centers or direct service providers. A brochure entitled "To Find the Way" outlines major sources of assistance for older Americans. For further information, contact

National Clearinghouse on Aging
Administration on Aging
330 Independence Avenue, S.W., Room 4146
Washington, DC 20201
(212) 245-2158

■ NATIONAL COUNCIL ON THE AGING, INC. (NCOA)
NCOA is a national, nonprofit organization dedicated to improving the lives of older persons. Its membership consists of voluntary agencies and associations and individuals. Although NCOA is geared to serve trained professionals, it does offer individuals some direct services.
   The editorial publications department publishes *Perspective on Aging,* a bimonthly magazine containing articles, columns, and book reviews. And the publication list includes items that may be of interest: *Facts and Myths About Aging; A Guide for Selection of Retirement Housing;* and *A Job Seeking Guide for Seniors.*
   There are conferences, seminars, and workshops sponsored by NCOA. For further information, contact

The National Council of the Aging, Inc.
600 Maryland Avenue, S.W.
West Wing 100
Washington, DC 20024
(202) 479-1200

■ NATIONAL COUNCIL OF SENIOR CITIZENS (NCSC)
The National Council of Senior Citizens is both a political advocate of older people's interests and a provider of health and recreation benefits. NCSC has more than 400 local clubs offering members a variety of activities and services:
   Legislative action • NCSC is currently working to increase Medicare coverage for glasses, hearing aids, drugs, and dentures; to eliminate deductibles and coverage gaps; for tax relief for those over sixty-five. (NCSC reports that they helped establish Medicare, several increases in Social Security benefits, the nutrition program providing inexpensive meals for older people, cheaper transportation, and more.)

Health insurance • members are eligible for group health insurance, individualized insurance to supplement Medicare coverage, and in-hospital plans for members under sixty-five or over sixty-five and ineligible for Medicare.

Discounts • Available on individual and group travel, lodging, and car rental.

The monthly *Senior Citizens News* covers legislative issues, information about Medicare and other federal programs, and other features.

NCSC administers a Nursing Home Information Service (NHIS) with a directory of long-term care available in the Washington, D.C. area containing information about residential care, day care, home health care, Meals-on-Wheels, hospice care, etc. NHIS can provide similar information about services around the country. It publishes the "Nursing Home Patient's Bill of Rights" and "Look, Listen, Smell, Question—How to Choose a Nursing Home," free on request.

For more information, contact

National Council of Senior Citizens
925 15th Street, N.W.
Washington, DC 20005
(202) 347-8800

■ NATIONAL INSTITUTE ON AGING

This institute, part of the National Institutes of Health, is devoted to conducting and supporting biomedical, social, and behavioral research related to the aging process, in addition to diseases and other special problems and needs of the aged.

NIA makes available, free of charge, to the general public, pamphlets such as *Q & A: Alzheimer's Disease* and *A Winter Hazard for the Old: Accidental Hypothermia.* NIA also offers *Age Pages,* which are informative sheets covering a wide range of topics of interest to the elderly, such as arthritis advice, sexuality in later life, and staying healthy after sixty-five. To get your free copy, contact

National Institute on Aging
National Institutes of Health
Building 31, Room 5C35
Bethesda, MD 20205
(301) 496-1752

■ NATIONAL SUPPORT CENTER FOR FAMILIES OF THE AGING

The organization seeks to help family members cope with their responsibilities to older relatives and to help people come to terms with their own aging. They publish materials for lay or professional caregivers and report they are currently assembling a national directory of support groups. For further information, write

National Support Center for Families of the Aging
P.O. Box 245
Swarthmore, PA 19081

■ STATE ADULT DAY CARE ASSOCIATIONS

Alabama Association of Adult Day
Care
Contact: Phil Ives
East Alabama Mental Health
P.O. Drawer 2426
Opelika, AL 36801-2426

Alaska Adult Daycare Association
Contact: Noel C. Matteson
Chugiak Senior Center
P.O. Box 414
Chugiak, AK 99567

Arizona Association of Adult Day
Care
Contact: Cynthia Brennan
Foundation for Senior Adult Living
1017 North 3rd Street, Suite 20
Phoenix, AZ 85004

California Association for Adult
Day Health Services
Contact: Linda Crossman
Marin Senior Day Services
P.O. Box 692
Mill Valley, CA 94942

Connecticut Association of Adult
Day Centers
Contact: Kathryn Katz
Director, Older Adult Day Care
Program
Jewish Home for the Elderly of
Fairfield County
175 Jefferson Street
Fairfield, CT 06432

Florida Association of Adult Day
Care
Contact: Laura A. Bivona
Medical Services Coordinator
Department of Aging Services
305 North Morgan Street
Tampa, FL 33602

Illinois Association of Adult Day
Care Providers
Contact: Mary Graber Hagarty
Suburban Adult Day Center
149 West Harrison
Oak Park, IL 60304

Indiana Adult Daycare Association
Contact: Katherine Williams, R.N.
6404 Castleway Court
Indianapolis, IN 46250

Iowa Association of Adult Day Care
Programs
Contact: Natalie Reese
Willis Adult Day Care
Sixth and University Avenue
Des Moines, IA 50314

Kansas Adult Day Care Association
Contact: Linda Cook Webb
6164 Charlotte
Kansas City, MO 64110

Louisiana Adult Day Care Associa-
tion
Contact: Elaine Marsh
New Directions
1523 North Dorgenois
New Orleans, LA 70130

Maryland Association of Adult Day
Care Programs
Contact: Marge Burba-Babbitt,
Director
Winter Growth Adult Day Center
P.O. Box 186
Sandy Spring, MD 20860

Massachusetts Association for
Adult Day Health Services, Inc.
Contact: Karen Laganelli
Jewish Home for the Aged Adult
Day Center
629 Salisbury Street
Worcester, MA 01609

Michigan Association of Senior Day
Care Centers
Contact: William S. Goodwill, Exec-
utive Director
Center for Independent Living, Inc.
1509 East Court Street
Flint, MI 48503

Ellen Tharp, Ph.D.
Senior Daytime Center
1201 West Oakland, Suite 101
Lansing, MI 48915

Minnesota Adult Daycare Association
Contact: Dorothy Ohnsorg
Wilder Adult Day Care Center
516 Humboldt
St. Paul, MN 55107

Missouri Adult Daycare Association
Contact: Mark Chapman
Research Downtown Adult Day Center
Research Downtown Health Care Center
Admiral Boulevard at Oak
Kansas City, MO 64106

Nebraska Adult Day Care Association
Contact: Paul Maginn
McAuley Bergan Center
3552 Farnam Street
Omaha, NE 68131

New Jersey Adult Day Care Association
Contact: Sister Winifred Kelly, S.C.
Paterson Adult Day Center
163 Graham Avenue
Paterson, NJ 07501

New Mexico Association of Adult Day Care
Contact: Maria Isela Gayton-Diaz
Cornucopia, Inc.
1734 Isleta Boulevard, S.W.
Albuquerque, NM 87105

New York State Adult Day Services Association
Contact: Cynthia Wishkovsky
Lockport Senior Citizens Center
57 Richmond Avenue
Lockport, NY 14094

North Carolina Adult Day Care Association
Contact: Suzi Kennedy
Life Enrichment Center
610 Charles Road
Shelby, NC 28150

Ohio Association of Adult Daycare
Contact: Andree Bognar
Today Center for Adults
711 Dayton-Xenia Road
Xenia, OH 45385

Pennsylvania Adult Day Care Association
Contact: Sister St. Gregory, Director
Adult Day Care Center
St. Joseph Villa
Wissahickon and Stenton Avenue
Flourtown, PA 19031

Rhode Island Directors Association for Senior Citizens Programs
Contact: Sister Ruth Crawley
Fruit Hill Adult Day Care
399 Fruit Hill Avenue
North Providence, RI 02911

Adult Day Care Association of Texas
Contact: Lisa Humes
North Texas Adult Day Health Care, Inc.
5012 Justin Avenue
Irving, TX 15060

Vermont Association of Adult Day Centers
Contact: Janet Gershaneck
Project Independence
40 South Main Street
Barre, VT 05641

Virginia Institute of Adult Daycare
Contact: Lory Osario, Executive Director
Stuart Circle Center
1605 Monument Avenue
Richmond, VA 23220

Washington State Association of Adult Day Centers
Contact: Nora Stabler
Norwest Day Center for Adults
9250-14th Street, N.W.
Seattle, WA 98117

Wisconsin Adult Daycare Association
Contact: June Cichowicz
Independent Living
1245 East Washington
Madison, WI 53703

Maria Alvarez
Adult Day Center
812 Wisconsin Avenue
Madison, WI 53703

■ STATE AND AREA AGENCIES ON AGING

The Select Committee on Aging of the U.S. House of Representatives offers a directory that identifies the agencies in each state and community that provide assistance and referral to millions of older Americans. It's called *Directory of State and Area Agencies on Aging,* and single copies are free. Write

Select Committee on Aging
House Annex No. 1, Room 712
Washington, DC 20515
Attn.: Publications

ARTHRITIS

■ ARTHRITIS FOUNDATION

The over seventy plus local chapters of the Arthritis Foundation serve as information resources about rheumatic diseases. Contacting your local chapter may provide a helpful referral for the physical, financial, and emotional problems that accompany rheumatic diseases. The local services that the chapters encourage and support include:

counseling and occupational therapy
support groups—a forum for sharing common problems and solutions
home visit programs for homebound arthritics
equipment loan services
telephone hot lines
education programs

The Foundation's publication list contains over thirty booklets, most of which are free. The Medical Information Series provides information about specific forms of arthritis and other rheumatic diseases. Other booklets include *Diet and Nutrition, Living and Loving, Good Treatment in Rheumatoid Arthritis, Self-Help Manual.* There is also a series of medication briefs that describe drugs used in treatment. The Foundation's newsletter, *National Arthritis News,* is printed in large type and carries practical and medical information. For the publications list, the location of a local chapter, or other information, contact

Arthritis Foundation
1314 Spring Street, N.W.
Atlanta, GA 30309
(404) 872-7100

■ ARTHRITIS HEALTH AND RESOURCE CENTER *(Massachusetts)*
The Arthritis Health and Resource Center has designed several programs to treat arthritic conditions, among them, support groups, physical therapy, stress management, exercise classes, and nutrition. For further information, contact

Arthritis Health and Resource Center
486 Washington Street
Wellesley, MA 02181
(617) 431-7080

■ NATIONAL INSTITUTE OF ARTHRITIS, DIABETES, AND DIGESTIVE AND KIDNEY DISEASES (NIADDK)
One of the eleven National Institutes of Health within the Department of Health and Human Services, the NIADDK is primarily a research-oriented institute and supports a number of multipurpose arthritis centers across the country.

Programs vary from center to center. They have included a pilot Home Visits Program at Boston University, arthritis patient clubs at the Dartmouth, New Hampshire, center, a study at the University of Michigan on arthritis and sexuality, and special children's clinics at the Dartmouth and Indiana University schools of medicine. To identify individual centers to contact, write or call

Multipurpose Arthritis Centers Program Director
Division of Arthritis, Musculoskeletal and Skin Disease
National Institute of Arthritis, Diabetes, and Digestive and Kidney Diseases
Westwood Building, Room 403
Bethesda, MD 20205
(301) 496-7495

BLINDNESS

■ AMERICAN COUNCIL OF THE BLIND
With national offices in Washington, D.C., and fifty-one state affiliates the American Council of the Blind is a national membership organization comprised primarily of blind and visually impaired people. Its monthly magazine, *Braille Forum* is available in braille, disc, cassette, and large print. Their services include the Washington Connection, a hotline on current legislative action, and educational, recreational, and social activities. Its pamphlet, *Facts About Blindness and Visual Impairment,* is informative and helpful. For further information, contact

American Council of the Blind
1211 Connecticut Avenue, N.W., Suite 506
Washington, DC 20036
(202) 833-1251 or 1-800-424-8666 (toll-free)

■ AMERICAN FOUNDATION FOR THE BLIND
This is *not* a membership organization but a group that works as a national
partner to local services for the blind and visually impaired people. The
American Foundation for the Blind offers some services directly to the consumer, including
> service information and referrals to public and private agencies
> educational information on blindness
> a lending library (at the New York City location), some material in braille
> a newsletter containing information on programs, products, and activi-
> ties, available free of charge
> *The Directory of Agencies Serving the Visually Handicapped in the U.S.*
> ($25)

For further information, contact

American Foundation for the Blind
15 West 16th Street
New York, NY 10011
(212) 620-2000

■ BETTER VISION INSTITUTE
The Better Vision Institute is a nonprofit organization composed of members
of the ophthalmic community and dedicated to increasing public awareness
for proper vision care. They publish numerous pamphlets (single copies are
free) on a variety of topics, including glaucoma, vision problems of the aging,
and eyeglasses for your special needs. Contact

Better Vision Institute
230 Park Avenue
New York, NY 10169
(212) 682-1731

■ GUIDE DOGS FOR THE BLIND, INC.
Guide Dogs for the Blind, Inc., is a nonprofit, charitable organization dedicated to providing highly trained guide dogs, and training in their use, to
qualified blind men and women, regardless of geographic area, over the age
of sixteen. To apply for a guide dog or receive a current list of other dog guide
schools in the United States, write

Guide Dogs for the Blind, Inc.
P.O. Box 1200
San Rafael, CA 94915
(415) 479-4000

■ NATIONAL ASSOCIATION FOR VISUALLY HANDICAPPED
This group acts as a clearinghouse and referral agency for public and private
services for the visually handicapped. The association prints and distributes
large-print books and has a free loan library of large print books. It publishes
a large-print newsletter and provides information about commercially avail-

able large-print publications and optical aids. For further information, contact

National Association for Visually Handicapped
305 East 24th Street, Room 17-C
New York, NY 10010
(212) 889-3141

■ NATIONAL BRAILLE ASSOCIATION
This is an international organization without local units. Instead, its volunteer members work through religious and community groups to produce and distribute braille, large-type and tape-recorded reading materials for visually impaired readers. Catalogs listing college textbooks, sheet music, and books of general interest are available on request, by contacting

National Braille Association, Inc.
422 South Clinton Avenue
Rochester, NY 14620
(716) 232-7770

■ NATIONAL FEDERATION OF THE BLIND
The National Federation of the Blind provides education and advocacy services for the blind. It is a membership organization with state and local chapters. The National Blindness Information Center answers questions about blindness and the rights of the blind. For state and local chapter addresses and blindness inquiries, contact

National Federation of the Blind
1800 Johnson Street
Baltimore, MD 21230
(301) 659-9314

■ NATIONAL INDUSTRIES FOR THE BLIND (NIB)
This is a private organization that acts as a liaison between the National Industries for the Blind, associated workshops, and the federal government. NIB has workshops in thirty-two states, Puerto Rico, and Washington, D.C. The workshops offer rehabilitation and vocational training. Contact NIB headquarters in New Jersey to learn of the workshop nearest you.

National Industries for the Blind
524 Hamburg Turnpike
Wayne, NJ 07470
(201) 595-9200

Note: If you contact your State Commission for the Blind, (check your local telephone directory under state offices), they will provide you with agencies near you providing rehabilitation and vocational training.

■ NATIONAL LIBRARY SERVICE FOR THE BLIND AND PHYSICALLY HANDICAPPED
Through a network of 160 local cooperating libraries and agencies, the National Library Service of the Library of Congress distributes braille and talking

books and magazines. Blind and physically handicapped persons who wish to borrow materials may contact them for the location of the nearest cooperating library. This service is free. Contact

National Library Service for the Blind and Physically Handicapped
Library of Congress
1291 Taylor Street, N.W.
Washington, DC 20542
(202) 287-5100

■ NATIONAL SOCIETY TO PREVENT BLINDNESS (NSPB)
The NSPB is a voluntary health agency working to prevent blindness. They offer annual glaucoma screenings and a variety of pamphlets promoting eye protection and safety. Titles include "Cataract: What It Is and How It's Treated," "TV and Your Eyes," and "The Aging Eye: Facts of Eye Care for Older Persons," all without charge. Contact

National Society to Prevent Blindness
79 Madison Avenue
New York, NY 10016
(212) 684-3505 or 1-800-231-3004 (toll-free)

Addresses and telephone numbers for the twenty-six state affiliates can be obtained from the national office or by consulting the telephone directory in a state's capital city.

■ RECORDING FOR THE BLIND
This is a national, nonprofit organization that provides recorded textbooks in cassette form to the visually, physically, or perceptually handicapped (free, on loan). Most of the recordings are educational. Recording for the Blind services students from every state and thirty-five foreign countries. Upon request, Recording for the Blind will send you "A Borrowers Application Kit," material describing the organization and eligibility requirements. Contact

Recording for the Blind
20 Roszel Road
Princeton, NJ 08540
(609) 452-0606

■ RETINITIS PIGMENTOSA FOUNDATION–FIGHTING BLINDNESS
This national organization is devoted to finding (through research) the cause, treatment, and prevention of retinitis pigmentosa. Upon request, the Foundation offers a booklet, *Answers to Your Questions on Retinitis Pigmentosa and Other Retinal Degenerative Diseases* and a quarterly newsletter, *Fighting Blindness News*. The confidential registry of persons affected by retinitis pigmentosa enables the Foundation to keep members posted regarding research developments and trial treatments. For further information, contact

Retinitis Pigmentosa Foundation–Fighting Blindness
8331 Mindale Circle
Baltimore, MD 21207
(301) 655-1011 (Maryland) 1-800-638-5682 (toll-free)

■ VISION FOUNDATION, INC.

The Vision Foundation is a self-help organization serving visually impaired people and their families and friends. The programs are run primarily by volunteers. The self-help groups meet regularly throughout the state of Massachusetts, but they do handle information and referral requests from all over the country. This service is free and covers such diverse subjects as transportation, guide dogs, adaptive aides, and mail order houses. A handbook, recently updated, entitled *Coping with Sight Loss: The Vision Resource Book,* is available in large print or voice-indexed cassette. For further information, contact

Vision Foundation
2 Mt. Auburn Street
Watertown, MA 02172
(617) 926-4232
1-800-852-3029 (toll-free)

■ *VOCATIONAL REHABILITATION SERVICES AND SERVICES FOR THE BLIND AND VISUALLY HANDICAPPED*

Vocational rehabilitation services are available to blind and visually impaired people within each state, either through the department of vocational rehabilitation or as a separate agency for the blind.

Each state determines the types and extent of services provided. All states offer some degree of vocational and other training services, including counseling, guidance, placement services, and postemployment services. There may be financial assistance for medically restorative services such as corrective surgery, eyeglasses, and visual services. Special services for the blind include reader services and orientation and mobility services. To obtain a listing of state rehabilitation agencies, contact

Rehabilitation Services Administration
Office of Special Education and Rehabilitative Services
Department of Education
330 C Street, S.W., Room 3431
Washington, DC 20202
(202) 245-0594

CANCER

■ AMERICAN CANCER SOCIETY (ACS)

ACS seeks to save more lives through research, education, and service and works through its 58 divisions and 3,000 local units located throughout the United States. The American Cancer Society's service and rehabilitation program provides practical help and emotional support to those affected by cancer. Services vary depending on the needs of the patient, available funds of ACS, and local facilities. The ACS provides the following services without

charge:
> information concerning ACS services, community health services, and resources that may help the patient
> loans of sickroom supplies and special comfort items for the homebound patient
> transportation to and from a doctor's office, clinic, or hospital for diagnosis and treatment

ACS utilizes Visiting Nurse Association and homemaker agencies for home health programs and provides trained volunteers—cancer patients themselves to help others. For the location of the division nearest you, contact the national headquarters:

American Cancer Society
90 Park Avenue
New York, NY 10016
(212) 599-8200

■ BREAST CANCER ADVISORY CENTER
The Breast Cancer Advisory Center disseminates information and maintains a library on breast cancer. Fact sheets are available (at nominal charge) on topics such as "How to Choose a Gynecologist for Breast Cancer," "If You've Had Breast Cancer," and "Breast Self-Exam." A book on breast cancer, *Alternatives,* by Rose Kushner, executive director of the Breast Cancer Advisory Center is available for $10 plus $1.50 postage and handling. For information, contact

Breast Cancer Advisory Center
P.O. Box 224
Kensington, MD 20895

■ CANCER CARE *(New York City, Long Island, New Jersey)*
Cancer Care "provides personalized, professional counseling and guidance to cancer patients and their families for as long as is needed, and at no cost to the patient." There are approximately fifty chapters of Cancer Care in New York City, Nassau, and Suffolk counties and New Jersey.
> Services to patients and their families include:
> individual counseling and group therapy for cancer patients
> counseling for family members
> social worker assistance to find homemaking/child care services
> possible supplementary financial support toward the cost of necessary home care services

For further information, contact

Cancer Care, Inc.
One Park Avenue
New York, NY 10016
(212) 679-5700
(516) 364-8130 (Long Island)
(201) 261-2003 (New Jersey)

■ CANCER CONNECTION

Based in Kansas City, Missouri, the Cancer Connection works as a support system that matches cancer victims with volunteers who have been cured, are in remission, or are being treated for the same type of cancer. Volunteers share personal experience and offer information and support to the newly diagnosed patient. For people living in Missouri and Kansas, the R. A. Bloch Cancer Management Center of the University of Missouri (Kansas City) provides a free second opinion by a multidisciplinary panel. The Cancer Connection accepts calls from anywhere in the United States, although beyond a certain geographical area, calls are returned collect. For further information, contact

Cancer Connection
4410 Mail Street
Kansas City, MO 64111
(816) 932-8453

■ CANDLELIGHTERS FOUNDATION

The Candlelighters Foundation is an international network of groups of parents with children in varying stages of cancer.

On a local basis, the Foundation acts as a very informal forum where parents share experiences and information on how they and their child live with cancer. Some groups sponsor crisis phone lines, parent-to-parent contacts, professional counseling, and self-help groups. Candlelighters also hold social functions where families can get together and relax. These groups also present speakers and panels on childhood cancer, maintain libraries, publish newsletters, and serve on community boards such as the American Cancer Society. The Candlelighters Foundation services are free. They can be contacted by writing to

Candlelighters Foundation
2025 I Street, N.W., Suite 1011
Washington, DC 20006

■ CITY OF HOPE

The patient care program of the City of Hope National Medical Center provides diagnosis and treatment for a broad spectrum of illnesses. Among the clinical areas in which services are provided are cancer, blood diseases and bone marrow transplantation, endocrine disorders, genetic diseases, and gastrointestinal diseases. Patients are accepted on referral from health professionals, and admission is based on an established set of criteria. Care is free. For further information, contact

Office of Referral and Admissions
City of Hope
National Medical Center
Duarte, CA 91010
(213) 359-8111
1-800-535-1390 (toll-free)

■ LEUKEMIA SOCIETY OF AMERICA

The Leukemia Society of America is a voluntary health agency supporting worldwide research into leukemia and related diseases, including lymphomas, Hodgkin's disease, and multiple myeloma, as well as sponsoring nationwide programs of patient assistance, public and professional education, and community service. Free information, including brochures, a bimonthly newsletter, and audiovisuals, is available through the Society's fifty-seven local chapters. Check your telephone directory for the chapter nearest you or write to

Leukemia Society of America
National Headquarters
733 Third Avenue
New York, NY 10017

■ MAKE TODAY COUNT

Make Today Count is an international membership organization (no dues) with 247 chapters in the United States, Canada, and Germany. They seek to provide information and support to people facing life-threatening illness: the patient, family, and friends. They publish a monthly newsletter and sponsor workshops and seminars. Their membership includes cancer victims, families, and friends, health professionals, clergy, and other interested persons. For further information, contact

Make Today Count
National Office
514 Tama Building
Burlington, IO 52601
(319) 753-6521

■ NATIONAL CANCER INSTITUTE

The National Cancer Institute is one of the Institutes of the National Institutes of Health, an agency within the U.S. Department of Health and Human Services. The National Cancer Institute supports substantive research in the areas of cancer detection and treatment at major medical centers around the country. They also screen patients for admission to research protocols conducted at their own center, the Warren Grant Magnuson Clinical Center in Bethesda, Maryland. Your doctor can write the director of the Clinical Center or call the patient referral services unit (310) 496-4891 for information.

The National Cancer Institute has a network of Cancer Information Services Offices. The Cancer Information Service provides information and confidential answers to callers' questions. By dialing 1-800-4-CANCER (800-422-6237), callers automatically reach the Cancer Information Service office serving their area.

For a National Institutes of Health publications list, write

(*Entry continued on following page*)

NIH Publications List
National Institutes of Health
Division of Public Information
Editorial Operations Branch
Building 31, Room 2B03
Bethesda, MD 20205

■ REACH TO RECOVERY
The Reach to Recovery Program (of the American Cancer Society) is a rehabilitation program for women who have had breast cancer. This program helps
women deal with the physical and emotional aspects related to the disease
and treatment.

Reach to Recovery works through trained volunteers who have experienced and adjusted to the surgery. Carefully selected volunteers who have
been through different forms of treatment can make a difference in helping
a woman adjust. In some cities, their program includes male volunteers to
help the man in their life cope. Some units conduct open forums for women
who have experienced breast cancer. Often there is a physician in attendance. There is no charge for any Reach to Recovery service. Contact

American Cancer Society
777 Third Avenue
New York, NY 10017
(212) 371-2900

COMMUNITY SERVICES (SOCIAL AND LEGAL)

■ AMERICAN ASSOCIATION OF RETIRED PERSONS (AARP)
Thousands of local AARP chapters across the country provide a variety of
services and programs to improve the lives of the nation's elderly. From consumer programs to widowed persons services, AARP activities address the
multiple issues and concerns with which the elderly must cope. (See page 513
in this Appendix.) For further information about programs and membership,
contact

American Association of Retired Persons
1909 K Street, N.W.
Washington, DC 20049
(202) 872-4700

■ AMERICAN RED CROSS
With more than 3,000 local chapters nationwide, the American Red Cross
offers a wide variety of services. Check with the Red Cross chapter in your
area to learn about services they offer. As an example, the New York chapter
will provide emergency housekeeping services for elderly patients discharged
from a hospital. People must be over sixty years old, able to move around by
themselves and administer their own medications, and have no one at home
to help them. Home care includes light shopping (food paid for by the patient),

light housekeeping, and meal preparation. For further information, look in the White Pages of your telephone directory under American Red Cross.

■ COMMUNITY COUNCIL OF GREATER NEW YORK
The Community Council of Greater New York issues a guide to social and health services in New York City. Entitled *How to Secure Help,* the guide lists emergency services, home care and home health care services, and more. For a copy, send a written request (and include a stamped [39¢ postage], self-addressed envelope)

Community Council of Greater New York
225 Park Avenue South
New York, NY 10003

■ COALITION OF SPANISH SPEAKING MENTAL HEALTH ORGANIZATIONS (COSSMHO)
COSSMHO is a coalition of agencies, organizations, and individuals dedicated to improving and expanding services to the Hispanic community. By directing inquiries to the appropriate agencies and services, COSSMHO helps members of the Hispanic community work through the system and "red tape" to obtain needed services. It may be help filling out forms or referral to an intergenerational program where young volunteers do errands for the elderly or referral to a Meals on Wheels program. A call or letter to COSSMHO's national office will put you in touch with your nearest COSSMHO affiliate or a Hispanic center in the National Association of Area Agencies. For further information, contact

COSSMHO
1030 15th Street, N.W., Suite 1053
Washington, DC 20005
(202) 371-2100

■ JEWISH BOARD OF FAMILY AND CHILDREN'S SERVICES *(Metro New York)*
The Jewish Board of Family and Children's services offers community-based services, residential and day treatment programs for disturbed children, confused couples, troubled families, new immigrants, people in crisis, and people suffering continuing emotional and social problems. They serve the five boroughs of New York City, Westchester, and Long Island. Services vary, depending on the needs of the community. The staff includes social workers, psychiatrists, psychologists, physicians, nurses, educators, and lawyers. For a directory of services, contact

Jewish Board of Family and Children's Services, Inc.
120 West 57th Street
New York, NY 10019
(212) 582-9100

■ LEGAL COUNSEL FOR THE ELDERLY *(Washington, D.C.)*
Legal Counsel for the Elderly provides a range of free legal services to residents of the nation's capital meeting certain income guidelines. They publish

a number of publications about Medicare, disability, and Social Security, which are available upon request. They also can refer you to similar groups around the nation. For further information, call or write

Legal Counsel for the Elderly
1909 K Street, N.W.
Washington, DC 20049
(202) 728-4333

■ MEALS ON WHEELS

Meals on Wheels is a program designed to help senior citizens over sixty who cannot prepare or shop for their own meals or are simply needy. Once you've enrolled in the program, someone will deliver to your home a meal that fulfills one-third of your daily nutritional requirements. Meals are delivered either five or seven times a week.

Senior citizens can initiate the process by contacting their local senior citizen center or the Department of Aging for the closest center. A social/case worker will visit them at home and determine eligibility. There is a voluntary contribution, but clients who cannot afford it are not turned away.

■ NATIONAL CONFERENCE OF CATHOLIC CHARITIES

The National Conference of Catholic Charities is not a direct provider of services; however, this national organization will refer you to your nearest Catholic Charity. Catholic charities provide a variety of social/human services to various segments of the population. Some services are offered free of charge; others are based on a sliding scale. For the disabled, chronically ill, or elderly, the following services are offered: counseling, foster family care, group home care, institutional care, homemaker services, day care, socialization activities, access services, emergency shelter, recreation, legal advice, and more. Not all services are available at every Catholic Charity. For further information, please contact

National Conference of Catholic Charities
Dupont Circle Building, Suite 307
1346 Connecticut Avenue, N.W.
Washington, DC 20026
(202) 785-2757

■ SELF-HELP CENTER

The Self Help Center is a clearinghouse on self-help and mutual aid groups and maintains a file of groups regionally and nationally. It has a twenty-four-hour hotline for locating self-help groups in your area. The center provides training and technical assistance to people setting up groups and sponsors workshops. For further information, contact

Self Help Center
1600 Dodge Avenue, Suite S-122
Evanston, IL 60201
(312) 328-0470 (24-hour line)

■ UNITED WAY

The United Way is an umbrella organization for regional and local offices of United Way. Funds that are raised by 2,100 local units are used to assist an estimated 37,000 health and social services agencies throughout the United States. Through United Way Community Services Program Grants, member agencies are better able to meet the needs of their community. The programs are diverse; for example, Richmond Senior Services, Inc., helps older adults find affordable housing, companionship, caregiving, and support in order to prevent institutionalization; and the 92nd Street YM-YWHA in New York has a program to provide 500 senior adults with educational, cultural, and recreational activities. For information regarding services provided and the location and telephone number of your local United Way, contact your regional office

(Northeast)
United Way
99 Park Avenue
New York, NY 10016
(212) 661-5666

(Southeast)
United Way
2150 Parklake Drive, Suite 310
Atlanta, GA 30345
(404) 938-5841

(Midwest)
United Way
10600 West Higgins Road, Suite 201
Rosemont, IL 60018
(312) 297-6160

(West)
United Way
410 Bush Street
San Francisco, CA 94108
(415) 772-4300

■ VOLUNTEERS OF AMERICA

The Volunteers of America is a national service organization operating in 150 communities around the country. Programs offered by each VOA do vary, but the following selected examples may represent services available near you.

For families: emergency financial aid or emergency shelters, a crisis hot line.

For the disabled: group homes/independent living programs for men-tally retarded adults; sheltered employment programs; respite care for families with disabled members; trained aids to assist people with disabilities.

For the elderly: home repair, homemaker assistance, transportation and senior center programs; group meals and meals on wheels; group homes; food cooperatives; foster grandparents programs.

To find out which programs your local Volunteers of America offers, look in the White Pages of your telephone book under Volunteers of America. Also see "Self-Help Groups and National Clearinghouses" in the Information Services section of this Appendix.

DEATH / DYING

■ CONCERN FOR DYING

Doctors, lawyers, educators, clergymen, and other interested individuals dedicated to helping people make their own decisions about dying are members of this educational council. The Concern for Dying office located in New York City publishes a quarterly newsletter and several other publications, including *A Legal Guide to the Living Will, Euthanasia—A Decade of Change,* and a report of the president's commission for the study of ethical problems in medical, biomedical, and behavioral research, *Deciding to Forgo Life Sustaining Treatment.* For further information, contact

Concern for Dying
250 West 57th Street
New York, NY 10107
(212) 246-6962

■ NATIONAL HOSPICE ORGANIZATION

The National Hospice Organization sets standards for hospice programs to ensure good-quality hospice care. They are a nonprofit membership organization dedicated to promoting the hospice concept of care and support for terminally ill patients and their families. In most cases a patient is referred to a hospice by the physician; however, referrals can also be made by family members, friends, clergy, or health professionals. For more information concerning hospice care or the locations of hospice programs in your state, contact

National Hospice Organization
1901 North Fort Meyer Drive, Suite 902
Arlington, VA 22209
(703) 243-5900

■ *STATE HOSPICE ORGANIZATIONS*

The following is a list of officially designated statewide organizations representing providers of hospice services. The list gives only the names of official state organizations. Where a state has only a few (two or so) hospices, we have listed the hospices themselves.

ALABAMA
Madeleine M. Hill, President
Alabama Hospice Organization
2211 Prince Avenue
Tuscaloosa, AL 35401
(205) 345-0067

ALASKA
Margaret R. Carter, Administrative Assistant
Hospice of Anchorage
3605 Arctic Boulevard #555
Anchorage, AK
(907) 272-0633
or

Mary Tonsmeire, Coordinator
Hospice of Juneau
P.O. Box 3-3000
Juneau, AK 99802
(907) 586-3414

ARIZONA
Phyllis Swanson, Secretary
Hospice of Yuma
P.O. Box 4211
Yuma, AZ 85364
(602) 343-2222

ARKANSAS
Sylvia Cheatham, President
Hospice of the Ozarks
906 Baker Street
Mountain Home, AK 72653
(501) 425-2797

CALIFORNIA
Pierre Salmon, M.D., President
Northern California Hospice Assn.
703 Market Street, Suite 550
San Francisco, CA 94103
(415) 543-9393
    or
Joyce Green, President
Hospice Organization of Southern
    California
637 South Lucas Avenue
Los Angeles, CA 90017
(213) 481-7340

COLORADO
Judy Schilling, President
3534 Kirwood Place
Boulder, CO 80302
(303) 449-7740

CONNECTICUT
Janice Casey, President
Hospice Council of Connecticut
Hospice of Stamford
461 Atlantic Avenue
Stamford, CT 06901
(203) 324-2592

DELAWARE
A. Murray Goodwin, Executive
    Director
3519 Silverside Road
Ridgeley Boulevard, Suite 100
Wilmington, DE 19810
(302) 478-5707

FLORIDA
Maryanne Jamerson, President
P.O. Box 449
Hospice of Central Florida
Winter Park, FL 32790
(305) 647-2523

GEORGIA
Elba Knavel, President
Hospice of the Golden Isles
1326 Union Street
Brunswick, GA 31520
(215) 265-4735

IDAHO
Judy Moyer, Secretary
Bannock Regional Medical Center
Memorial Drive at ISU Campus
Pocatello, ID 83201
(208) 232-6150

ILLINOIS
Anne Rooney, R.N., President
Coordinator Hospice of Proviso-
    Leyden
330 Eastern Avenue
Bellwood, IL 60104
(312) 547-8282

INDIANA
Steve Arter, President
Parkview Memorial Hospice
2200 Randolph Drive
Fort Wayne, IN 46805
(219) 484-6636 ext. 4183

IOWA
Dr. Marilyn Story, President
205 Loma Street
Waterloo, IA 50701
(319) 273-2814 (work)
(319) 291-6767 (home)

KANSAS
Nancy Solscheid, President
Association of Kansas Hospices
7540 Aberdeen
Praire Village, KS 66208
(913) 341-7844

KENTUCKY
Gretchen Brown, President
Community Hospice of Lexington
465 East High Street
Lexington, KY 40508
(606) 252-2308

LOUISIANA
Ruth Sherwood, Chairperson
3901 Tulane Avenue
New Orleans, LA 70119
(504) 482-1113

MAINE
Val Gates, President
Coalition of Maine Hospices
Coastal Family Hospice
RFD 1, Box 360A
6 Seaport Drive
Rockport, ME 04856
(207) 236-4849

MARYLAND
Susan Riggs, President
Maryland State Hospice Network
Sinai Hospital of Baltimore Home
    Care Hospice
Belvedere at Greenspring
Baltimore, MD 21215
(301) 578-5600

MICHIGAN
Karl L. Zeigler, President
Michigan Hospice Organization
1825 Watson Road
Item Lock, MI 48626
(517) 642-8121

MINNESOTA
Anne O'Brien, President
Minnesota Hospice Organization
c/o Metro Medical Center
900 South 8th Street
Minneapolis, MN 55404
(612) 347-4377

MISSOURI
Karen Beckman Pace, President
Missouri Hospice Organization
527 West 39th Street
Kansas City, MO 64101
(816) 531-1200

MONTANA
Sheila Gapay, President
Montana Hospice Exchange Council
St. Joseph's Mission Mountain Hos-
    pice
P.O. Box 1010
Polson, MT 59860
(406) 883-5377

NEBRASKA
Tom Perkins, President
Nebraska Hospice Assn.
1010 East 35th Street
Scotts Bluff, NE 69361
(308) 635-3171

NEW HAMPSHIRE
Byll Reeve, President
Chris Chatfield, Secretary
Hospice Affiliates of New Hamp-
    shire, Inc.
P.O. Box 1221
Concord, NH
(603) 225-4903

NEW JERSEY
Maureen Eng. Executive Director
New Jersey Hospice Organization
760 Alexander Road
Princeton, NJ 08540
(609) 452-9280

NEW MEXICO
Bette Betts, Hospice Coordinator
Santa Fe Visiting Nurse Service
P.O. Box 1951
Santa Fe, NM 87501
(505) 471-9201
    or
Kathleen Hart, Director
Hospital Home Health / Hospice
    Care
500 Walter N.E., Room 316
Albuquerque, NM 87102
(505) 842-5967

NEW YORK
Charlotte Shedd, President
New York State Hospice Assn., Inc.
% Hospice Buffalo
2929 Main Street
Buffalo, NY 14314
(716) 838-4438
    or
Carol Selinske, Executive Director
469 Rosedale Avenue
White Plains, NY 10605
(914) 946-7699

NORTH CAROLINA
Judi Lund, Executive Director
Hospice of North Carolina, Suite
    401
800 St. Mary's Street
Raleigh, NC 27605
(919) 829-9588

NORTH DAKOTA
Ruth Dzik
North Dakota / NW Minnesota Hos-
    pice Coordinators
% Riveredge Hospice of St. Francis
415 Oak Street
Breckenridge, MN 56502
(218) 643-6641

OHIO
Linda Proffiit
Hospice Council for N. Ohio
1001 Huron Road, Suite 516
Cleveland, OH 44115
(216) 771-1797

OKLAHOMA
Linda Duncan
Hospice of Central Oklahoma
4500 North Lincoln
Oklahoma City, OK 73105
(405) 424-7263

OREGON
Valerie Ivey
Oregon Council of Hospices
Washington Country Home Health
    Assn.
1809 Maple Street
Forest Grove, OR 97116
(503) 640-2737

PENNSYLVANIA
Frances Cohen, President
Pennsylvania Hospice Network
% South Hills Family Hospice
1000 Bower Hill Road
Pittsburgh, PA 15243
(412) 561-4900

RHODE ISLAND
Robert J. Canny, Executive
    Director
Hospice Core of Rhode Island, Inc.
1240 Pawtucket Avenue
Rumford, RI 02916
(401) 434-4740

TENNESSEE
Sheridan Montgomery, President
Hospice of Tennessee
% Hospice of Chatanooga
921 East 3rd Street
Chattanooga, TN 37403
(615) 267-6828

TEXAS
Elaine Magruder, President
Texas Hospice Organization
2525 Walling Wood, Room 104
Timberline Office Park
Austin, TX 78746
(512) 327-9149

UTAH
Helen Rollins, Secretary
Hospice of Salt Lake
1370 Southwest Temple
Salt Lake City, UT 84115
(801) 486-5131

VERMONT
Patricia Healy-Sullivan, President
P.O. Box 544
Adams Mill Road
Moscow, VT 05662
(802) 253-7360

VIRGINIA
Dr. John Q. Mattern, President
15 Garland Drive
Newport News, VA 23606
(804) 599-6900

WASHINGTON
Grant Howarth, President
Seattle King County Visiting Nurse
    Service
909 University Street
Seattle, WA 98101
(206) 382-9700

WEST VIRGINIA
Margaret Kerney, President
Morgantown Hospice Inc.
P.O. Box 4222
Morgantown, WVA 26505
(304) 598-3424

(*Continued*)

WISCONSIN
James Ewens, President
Milwaukee Hospice Home Care
1022 North 9th Street
Milwaukee, WI 53233
(414) 271-3686

WASHINGTON, D.C. (*Metro area*)
Dale Lupu
Hospice Care Providers of Metro-
    politan Washington
(202) 951-9009
Dorothy Moga
(703) 525-7070

DENTISTRY

■ NATIONAL FOUNDATION OF DENTISTRY FOR THE HANDICAPPED
To meet the special needs of handicapped children and adults, the National Foundation of Dentistry for the Handicapped has a dentistry program for the homebound. A specially designed van can be used to reach people confined to their homes or nursing homes. If necessary, treatment can be provided while a person remains in bed. Consult your telephone directory to see if there is a Foundation affiliate in your area. If not, contact your local dental society to identify dentists who make housecalls, or contact

National Foundation of Dentistry for the Handicapped
1726 Champa, Suite 422
Denver, CO 80202
(303) 573-0264

DIABETES

■ AMERICAN DIABETES ASSOCIATION
The American Diabetes Association, through its nationwide affiliates, works to teach people with diabetes to live full lives despite the restrictions of the illness. Education programs, in-hospital orientation programs, seminars, and twenty-four-hour hotlines seek to show people how to become partners in health care with health professionals helping to control the disease. The ADA publishes a cookbook and a magazine, *Diabetes Forecast,* which features medical information, current research, recipes, and reports of affiliate activities. For the affiliate or chapter in your area, consult the White Pages of your telephone directory, or contact

American Diabetes Association
2 Park Avenue
New York, NY 10016
(212) 683-7444

■ DIVISION OF DIABETES CONTROL
Through the Center for Disease Control, the U.S. Department of Health and
Human Services has established diabetes control programs in twenty states.
Most of these programs conduct educational programs to teach people with
diabetes about proper care of the disease. The cost for enrollment is often
covered by Medicare, Medicaid, Blue Cross/Blue Shield, or other third party
reimbursement. The states with listed programs are California, Colorado,
Georgia, Illinois, Kentucky, Louisiana, Maine, Michigan, Minnesota, Mississippi, Missouri, Nebraska, New Jersey, New York, Ohio, Pennsylvania, South
Carolina, Utah, and Washington. To find out about a program near you, contact

Division of Diabetes Control
Centers for Disease Control
Atlanta, GA 30333
(404) 329-1851

■ JUVENILE DIABETES FOUNDATION
The Juvenile Diabetes Foundation is a worldwide voluntary organization that
supports research and conducts programs aimed at treatment, care, and control of diabetes. One program, the Association of Insulin-Dependent Diabetics, is a peer support group that helps members face the problems of living
with diabetes. To find out about the programs your local chapter offers, check
your telephone directory, or contact

Juvenile Diabetes Foundation
23 East 26th Street
New York, NY 10010
(212) 889-7575

■ NATIONAL DIABETES INFORMATION CLEARINGHOUSE
This clearinghouse answers requests for information about diabetes from health
professionals, people with diabetes, their families, and the general public.
They have bibliographies by topic, a resource directory, and numerous other
publications. On-line access to an automated file of brochures, books, articles,
fact sheets, etc., will soon be available to people in the diabetes community.
To add your name to their mailing list, or to obtain a list of materials in
specific topic areas, contact

National Diabetes Information Clearinghouse
P.O. Box NDIC
Bethesda, MD 20205
(301) 468-2162 or 496-7433

538   DIGESTIVE DISORDERS

DIGESTIVE DISORDERS

■ CYSTIC FIBROSIS FOUNDATION
The Cystic Fibrosis (CF) Foundation is a nationwide voluntary health organization that supports programs in over 125 CF treatment centers around the country that provide specialized diagnosis and medical care for patients. In addition, there are financial, educational, and social services offered to the patient, the family, and or the caregiver. For the location and telephone number of the Cystic Fibrosis Foundation chapter nearest you, contact

Cystic Fibrosis Foundation
6000 Executive Boulevard
Rockville, MD 20852
(301) 881-9130

■ NATIONAL DIGESTIVE DISEASES EDUCATION AND INFORMATION
CLEARINGHOUSE
A service of the National Institute of Arthritis, Diabetes, and Digestive and Kidney Diseases of the National Institutes of Health, this clearinghouse is mandated by Congress to educate physicians, other health care providers, patients, their families, and the public to promote greater understanding of digestive diseases. They publish a *Digestive Disease Directory*—a guide to the organization that can help, respond to inquiries, and distribute educational materials. For further information, contact

National Digestive Diseases Education and Information Clearinghouse
1555 Wilson Boulevard, Suite 600
Rosslyn, VA 22209
(301) 496-9707

■ NATIONAL FOUNDATION FOR ILEITIS AND COLITIS
The National Foundation for Ileitis and Colitis offers information and assistance to members and other interested people about inflammatory bowel disease. They publish a quarterly newsletter, conduct educational programs, and guide mutual help groups designed for patients and their families. Many of their eighteen chapters can refer you to doctors knowledgeable about inflammatory bowel disease. For chapter locations, contact

National Foundation for Ileitis and Colitis
295 Madison Avenue
New York, NY 10017
(212) 685-3440

■ UNITED OSTOMY ASSOCIATION
The United Ostomy Association is dedicated to helping ostomy patients return to normal living through mutual help and moral support. There are more than 625 chapters of UOA; the majority of its members are ostomates, who supplement the work of the surgeon and the enterostomal therapist by offer-

ing mutual aid and moral support. Members exchange practical, personal experiences about their ostomies at monthly meetings of local chapters. In addition, ostomy equipment and supplies are often displayed, and speakers knowledgeable about ostomy are often featured. A list of chapters is available upon request from the UOA office. Contact

United Ostomy Association
2001 West Beverly Boulevard
Los Angeles, CA 90057
(213) 413-5510

EQUIPMENT AND SUPPLIES

Your local pharmacist may carry some of the products and supplies that you need; he may be able to order them for you or send you to another pharmacy specializing in home health care products and supplies. Large drugstores with home health care departments can now be found in many parts of the country, and surgical supply dealers may also have a retail division. Check your Yellow Pages under "Pharmacies" and "Surgical Supplies."

In addition, the following companies represent a selection of mail order firms that sell a variety of home care products. Many sell aids for daily living; some sell medical equipment and supplies. Contact them for brochures and catalogs, if available. They may also tell you of local stores which sell their products:

Anik, Inc.
P.O. Box 3232
San Rafael, California 94912
(415) 461-1477

Brookstone Company
Vose Farm Road
Peterborough, New Hampshire
  03458
(603) 924-9511

Cleo, Inc.
3957 Mayfield Road
Cleveland, Ohio 44121
(216) 382-9700

Comfortably Yours
Aids for Easier Living
53 West Hunter Avenue
Maywood, New Jersey 07670
(201) 368-0400

Fashion-Able
5 Crescent St.
Rocky Hill, New Jersey 08553
(609) 921-2563

Independent Living Aids, Inc.
11 Commercial Court
Plainview, N.Y. 11803

Maddak, Inc.
Pequannock, New Jersey 07440
(201) 694-0500

Miles Kimball
41 West Eighth Avenue
Kimball Building
Oshkosh, Wisconsin 54901
(414) 231-3800

J. A. Preston Corporation
60 Page Road
Clifton, New Jersey 07012
1-800-631-7277

Fred Sammons, Inc.
Box 32
Brookfield, Illinois 60513-0032
1-800-323-5547

(Continued)

Sears Roebuck & Co.
Home Health Care
Sears Tower
Chicago, Illinois 60684
(312)875-2500

Travenol Home Therapy
Travenol Laboratories
1 Baxter Parkway
Deerfield, Illinois 60015
(312) 948-2000
(Hightech home therapies such as
total parenteral nutrition, antibiotic therapy dialysis.)

HEARING DISORDERS

■ AMERICAN HEARING RESEARCH FOUNDATION
Although primarily devoted to research, the American Hearing Research
Foundation does publish two pamphlets of interest to the lay person: "Facts
and Fancies About Hearing Aids" and "Care of the Ears and Hearing for
Health." Contact

American Hearing Research Foundation
55 East Washington Street
Chicago, IL 60602
(312) 726-9670

■ BETTER HEARING INSTITUTE
The Better Hearing Institute is an educational institution offering information about hearing loss and available medical, surgical, hearing aid rehabilitation, and other amplification assistance. The Institute publishes several
consumer pamphlets, a newsletter, reprints of magazine and newspaper articles, and several audiovisual presentations. They have a toll free HelpLine,
which offers suggestions and handles complaints about hearing aid services.
For further information, contact

Better Hearing Institute
1430 K Street, N.W., Suite 700
Washington, DC 20005
1-800-424-8576 Helpline

■ NATIONAL HEARING AID SOCIETY
The principal public service of the National Hearing Aid Society is the Hearing Aid Helpline, which you can call with questions about hearing loss. To
help you proceed when hearing loss is suspected, the Helpline will send you
a consumer kit containing a directory of National Hearing Aid Society members, arranged geographically, and a Better Business Bureau booklet, "Facts
About Hearing Aids." The Helpline has a variety of other pamphlets and
booklets, all of them free. Contact

National Hearing Aid Society
20361 Middlebelt
Livonia, MI 48152
1-800-521-5247 Helpline

■ NATIONAL INFORMATION CENTER ON DEAFNESS
This information center is run by Gallaudet College, an independent institution of higher education serving deaf people by providing instruction, public service, and research. The resource center provides feedback to questions via personal letters, brochures, fact sheets, bibliographies, and referrals. A variety of topics are covered, such as education, research, demographics, law, and technology. A professional staff and highly trained volunteers are on hand to respond to all information requests. Parents, professionals, and the general public are welcome to utilize this service. Written requests should be addressed to

National Information Center of Deafness
Gallaudet College
Kendall Green
Washington, DC 20002
(202) 651-5109

■ PHONE TTY
Phone TTY (TTY means teletype) is devoted to the manufacture and distribution of telephone equipment and signaling devices for the deaf or deaf-blind, who cannot use ordinary telephone equipment. For more information about equipment and their prices, contact

Phone-TTY
202 Lexington Avenue
Hackensack, NJ 07601
(201) 489-7889

■ SELF HELP FOR THE HARD OF HEARING
Self Help for the Hard of Hearing is a membership organization with 120 chapters nationwide, working to create awareness and understanding about hearing loss (not deafness) and effective coping strategies. Local chapters have self-help programs, newsletters, and social and recreational programs. On the national level, Self Help for the Hard of Hearing provides representation for the hearing disabled at the National Institutes of Health, the Veterans Administration, and other government agencies. For further information about membership, contact

Self Help for Hard of Hearing, Inc.
4848 Battery Lane, Suite 100
Bethesda, MD 20814
(301) 657-2248
(301) 657-2249(TTY)

■ TELECOMMUNICATIONS FOR THE DEAF
Telecommunications for the Deaf is comprised of more than 9,000 people with hearing impairments, their families, and organizations using teletypewriter machines and other special equipment for communication with deaf people. They publish a nationwide directory of TTY/TDD (Teletype/Telecom Device for the Deaf) users and help distribute donated surplus machines to people who need them. For a copy of the directory, or for further information, contact

Telecommunications for the Deaf
814 Thayer Avenue
Silver Spring, MD 20910
(301) 589-3006

HEART DISEASE AND STROKE

■ AMERICAN HEART ASSOCIATION
The American Heart Association through its 55 affiliates and 1,100 chapters sponsors community programs designed to meet the needs and concerns of the health professional community and the public. Local heart associations may provide guidance or referral to facilities and community agencies. The AHA has an active public education program, which seeks to build awareness about risk factors, prevention, early detection, and treatment of cardiovascular disease and stroke. For more information and/or the address of your nearest AHA chapter, contact

American Heart Association
7320 Greenville Avenue
Dallas, TX 75231
(214) 750-5300

■ MENDED HEARTS
The Mended Hearts is a mutual help organization composed of people who have successfully undergone heart surgery (and their families and friends). They are often eager to help others by providing them with information, encouragement, and support for people facing or recovering from heart surgery. For information about membership and local chapters, contact

Mended Hearts, Inc.
7320 Greenville Avenue
Dallas, TX 75231
(214) 750-5442

HOME CARE SERVICES

The discharge planner at your local hospital probably has a listing of Medicare-certified home health agencies in your area. In addition, the Yellow Pages of your telephone directory lists various services under at least two headings: "Home Health Agencies" and "Nursing."

■ NATIONAL ASSOCIATION FOR HOME CARE
The National Association for Home Care is a Washington D.C., based trade association representing and serving the interests of home health care agencies. Should you wish to learn about legislative and regulatory issues concerning home health care, of if you seek the names of home health care agencies in your community, contact

National Association for Home Care
519 C Street, N.E.
Washington, DC 20002
(202) 647-7424

■ NATIONAL HOMECARING COUNCIL
The mission of the National HomeCaring Council is to promote, develop, and ensure provision of responsible homemaker, home health aide, and related services of high quality for families and individuals in need of service. Among the many programs of the National HomeCaring Council are training guides for professionals working with homemaker–home health aide services and an accreditation program for home health agencies. For consumers, they have published a booklet, *All About Home Care,* which offers a guide to wise selection of home care services. It describes common problems that consumers face when they seek good home care—and ways to overcome them. For more information, contact

National HomeCaring Council
235 Park Avenue South
New York, NY 10003
(212) 674-4990

■ *INVESTOR-OWNED (PROPRIETARY) COMPANIES*
The following companies are investor-owned (proprietary) organizations that provide home care services and supplemental nursing services through networks of offices in cities throughout the United States. Check the White Pages of your telephone directory to locate an office in your town, or write or call the corporate offices for further information

Beverly Home Health Services
23639 Hawthorne Boulevard
Torrance, CA 90505
(213) 378-9263

Kimberly Services, Inc.
8500 West 110th Street
Overland Park, KS 66212
(913) 642-9380

Medical Personnel Pool
303 Southeast 17th Street
Ft. Lauderdale, FL 33316
(305) 764-2200

Olsten Corporation
One Merrick Avenue
Westbury, NY 11590
1-800-645-6570 (toll-free)

Quality Care Nursing Services, Inc.
100 North Centre Avenue
Rockville Centre, NY 11570
1-800-645-3633 or
1-800-632-3201 (New York)

Staff Builders, Inc.
122 East 42nd Street
New York, NY 10018
(212) 867-2345

Upjohn Healthcare Services, Inc.
2065 East Kilgore Road
Kalamazoo, MI 49002
(616) 342-7000

■ PROPRIETARY REHABILITATION SERVICES

The following company has offices in major cities.

Travenol Physical Therapy Services
Suite 109, 1100 Woodfield Road
Schaumberg, Illinois 60195
(312) 861-0060

■ STATE HOMEMAKER / HOME HEALTH AIDE ORGANIZATIONS

The following is a list of officially designated statewide organizations for providers of homemaker/home health aide services. (H-HHA)

IOWA COUNCIL FOR H-HHA SERVICES
Judy Klemm, President
Hancock Winnebago County
H-HHA Service
Court House Annex
Garner, IA 50438
    or
Mary Helen Cogley, Secretary
Iowa Department of Social Services
Hoover Building
Des Moines, IA 50319

H-HHA COUNCIL OF MAINE
Mrs. Kaye Flanagan, State Repre-
    sentative
Administrative Director
Holy Innocents' Home Care Service
P.O. Box 797
83 Sherman Street
Portland, ME 04104
    or

James L. Gorman, President
Program Director
Kennebec-Somerset Home Aide
    Service
224 Main Street
Waterville, ME 04901
(207) 837-1146
    or
Ray Beale, Vice President
Program Director
Department of Human Relations
    Service
Washington County Homemaker
    Service
Jonesport, ME 04649

MASSACHUSETTS COUNCIL FOR
H-HHAS
Ina Resnikoff, President
Director of H-HHA Department
Family Service Association of
    Greater Boston
34½ Beacon Street
Boston, MA 02108
or
Peggy Munro, Executive Director
Massachusetts Council for Home-
    maker–Home Health Aide
    Services
34½ Beacon Street
Boston, MA 02108
(617) 523-6400 Ext. 559

MISSOURI COUNCIL FOR HOMEMAKER
SERVICES
Carol Schultz, President
SERVE, Inc.
2 St. Louis Avenue
Fulton, MO 65251

HOMEMAKERS GUILD OF NEW
HAMPSHIRE
Eldora Clogston, President
Homemakers Guild of New Hamp-
    shire
Route 2, Beauregard Street
Claremont, NH 03743
(603) 542-2039
or
Patrick T. Eisenhart, Executive
    Director
Strafford County Homemaker–
    Home Health Aide Association
34 South Main Street
Rochester, NH 03867
(603) 335-1770

THE HOME CARE COUNCIL OF NEW
JERSEY
Mrs. Jeanne Locke, President
or

Kenneth Dolan, Executive Director
60 South Fullerton Avenue
Montclair, NJ 07042
(201) 744-8103

OHIO COUNCIL FOR H-HHA SERVICES
Alfred Liming, President
Executive Director
Family Service Agency of Spring-
    field and Clark County
Tecumseh Building, 10th Floor
34 West High Street
Springfield, OH 45502
(513) 325-5564

OREGON COUNCIL OF HOMEMAKER
SERVICES
Joanne Gulsvig, President
Family Counseling Homemaker
    Service
1432 Orchard
Eugene, OR 97403
(503) 485-5113
or
Carol Mills, Vice President
Central Oregon Council on Aging
324 NE Irving Avenue
Bend, OR 97707
(503) 389-3311

PENNSYLVANIA COUNCIL FOR
H-HHAS, INC.
John Buck, Executive Director
Central Pennsylvania Homemaker
    Service
2001 North Front Street
Harrisburg, PA 17102
(717) 233-6479
or
Hugh W. Ransom
403 Candlewyck Road
Camp Hill, PA 17011
(717) 737-7122

■ VISITING NURSE ASSOCIATIONS
These are voluntary agencies that provide nursing and other services in the
home, including health supervision, education, and counseling, bedside care,

a homemaker or home attendant, and Meals on Wheels. Although most of their services are paid for by Medicaid, Medicare, and private insurance, last year, the VNA provided $2.8 million worth of home health care at no cost. For more information, consult your phone book for the Visiting Nurse Association nearest you.

INFORMATION SERVICES

■ CENTER FOR MEDICAL CONSUMERS
The Center, located in New York City, is a resource center to help consumers become better educated about their health care. It is, in essence, a medical library for lay people. With over a thousand books and periodicals available for use, you can, for example, look up side effects of prescription drugs, or look up your doctors' training and experience. The Center publishes a monthly newsletter, *Health Facts,* which covers a single health topic in each issue. For a publications list, or to find out more about the Center, contact

Center for Medical Consumers
237 Thompson Street
New York, NY 10012
(212) 674-7105

■ FEDERAL TRADE COMMISSION
The Federal Trade Commission offers a varied list of publications that are available free on request. Consumers may select from two publications listings: The FTC Best Seller List or the more comprehensive Publications List. Contact

Federal Trade Commission
Public Reference Room 130
6th and Pennsylvania Avenue, N.W.
Washington, DC 20580

■ NATIONAL CLEARINGHOUSE ON AGING
The National Clearinghouse on Aging collects, analyzes, and disseminates information on the problems of the aging. It responds to inquiries by sending fact sheets, bibliographies, and other publications or by making referrals to other information centers or direct service providers. A brochure entitled "To Find the Way" outlines major sources of assistance for older Americans. For further information, contact

National Clearinghouse on Aging
Administration on Aging
330 Independence Avenue, S.W.
Washington, DC 20201
(202) 245-2158

■ NATIONAL HEALTH INFORMATION CLEARINGHOUSE

The Clearinghouse will assist you in locating specific sources of health information. Inquiries can be made by toll-free telephone or by mail. A free directory, describing seventy-six resources, *Health Information Resources in the Department of Health and Human Services,* is available to written inquiries providing a self-addressed mailing label. For information, contact

National Health Information Clearinghouse
P.O. Box 113
Washington, DC 20013
(703) 522-2590 (in Virginia)
(800) 336-4797 (outside Virginia)

■ *SELF-HELP GROUPS AND NATIONAL CLEARINGHOUSES*

Self-help organizations are mutual aid groups that provide assistance to patients and their families who are trying to cope with stress brought on by a specific disease, chronic illness, or disability. The members of a group offer each other support and encouragement in dealing with such matters as emotional, social, and medical problems and questions concerning prescribed treatments. By sharing experiences and knowledge, the group helps to create positive attitudes and to strengthen patients and families for the difficulties that lie ahead.

Currently, about 500,000 self-help and support groups are working nationwide. Many publish newsletters and other material that keep patients, families, and physicians up to date on available services and supplies.

There are twenty-seven clearinghouses in the nation, as indicated in the following list. They are valuable sources for those in need of information on self-help groups, publications, diseases, and other relevant matters. In addition to directing those in need to an existing self-help group, the clearinghouses can be instrumental in forming new groups. A National Self-Help Clearinghouse at the City University of New York (33 West 42nd Street, New York, NY 10036) maintains a current listing of mutual aid organizations throughout the country.

California		New Jersey	(201) 625-7101
Statewide	1–800-222-LINK	Statewide	(518) 474-6293
Merced Co.	(209) 723-5111	New York	(212) 852-4290
Sacramento	(916) 456-2070	Statewide	(518) 474-6293
San Diego	(619) 275-2344	New York City	(212) 852-4290
San Francisco	(415) 921-4401	Brooklyn	(212) 834-7373
Santa Maria	(805) 922-2165	Long Island	(516) 499-8800
Connecticut	(203) 789-7645	Westchester Co.	(914) 347-3620
Illinois	(312) 328-0470	Ohio	(216) 696-4262
Kansas	(316) 686-1205	Oregon	(503) 222-5555
Michigan	(616) 983-7781	Pennsylvania	
Minnesota	(612) 642-4060	Philadelphia	(215) 568-0860
Nebraska	(402) 476-9668	Scranton	(717) 961-1234

Tennessee	(615) 588-9747	Washington, D.C.	(703) 536-4100
Texas		Wisconsin	(414) 461-1466
Dallas	(214) 748-7825		
Ft. Worth	(817) 335-5405		

■ TEL-MED, INC.
Tel-Med is a telephone information service providing consumers with information on preventive medicine, health maintenance, and adjustment to illness. All messages are prerecorded. Tel-Med Centers maintain a library of tapes that are played upon telephone request. To obtain the telephone number of your local Tel-Med licensee, consult the White Pages of your telephone book, or contact

Tel-Med, Inc.
952 South Mt. Vernon Avenue
P.O. Box 1500
Colton, CA 92324
(714) 825-6034

■ U.S. GOVERNMENT PRINTING OFFICE
The U.S. Government Printing Office publishes books, pamphlets, and other publications in numerous subject areas. The health category is large and varied. Some publications are written for health professionals; others for the lay person. Request a catalog and order form from

Superintendent of Documents
U.S. Government Printing Office
Washington, DC 20402

INSTITUTIONALIZED PATIENT SERVICES

■ CONCERNED RELATIVES OF NURSING HOME PATIENTS
This is a nonprofit organization with members in twenty-eight states. They aim to monitor quality of care in nursing homes and to be an advocacy group for patients' rights. Members consist of family and friends of nursing home patients. There are no dues. The organization publishes a newsletter, which includes updates of new legislation affecting nursing home patients and changes in Medicare/Medicaid. They also publish a booklet, *Selecting a Nursing Home,* which contains questions and tips for families about how to place a relative in a nursing home. For further information, contact

Concerned Relatives of Nursing Home Patients
P.O. Box 18820
Cleveland Heights, OH 44118
(216) 321-0403

■ FRIENDS AND RELATIVES OF INSTITUTIONALIZED AGED, INC. *(New York City)*
This is an independent consumer watchdog organization made up of the friends
and families of residents of long-term care facilities. Their membership fee
obtains a copy of *A Consumer's Guide to Nursing Home Care in New York,* a
nursing home checklist, and a subscription to a monthly newsletter. FRIA
counsels family members considering nursing home placement for an elderly
relative and assists in resolving complaints about care. For further information, contact

FRIA, Inc.
425 East 25th Street
New York, NY 10010
(212) 481-4422

KIDNEY DISEASES

■ NATIONAL ASSOCIATION OF PATIENTS ON HEMODIALYSIS AND
TRANSPLANTATION
Through thirty local chapters, the National Association of Patients on Hemodialysis and Transplantation informs the public and patients about kidney
diseases, treatments, and patients' rights issues. They maintain a list of dialysis
centers worldwide that accept patients. In addition, they work to encourage
organ donation. The Association publishes a number of free pamphlets, available from the national office, including "Living with Renal Failure," "Dialysis
Worldwide for the Traveling Patient," "Na-K (Sodium-Potassium) Counter:
A Ready Dietetic Reference for the Dialysis Patient," and "State Renal Programs." For further information, contact

National Association of Patients on Hemodialysis and Transplantation
505 Northern Boulevard
Great Neck, NY 11021
(516) 482-2720

■ NATIONAL KIDNEY FOUNDATION
The National Kidney Foundation provides a variety of services through their
fifty-four affiliates, among them information and referral programs for patients
and families and counseling programs for patients and families of patients
with end-stage renal disease. They also support blood banks for dialysis
patients, publish a book list, a film list, and other educational brochures. For
further information and/or the address of your nearest affiliate, contact

National Kidney Foundation
2 Park Avenue
New York, NY 10016
(212) 889-2210

■ *RENAL DISEASE PROGRAMS*
The Renal Disease Programs are operated by The Health Care Financing Administration of the Department of Health and Human Services. People covered by Medicare are entitled to a full range of services. Under the renal disease provision of Medicare, dialysis services are covered in a hospital, outpatient facility, or patient's home. When dialysis takes place in the home, Medicare covers the rental/purchase of home dialysis equipment along with most supplies necessary for its effective use. People with end-stage renal disease and chronic kidney disease (requiring dialysis/transplant) are covered under the Medicare renal disease provision, regardless of age. In addition, thirty-seven states have renal programs that supplement Medicare, for persons who are not covered. Many states pay for portions of dialysis services, and most help cover costs of kidney transplants. Other services provided by various states include home dialysis training, equipment rental or purchase, physicians fees, drugs, laboratory fees. For further information, contact

Office of End State Renal Disease
6401 Security Boulevard
1-C-c Dogwood West
Baltimore, MD 21235
(301) 934-6533

Kidney Disease Activity
Chronic Disease Activity
C-JA
Center for Disease Control
Atlanta, GA 30333
(404) 329-3311

MENTAL HEALTH

■ *COMMUNITY MENTAL HEALTH CENTERS (CMHC)*
There are more than 750 community mental health centers across the country, which provide a variety of services to individuals in their own communities. Services include inpatient and outpatient care, emergency treatment, and special programs for children, the elderly, and people who abuse drugs and alcohol. More than 100 community mental health centers are affiliated with community health centers to coordinate physical and emotional care. For further information, contact your local health department, or contact

National Institute of Mental Health
Public Inquiries
5600 Fishers Lane,
Room 11A-21
Rockville, MD 20857
(301) 443-2403

■ NATIONAL CONFERENCE OF CATHOLIC CHARITIES
The National Conference of Catholic Charities is not a direct provider of services; however, this national organization will refer you to your nearest Catholic Charity; Catholic Charities provide a variety of social/human services to

various segments of the population including, counseling, socialization activities, and more. For further information, contact

National Conferences of Catholic Charities
Dupont Circle Building, Suite 307
1346 Connecticut Avenue, N.W.
Washington, DC 30026
(202) 785-2757

■ UNITED WAY
The United Way is an umbrella organization for regional and local offices of United Way. Funds that are raised by 2,100 local units are used to assist an estimated 37,000 health and social service agencies throughout the United States. Through United Way community service program grants, member agencies are better able to meet the needs of their community. For information regarding services provided and the location and telephone number of your local United Way, contact your regional office.

(Northeast)
United Way
99 Park Avenue
New York, NY 10016
(212) 661-5666

(Southeast)
United Way
2150 Parklake Drive, Suite 310
Atlanta, GA 30345
(404) 938-5841

(Midwest)
United Way
10600 West Higgins Road, Suite 201
Rosemont, IL 60018
(312) 297-6160

(West)
United Way
410 Bush Street
San Francisco, CA 94108
(415) 772-4300

MISCELLANEOUS

■ MEDIC ALERT
Medic alert is an emergency medical identification system. The Medic Alert emblem, worn as a bracelet or necklace, alerts people that you have a special medical condition, such as epilepsy, glaucoma, diabetes, an allergy to certain drugs. Emergency and health care personnel are trained to look for the Medic Alert emblem in the event of an accident or other emergency. For more information, contact

Medic Alert
P.O. Box 1009
Turlock, CA 95381-1009
(209) 668-3333 (California)
1-800-344-3226 (toll-free)

■ NATIONAL ORGANIZATION FOR RARE DISORDERS
The National Organization for Rare Disorders works as a clearinghouse for

the more than 2,000 "orphan diseases" and their accompanying "orphan drugs." Orphan diseases are rare, debilitating illnesses that strike small numbers of people (fewer than 2 million), and orphan drugs are therapies for these illnesses, many of which have not been developed by the pharmaceutical industry because they are unprofitable. NORD seeks to provide patients and their families with the best available resources to assist them in coping with a rare illness. For more information, contact

National Organization for Rare Disorders
1182 Broadway, Suite 402
New York, NY 10001
(212) 686-1057

■ VETERANS ADMINISTRATION (VA)
The VA provides a wide range of benefits to eligible veterans and their dependents and beneficiaries. Its programs include medical care, rehabilitation, and financial assistance. VA field offices are located in many cities throughout the United States. A booklet, *Federal Benefits for Veterans and Dependents,* is available free. Contact your local VA office or

Veterans Administration
810 Vermont Avenue, N.W.
Washington, DC 20420

NEUROLOGICAL / NEUROMUSCULAR DISEASES

Alzheimer's Disease

■ ALZHEIMER'S DISEASE AND RELATED DISORDERS
This organization has fifty-eight chapters in twenty-six states providing information and other resources to members. They also provide information about support groups for patients and their families, which serve as a source of practical and emotional assistance. Local chapters and support groups may help you find services, specialists, and other helpful resources. Check the White Pages of your telephone book, or contact

Alzheimer's Disease and Related Disorders
360 Michigan Avenue
Chicago, IL 60602
(312) 853-3060

Amyotrophic Lateral Sclerosis (ALS)

■ AMYOTROPHIC LATERAL SCLEROSIS SOCIETY OF AMERICA
The ALS Society of America has 55,000 members, mostly patients, their rel-

atives, and friends. The organization raises money to fund ALS clinics and can refer you to whichever place will best meet your need. The ALS Society has a variety of fact sheets to answer the most frequently asked questions about ALS. Topic areas include activities of daily living, breathing, communications techniques, treatment possibilities. The ALS Society may refer you to the Muscular Dystrophy Association, which provides free medical and recreational services for ALS patients. For more information, contact

ALS Society of America
15300 Ventura Boulevard, Suite 315
P.O. Box 5951
Sherman Oaks, CA 91403
(213) 990-2151

■ NATIONAL ALS FOUNDATION
The National ALS Foundation offers a variety of services to ALS families and patients. Clinical services are available at Mt. Sinai Medical Center, New York; University of Chicago Medical Center; and Jackson Memorial Hospital, University of Miami Medical Center. The staff at these centers are a multidisciplinary team of health professionals seeking to help ALS patients and their families cope with the physical and emotional effects of the disease. In addition, the National ALS Foundation maintains a national referral list of home health care agencies, a reference list of equipment for the handicapped, and equipment for loan to ALS patients. A series of publications about ALS is also available. For information about these services, or for chapter locations, contact

National ALS Foundation
185 Madison Avenue
New York, NY 10016
(212) 679-4016

Huntington's Disease

■ HUNTINGTON'S DISEASE FOUNDATION OF AMERICA
This foundation is a primary resource for Huntington's disease information and assistance. There are forty-two chapters and affiliates in communities across the country working to support research into the causes and cures of Huntington's disease. The foundation publishes a newsletter and other educational materials, including: "Caring for the Huntington's Disease Patient at Home." Its genetic counseling, information, and referral services tap a nationwide network of physicians, scientists, social workers, and other health professionals. For further information, contact

Huntington's Disease Foundation of America
250 West 57th Street
New York, NY 10107
(212) 757-0443

■ NATIONAL HUNTINGTON'S DISEASE ASSOCIATION
Local chapters of the National Huntington's Disease Association maintain hotline services to help patients and families with a variety of problems, from finding financial assistance to locating professionally led support groups. Several booklets on Huntington's disease are published by the Association, including *Support Groups for Huntington's Disease Families, A Neurologist Speaks with Huntington's Disease Families.* For further information, contact

National Huntington's Disease Association
128 A East 74th Street
New York, NY 10021
(212) 684-2781

Multiple Sclerosis

■ NATIONAL MULTIPLE SCLEROSIS SOCIETY
The National Multiple Sclerosis Society offers a comprehensive range of services designed to provide practical assistance, emotional support, and reliable information to patients and their families. While services vary among the over 150 chapters and branches, they usually include publications, reprints and books, counseling, information about medical and self-help equipment, financial aid, and recreation and physical fitness programs. The Society sponsors a network of sixty-seven clinics in twenty-nine states. A sample of the pamphlets available: "What Everyone Should Know About Multiple Sclerosis" (Spanish version also available), "Home Exercises," "Sexuality and MS," "Careers for the Homebound." Check the White Pages of your telephone book for a local chapter, or contact

National Multiple Sclerosis Society
205 East 42nd Street
New York, NY 10017
(212) 986-3240

Muscular Dystrophy

■ MUSCULAR DYSTROPHY ASSOCIATION
This is the nation's largest voluntary health agency, providing services to thousands of people with neuromuscular diseases such as amyotropic lateral sclerosis, Friedrich's ataxia, muscular dystrophy, and over thirty other related diseases.

In more than 230 MDA clinics across the country, patients are diagnosed, treated, and provided with orthopedic aids, transportation assistance, and recreation at MDA summer and winter camps—without charge. Upon diagnosis of a neuromuscular disease covered by MDA's medical services program, the clinics provide a variety of services, including follow-up examinations for periodic reevaluation, a limited number of sessions of physical, occupational, and respiratory therapy, genetic counseling (if appropriate), aids such as walkers, wheelchairs, orthopedic shoes, hospital beds and accessories, and bath aids. In addition, MDA helps patients find assistance from other community agencies for services it cannot provide. To find your local MDA chapter, check the White Pages of your telephone book, or contact

Muscular Dystrophy Association
810 Seventh Avenue
New York, NY 10019
(212) 586-0808

Myasthenia Gravis

■ MYASTHENIA GRAVIS FOUNDATION
The Myasthenia Gravis Foundation has fifty-one chapters and branches nationwide. The foundation publishes several pamphlets available free, including: "Myasthenia Gravis: A Manual for the Nurse," "Help Is on the Way: A Patient Handbook." To find the chapter nearest you or for more information, contact

Myasthenia Gravis Foundation
15 East 26th Street
New York, NY 10010
(212) 889-8157

Parkinson's Disease

■ AMERICAN PARKINSON DISEASE ASSOCIATION
This is a national organization, affiliated with several hospitals and universities, with chapters across the country. There are information and referral centers which offer patients referral to neurologists or hospitals in your area specializing in the treatment of Parkinson's or to a self-help support group. In addition the Foundation offers a variety of literature including suggestions for aids and equipment to be used in the home. For a list of local chapters, contact

American Parkinson Disease Foundation
116 John Street
New York, NY 10038
(212) 732-9550

■ NATIONAL PARKINSON FOUNDATION, INC.
The Foundation supports clinical research as well as the National Parkinson Institute, associated with the University of Miami School of Medicine. This Institute offers patients a multidisciplinary team approach for diagnosis, treatment, care, and rehabilitation. The National Parkinson Foundation publishes a number of booklets, including: *The Parkinson Handbook, What*

the Patient Should Know About Parkinson's Disease, and *Psychological Factors in the Management of Parkinson's Disease.* For more information, contact

National Parkinson Foundation, Inc.
1501 N.W. 9th Avenue
Miami, FL 33136
(305) 547-6666 (in Florida)
1-800-327-4545 (toll-free)

■ PARKINSON'S DISEASE FOUNDATION
The Parkinson's Disease Foundation, located at Columbia University Medical Center, serves as a source of information to patients and physicians about Parkinson's disease and some other neurological diseases (cerebral palsy, Alzheimer's, Huntington's disease, dystonia, etc.). They offer referral to specialists or self-help groups in your area. Information and publications include: *The Parkinson Patient at Home, Exercises for the Parkinson Patient with Hints for Daily Living.* There are no dues. A request for information will result in an information package with a variety of pamphlets and articles. Contact

Parkinson's Disease Foundation
Columbia University Medical Center
640 West 168th Street
New York, NY 10032
(212) 923-4700

■ PARKINSON'S EDUCATIONAL PROGRAM
This group provides information to educate the public about Parkinson's and to help patients and their families with the disease. Their publications and products list includes books and pamphlets and other practical tips. *The PEP Exchange* is a newsletter written by and for Parkinson patients and families, serving as a vehicle for members to share information and experiences. For more information, contact

Parkinson's Educational Program
1800 Park Newport, Room 302
Newport Beach, CA 92660
(714) 640-0218

■ UNITED PARKINSON FOUNDATION
The United Parkinson Foundation offers a variety of services to Parkinson's patients, most of which are available free of charge, including an extensive referral service, educational meetings held in different locations in the United States and Canada, a quarterly newsletter, publications, and a mail order pharmacy program. For more information, contact

United Parkinson Foundation
220 South State Street
Chicago, IL 60604
(312) 922-9734

NUTRITION

■ AMERICAN DIABETES ASSOCIATION
The American Diabetes Association, through its nationwide affiliates, works to teach people with diabetes to live full lives despite the restrictions of the illness. The ADA publishes a cookbook, and your local chapter can provide you with other nutritional information. For the chapter in your area, consult the White Pages of your telephone directory, or contact

American Diabetes Association
2 Park Avenue
New York, NY 10016
(212) 683-7444

■ AMERICAN DIETETIC ASSOCIATION
The American Dietetic Association is the nation's largest organization of nutrition professionals. They seek to educate the public by providing the latest nutritional information. They publish cookbooks, recipes for allergy sufferers, exchange lists for meal planning. To request a catalog and price list, contact

American Dietetic Association
430 North Michigan Avenue
Chicago, IL 60611
(313) 280-5012

■ AMERICAN HEART ASSOCIATION
Nutrition information materials—cookbooks, pamphlets, posters—of all sorts are available from local chapters of the American Heart Association or from the National Center in Dallas, Texas. The American Heart Association Cookbook, 3rd edition (David McKay, NY, 1979), is an excellent resource for recipes and tips on low-fat, low-salt, tasty recipes, and it's available at your library or bookstore. For the AHA chapter near you, check the White Pages of your telephone directory, or contact the National Center

American Heart Association
7320 Greenville Avenue
Dallas, TX 75231
(214) 740-5300

■ LIFELINE FOUNDATION, INC.
In order to provide peer support to individuals who receive their nourishment via one of two nontraditional methods, enterally (by tube) or parenterally (by vein), Lifeline Foundation offers a publication and a number of services without charge. *Lifeline Letter* is their bimonthly newsletter. Regional get-togeth-

ers are arranged and a visiting program offering in-person support to prospective Lifeliners is planned. For Further information, contact

Lifeline Foundation, Inc.
30 East Chestnut Street
Sharon, MA 02067
(617) 784-3250

■ U.S. DEPARTMENT OF AGRICULTURE
The USDA offers a number of helpful publications. Among them, *Nutrition and Your Health: Dietary Guidelines for Americans* is available free from the Human Nutrition Information Services. Write

USDA
6505 Belcrest Road
Hyattsville, MD 20782

■ *BUREAU OF NUTRITION/HEALTH DEPARTMENT*

Check with your local health department. They may have a nutrition bureau with nutrition programs and information available.

■ *FOOD PRODUCTS AND INGREDIENTS*

Most food manufacturers have a consumer affairs specialist on staff. Contact them directly with any questions about a particular product, its ingredients or preservatives. The name and address of the manufacturer can be found right on the label of the food product. Address your correspondence to the department of consumer services, and be sure to identify the product as it is listed on the label.

PAIN

■ NATIONAL COMMITTEE ON THE TREATMENT OF INTRACTABLE PAIN
The National Committee on the Treatment of Intractable Pain is a diverse group of professionals and consumers committed to pain prevention and control. The Committee acts as a clearinghouse for information on research and publishes a newsletter. They offer a free booklet (include 39¢ postage), *Chronic Pain: Hope Through Research.* For further information, write

National Committee on the Treatment of Intractable Pain
P.O. Box 9553
Friendship Station
Washington, DC 20016-1553

PHYSICAL DISABILITY

■ CLEARINGHOUSE ON THE HANDICAPPED
Part of the Department of Education, the Clearinghouse responds to inquiries directly or refers you to other sources. (There is no charge for this service.) They offer information on a variety of topics concerning handicapping conditions, rehabilitation and vocational programs, and related services. They are knowledgeable about federal legislation and federal funding of programs for the handicapped. The Clearinghouse publishes a bimonthly newsletter and *The Directory of National Information Sources on Handicapping Conditions and Related Services,* which describes the scope and services of numerous organizations, agencies, and clearinghouses. Publications are free. Contact

Clearinghouse on the Handicapped
Department of Education
Switzer Building, Room 3106
Washington, DC 20202
(202) 245-0080

■ INFORMATION CENTER FOR INDIVIDUALS WITH DISABILITIES
This is a private, nonprofit information and referral service to assist individuals with disabilities. Although the majority of users are Massachusetts residents, requests come in from across the United States. The Center gathers information in such areas as housing, recreation, access, equipment, law, transportation, and travel. There are no fees for their services. For further information, contact

Information Center for Individuals with Disabilities
20 Park Plaza, Room 330
Boston, MA 02116
(617) 727-5540

■ JUST ONE BREAK
Just One Break is a placement service representing the disabled in their search for employment in the public and private sectors. At present JOB serves New York City, Toronto, Boston, and Hackensack and West Orange, New Jersey. JOB provides individual counseling, group workshops, and other support services to improve the chances of finding and keeping a job. There is no fee for this service to either employer or applicant. To learn more about JOB, contact

Just One Break
373 Park Avenue South
New York, NY 10016
(212) 725-2500

■ NATIONAL ASSOCIATION OF THE PHYSICALLY HANDICAPPED
The National Association of the Physically Handicapped is a self-help action

membership group working to improve the social, economic, and physical welfare of all physically handicapped people. Through a network of local autonomous chapters, NAPH offers its members a wide variety of activities and opportunities for exchange of ideas, experiences, and information. For further information and to learn the location of your local chapter, contact

National Association of the Physically Handicapped, Inc.
Business Office
76 Elm Street
London, OH 43140
(614) 852-1664

■ NATIONAL EASTER SEAL SOCIETY

The National Easter Seal Society is the country's oldest health care agency providing direct services to people with disabilities. Services are provided by 876 state and local affiliates operating approximately 2,000 facilities and programs. Programs and services go beyond physical disability and include hearing disorders, learning disabilities, stroke, and rehabilitation. For the physically disabled person, many Easter Seals Society affiliates offer information about and access to physical therapy, escorted transportation, and other support services. There is an extensive library of pamphlets and information brochures available at a nominal charge (and a publications listing and order form is available). Titles of interest include: *Handy, Helpful Hints for Independent Living After Stroke, What Is Rehabilitation, Psychological Considerations in the Adjustment to Spinal Cord Injury.* For further information or the location of your nearest affiliate, contact

National Easter Seal Society
2023 West Ogden Avenue
Chicago, IL 60612
(312) 243-8400 (voice)
(312) 243-8880 (TTY)

■ NATIONAL REHABILITATION INFORMATION CENTER (NARIC)

NARIC is an information services center with specialists on staff to answer questions about products, services, and research. NARIC information specialists will respond to telephone or written requests with either an on-the-spot answer or through a computer search through one of two data bases that they maintain.

One data base focuses on products and sources for products that are of interest to (or needed by) disabled persons. Called Able Data, it offers information on rehabilitation equipment and aids and identifies the manufacturing source. Able Data stores information on over 4,000 items: ambulatory devices, orthotics, transportation, rehabilitation counseling programs, and much more.

The other data base, Rehab Data, catalogs books, publications, and other reference material about rehabilitation of interest to researchers, therapists, and consumers. Sample questions asked of NARIC may include: Who manufactures air flotation seat cushions for wheelchairs and what are their addresses? Are there any government-funded spinal cord research projects, and where are they located?

There is no charge for on-the-spot information, and a nominal fee is charged for computer searches. Call or write NARIC with your questions or for further information

National Rehabilitation Information Center
4407 8th Street, N.E.
Catholic University of America
Washington, DC 20017
(202) 635-5826
(202) 635-5884 (TDD-Telecommunications for the Deaf)

■ NATIONAL SPINAL CORD INJURY ASSOCIATION
The Association is a membership organization with forty-one local chapters serving individuals and their families, friends, and many others interested in overcoming the problems involved in a spinal cord injury. Service programs are available through local chapters to assist the newly injured, their family, and their friends and to support the needs of the community. Membership fees are nominal; members receive the publication *Spinal Cord Injury Life*. For more information, contact

National Spinal Cord Injury Association
149 California Street
Newton, MA 02158
(617) 964-0521

■ PROMOTE REAL INDEPENDENCE FOR THE DISABLED AND ELDERLY (PRIDE)
PRIDE is an organization dedicated to solving clothing problems for the physically disabled person. They offer information resources and a guide for the adaptation and/or modification of clothing. They seek to design or redesign clothing and accessories to enable people to dress more easily yet wear attractive garments. The PRIDE Foundation offers a traveling truck show filled with clothing that has been modified. Organizations and small groups can rent the show to display to their members. They sell a 116-page book, *Dressing with Pride*, which demonstrates modifications to store-bought clothing and includes other wardrobe tips. For more information, contact

PRIDE
1159 Poquonnock Road
Groton, CT 06340
(203) 447-7433 (Connecticut)
1-800-962-0707 (toll-free)

RECREATION

There are numerous recreation programs and activities operating all over the country. Many are designed for special interests: crafts, arts, travel, bowling, sports. Others are directed to special groups, such as elderly, blind, physically disabled people.

You will need to do some homework to find the programs and activities available in your community. Check with the special education department of your city or county education department. Talk with the recreation specialist or director of volunteer services at your local hospital; contact your local recreation and parks department; or check with churches, synagogues, and community centers in your area.

Listed below are a few national organizations which may be of interest and assistance.

■ AMERICAN RED CROSS

The American Red Cross offers training in swimming for special populations. Check with your local group for information on courses, or contact

American Red Cross
National Headquarters
17th and D Street, N.W.
Washington, DC 20006
(202) 737-8300

■ AMERICAN FOUNDATION FOR THE BLIND, INC.

The American Foundation for the Blind has pioneered recreation services for the blind. They offer books, equipment, and games and conduct a series of special projects. For more information, contact

American Foundation for the Blind, Inc.
16 West 16th Street
New York, NY 10011
(212) 924-0402

■ ELDER CRAFTSMEN

This Manhattan-based shop offers skilled persons over sixty years of age the opportunity to show and sell their wares at a profit to the individual. Although the Elder Craftsmen maintain only one location, more than 700 craftspeople from nearly forty states consign their wares to the shop. There is a Craft Selection Committee that reviews and accepts products for sale at the shop. In addition, craftspeople are hired to make items that are known to sell well in the shop. They are paid on a piecework basis. For more information, contact

Elder Craftsmen
135 East 65th Street
New York, NY 10021
(212) 861-5260

■ HOSPITAL AUDIENCES, INC.

Hospital Audiences, Inc., works to serve the cultural needs of New York City's homebound and institutionalized. Each year, Hospital Audiences, Inc., arranges reserved seating, wheelchair-accessible bathrooms, and transportation for thousands of people to attend various cultural events in New York City. Theater parties, museum visits, and outdoor concert attendance are a few of the events organized by Hospital Audiences, Inc. For more information, contact

Hospital Audiences, Inc.
1540 Broadway
New York, NY 10038
(212) 575-7676

■ INTERNATIONAL MAILBAG CLUB, INC.
The International Mailbag Club's established chapters are located in Ohio and Indiana, with other chapters organizing in cities and towns in the Midwest. They are dedicated to bringing cheer, diversion, and assistance to the homebound and institutionalized person. For more information, contact

Mrs. Isabelle Shepard
International Mailbag Club, Inc.
130 Center Street
Findlay, OH 45840
(419) 422-2362

■ NATIONAL COMMITTEE ARTS FOR THE HANDICAPPED (NCAH)
NCAH provides lists of national, state, and local organizations with art programs for the handicapped, model special arts programs, and other programs of interest. For more information, contact

National Committee Arts for the Handicapped, Inc.
1825 Connecticut Avenue, N.W.
Washington, DC 20009
(202) 332-6960 (voice or TDD)

■ NATIONAL EASTER SEAL SOCIETY
National Easter Seal Society includes special recreation as part of its programs, among them, Easter Seal Camps for Handicapped children and adults. For more information, contact

National Easter Seal Society
2023 West Odgen Avenue
Chicago, IL 60612
(312) 243-8400 (voice)
(312) 243-8880 (TDD)

■ NATIONAL ENDOWMENT FOR THE ARTS
There is an Office for Special Constituencies of the National Endowment for the Arts, which provides information and technical assistance to art organizations and programs designed for the disabled and the elderly. Individuals contacting the Office for Special Constituencies will be referred to an arts program in their community.
    For further information, contact

Office of Special Constituencies
National Endowment for the Arts
1100 Pennsylvania Avenue, N.W.
Washington, DC 20506
(202) 682-5531

■ NATIONAL HANDICAPPED SPORTS AND RECREATION ASSOCIATION
With its focus on skiing, the National Handicapped Sports and Recreation Association conducts ski clinics and sponsors the U.S. Handicap Ski Team.
   For more information, contact

National Handicapped Sports and Recreation Association
10085 West 18th Avenue
Denver, CO 80218
(303) 232-4575

■ NATIONAL WHEELCHAIR ATHLETIC ASSOCIATION
This organization sponsors the National Wheelchair Games. Contact

National Wheelchair Athletic Association
2107 Templeton Cap Road
Colorado Springs, CO 80907
(303) 632-0698

■ NORTH AMERICAN RIDING FOR THE HANDICAPPED ASSOCIATION
There are more than 200 riding for the handicapped centers nationwide. North American Riding for the Handicapped Association will refer you to a center in your area. For more information, contact

North American Riding for the Handicapped Association
Leonard Warner, Executive Director
P.O. Box 100
Ashburn, VA 22011

■ SOCIETY FOR THE ADVANCEMENT OF TRAVEL FOR THE HANDICAPPED
Members tend to be travel agents, car rental firms, sightseeing companies, etc., with a special interest in easing travel for the handicapped, elderly, and retired. The Society has information on travel and will refer you to the SATH travel agent near you. They publish a newsletter, *SATH News,* which contains information of interest to the handicapped traveler. For more information, contact

Society for the Advancement of Travel for the Handicapped
International Head Office
26 Court Street, Suite 1110
Brooklyn, NY 11242
(212) 858-5483

■ SPECIAL RECREATION, INC.
This is a resource and consulting group that publishes *Special Recreation Digest,* a quarterly publication that provides up-to-date information on spe-

cial recreation-related programs and services, reporting on the full range of organizations providing special recreation. For more information, contact

Special Recreation, Inc.
362 Koser Avenue
Iowa City, IO 52240

RESPIRATORY PROBLEMS

■ EMPHYSEMA ANONYMOUS, INC.
Emphysema Anonymous is a voluntary organization dedicated to helping victims of emphysema through education, encouragement, and mutual assistance. They publish a quarterly newsletter as well as a number of informative pamphlets on emphysema: "Our Daily Breath," "If You Have Emphysema or Chronic Bronchitis." For further information and the location of the chapter nearest you, contact

Emphysema Anonymous, Inc.
P.O. Box 66
Ft. Myers, FL 33902
(813) 334-4226

SEXUALITY

■ SEX INFORMATION AND EDUCATION COUNCIL OF THE UNITED STATES (SIECUS)
SIECUS maintains a resource center and library that houses a noncirculating collection of books and periodicals for use by individuals interested in the many aspects of human sexuality. Materials for sale include SIECUS publications, consumer pamphlets recommended by SIECUS, and duplicate books. The library is located on the campus of New York University. For further information, contact

SIECUS
715 Broadway, Room 213
New York, NY 10003
(212) 673-3850

SKIN

■ AMERICAN LUPUS SOCIETY
Through its thirty-three chapters in the United States, the American Lupus Society assists families in coping with the daily problems associated with the

disease. Chapters hold meetings and occasional medical seminars to keep members informed of new developments or knowledge about lupus. For a list of local chapters, or for further information, contact

American Lupus Society
23751 Madison Street
Torrence, CA 90505
(213) 373-1335

- LUPUS FOUNDATION OF AMERICA
There are more than eighty chapters of the Lupus Foundation of America, providing information, referral service, and support to people with lupus and their families. The chapters conduct education programs, distribute literature, and provide person-to-person contact among members. They have a number of publications, including: *Lupus and You, Lupus Erythematosus: A Handbook for Physicians, Patients and Their Families.* For the publications list or the location of your local chapter, contact

Systemic Lupus Erythematosus Foundation, Inc.
95 Madison Avenue
New York, NY 10016
(212) 685-4118

- NATIONAL PSORIASIS FOUNDATION
The National Psoriasis Foundation provides educational literature on psoriasis to the public and raises funds for psoriasis research. For further information, contact

National Psoriasis Foundation
6415 Southwest Canyon Court
Portland, OR 97221
(503) 297-1545

- PHOENIX SOCIETY
The Phoenix Society is a nationwide self-help organization for people who have been severely burned and their families. They produce and distribute a number of publications, films, and other audiovisual materials on burn prevention, treatment, and rehabilitation. For a publications list or the location of local chapters, contact

Phoenix Society
11 Rust Hill Road
Levittown, PA 19056
(215) 946-4788

SPEECH

■ AMERICAN SPEECH-LANGUAGE-HEARING ASSOCIATION
This is the national professional and scientific association for speech language pathologists and audiologists in this country. Their consumer affiliate, the National Association for Hearing and Speech Action is a membership organization representing the communicatively handicapped. Their activities include:

advocacy, legislation, and public information

insurance updates

an information resource center

a quarterly newsletter

information materials and brochures such as: "Do your Health Insurance Benefits Cover Speech, Language and Hearing Services," "Hearing Aids and Hearing Help," "Communication Disorders and Aging"

a helpline toll-free telephone service providing consumers with information concerning their own speech/hearing problem as well as referrals to speech pathologists or audiologists.

If you would like to join NAHS, or would like more information, contact

National Association for Hearing and Speech Action
10801 Rockville Pike
Rockville, MD 20852

For helpline/membership information in Maryland, Alaska, or Hawaii, call collect: (301) 897-8682 (voice or TTY)

For helpline/membership information from anywhere else, call toll-free: (800)-638-8255 (voice or TTY)

Index

abuse, elder, 315–18
acetaminophen, 268
acetylcholine deficiency, 369
aches and pains:
    exercise and, 222–23
    topical analgesics for, 217
actinic kerotoses, 234
"activity to tolerance," 504
addictions, narcotic, 266
adrenaline, 266
adult nurse practitioners, 63
aerobic exercises, 229–32
agencies, home health care, 59–63
    aides trained by, 64–65
    Blue Cross and, 92
    certification of, 61
    fees charged by, 59–61
    high-tech home care and, 286–87
    homemakers screened by, 81
    information resources on, 542–45
    licensure requirements and, 60, 62
    number of, 59
    questions in evaluation of, 61–62
    rehabilitation therapists and, 69
    services offered by, 59
    variety of, 60
aging process, 309–18
    dementia associated with, 361–62
    falling and, 313
    hearing loss and, 310–11, 338–39
    heat stress and, 313–14
    hypothermia and, 314–15
    incontinence and, 238, 240
    information resources on, 513–19
    memory loss and, 311–12
    mental activity and, 315
    skin and, 233–34, 242
    sleep requirements and, 259
    vision and, 220–21, 312
    see also elderly

alcohol intake:
    drug interactions and, 210–11
    stress and, 115
allergic reactions:
    to medication, 205–6, 212
    skin and, 233, 236
ALS (amytrophic lateral sclerosis), 75–76, 159, 373–81
    average course of, 376
    causes of, 379
    definition of, 373–74
    feeding methods in, 375
    home health aides for, 380–81
    information resources on, 551–52
    insurance and, 380
    intellectual capacity and, 376
    in men vs. women, 374
    onset of, 374
    patients' spirits in, 381
    pressure sores in, 378
    progression of, 374–75
    respiratory assistance in, 378–79
    symptoms of, 374
    treatment of, 377–80
    viral origins of, 379
    voluntary muscles in, 373–74
    work and, 376
ALS Society of America, 379–80, 381
Alzheimer's disease, 159, 360–73
    acetylcholine deficiency in, 369
    aluminum concentrations in, 369
    care guidelines for, 369–70
    caretakers' needs in, 370–71
    day care and, 372
    denial in, 365–66, 368
    description of, 360–61
    diagnosis of, 362–63
    diseases similar to, 362–63
    early confusion in, 364–65
    early dementia in, 365–66

Alzheimer's disease (*continued*)
  exercise and, 223
  genetics in, 369
  incontinence in, 366–68
  information resources on, 551
  insurance and, 367
  late confusion in, 365
  late dementia in, 368
  middle dementia in, 366–68
  normal level in, 364
  nursing home care and, 372
  professional assistance and, 371–73
  prevalence of, 361, 362
  research in, 363–64
  support groups for, 370–71
  symptoms of, 363
  viral origins of, 369
Alzheimer's Disease and Related Disorders Association, 370–71
amantadine hydrochloride, 393
ambulating capabilities, 71
ambulation aids, 162–63, 190–91
American Association of Homes for the Aging, 37
American Cancer Society, 35, 330
American Diabetes Association, 35, 345, 536
American Dietetic Association, 345
American Heart Association, 415–16, 422–24, 438, 444, 459
American Hospital Association, 28–29
American Medical Association, 28
American Occupational Therapy Association, 161
American Paralysis Association, 411–12
Amsler grid tests, 222
analgesics, 266–67
  see also aspirin
analgesics, topical, 217
  in cancer treatment, 328
Anatomy of an Illness (Cousins), 145–50, 272
anesthetic analgesics, 217
aneurysms, 414
anger, 67–68
  terminal illness and, 289, 294–95
angina pectoris, 446–51
  prevention of, 447–50
  surgery for, 450–51
angiography, fluorescein, 353
angioplasty, 451
ankle movement, exercise for, 226

antibiotics:
  intravenous, 281, 283
  potentiation of, 211
anticholinergic drugs, 393
anticoagulants, 215
antihistamines, 393
antihypertensive drugs, 458, 459–63
anti-inflammatory drugs, 470
antiparkinsonism drugs, 391–96
aphasia, 420–22
apnea, sleep, 259–60
aprons, 184
aqueous humor, 334
arthritis, 468–86
  aspirin and, 478, 479, 480
  cold therapy and, 475
  definition of, 469
  energy conservation in, 476–78
  exercise and, 223, 230, 474–76
  gout, 214, 460, 473–74
  heat therapy and, 475
  incidence of, 468, 473
  information resources on, 519–20
  kinds of, 468
  medications for, 267, 468, 470–71, 478–85
  "miracle cures" for, 479
  nutrition and, 479
  osteoarthritis, 471–72
  positive attitudes in, 486
  replacement joints in, 468, 472–73
  research in, 468
  rest and, 476–78
  rheumatoid, 469–71
  self-treatment of, 468–69
  sexual activity and, 253
  skin care and, 235
  support groups for, 486
Arthritis Foundation, 35, 486
Arthritis Helpbook, The (Loring and Fries), 470, 471
"Arthwriters," 188
aspirin, 216, 269
  arthritis and, 478, 479, 480
  pain relieved by, 266
Assisto-seats, 190
asthma, 501–3
  incidence of, 501
  "outgrowing" of, 503
  respiratory therapy for, 77–78
  symptoms of, 502
  treatment of, 503

types of, 502–3
see also respiratory diseases
atherosclerosis, 413–14, 415, 453
audiologists, 337, 340–41
"augmentative communication," 76
auto forks, 179
autoimmune system, Alzheimer's disease
    and, 369
automobiles:
    modified controls in, 189
    parking spaces reserved for, 190

back rests, 190
bathing, baths, 70–71
    excessive, 234
    warm, pain control and, 271
bathrooms, 117–23
    accidents in, 367
    cabinets in, 123
    calling devices in, 123
    clutter in, 121
    dangers in, 117–18
    doors to, 118–19
    faucets in, 119, 121
    floor surfaces in, 119
    grab bars in, 120, 122, 123, 171
    grooming devices in, 166–71
    Parkinson patients in, 401
    sinks in, 119
    smallness of, 118
    transfer benches in, 120–21
bathtubs, 119–21
    grab bars in, 120, 171
    shower heads in, 121, 171
Batting the Breeze, 508
bedbound patients, 164–65
    oral care for, 246–47
bed linens, 124, 128
bedrooms, 123–29
    bedside caddies in, 125
    calling devices in, 127
    chairs in, 124–26
    privacy in, 126
    range of mobility in, 126–27
    tables in, 125, 126
    wastebaskets in, 126
beds:
    bedsore prevention and, 278–79
    guardrails on, 124
    hospital vs. conventional, 124
    linens for, 124, 128

in living rooms, 134–35, 153–54
making of, 184
mattresses for, 127, 257
motorized adjustable, 127
Parkinson's patients and, 400–401
sleep difficulties and, 257–58
trapeze bars for, 128, 185
wedges for, 128, 190
bedsores, *see* pressure sores
Bedspecs Prism glasses, 189
beta blockers, 460
Better Hearing Institute (BHI), 336
bidets, 169, 170
bioavailability, drug, 212–13
biofeedback, pain control and, 273
blindness, 220, 221–22
    glaucoma and, 334–35
    information resources on, 520–24
blood glucose monitors, 284
Blue Cross health insurance, 86
    visits covered by, 91–92
bone strength, exercise and, 231
boot jacks, 174
boredom, patient's, 151–52
bottles, opening of, 176–77
Bradley, Walter, 379
bradykinesia, 390, 393
breathing:
    correct, exercise for, 499
    normal process of, 496
Brody, Jane, 196
Brompton cocktails, 301
bronchitis, chronic, *see* respiratory dis-
    eases
brushes, 168
burn patients, 72
bypass surgery, 450–51

calling devices, 123, 127
Cancer Information Service, 320
cancer treatment, 319–33
    chemotherapy in, 281, 285–86, 324–25
    coordinating care in, 320
    cures affected by, 329–30
    information resources on, 524–28
    massage in, 329
    nausea in, 326
    nutrition in, 323–24, 326–27
    oral care in, 246, 326
    pain control in, 327–28
    patients' activities in, 328–29
    questions asked before, 325–26

cancer treatment (*continued*)
  radiation in, 323–24
  second opinion and, 319–20
  sexuality and, 330
  skin care in, 236
  specialists in, 319, 320
  surgery in, 322–23
  TPN in, 324, 327
  various cancers responsive to, 319, 321
  warlike nature of, 321–22
canes, 162–63, 190–91, 313
cans, opening of, 176
CAPD (continuous ambulatory peritoneal
    dialysis), 490
caregivers, 34–35, 49–83
  for aging couples, 309–10
  critical role of, 49–50
  day care centers and, 82
  discharge planning and, 52–54
  elder abuse and, 315–18
  guilt experienced by, 55, 114–15, 159–
    60
  health care associations consulted by,
    35, 55, 57
  hearing loss and, 340
  high-tech home care and, 280–82
  home care agencies and, 59–63
  home care team and, 50–52
  homemakers / housekeepers and, 79–82
  illness or disease studied by, 111
  incontinence and, 239–40
  insurance considered by, 55, 56–57
  listening skills of, 112–13
  massages given by, 272–73
  meals-on-wheels arranged by, 35, 66,
    82–83
  objectivity as difficult for, 110–12, 141
  observation skills of, 74
  occupational therapists and, 74–75
  patients' closeness to, 110–12
  patients' depression and, 37–38, 67–68
  patients' independence and, 112–13
  patients' needs outlined by, 55–56
  patients' transportation and, 82, 83–84
  personal lives of, 139, 141, 159–60
  physicians and, 54, 78–79
  psychological counseling and, 67–68
  records kept by, 57–58
  references requested by, 61–62
  stress experienced by, 113–16
  tasks of, 111
  time invested by, 61

carts, wheeled, 157–58, 180, 185
  laundry, 182
CAT (computerized axial tomography)
    scans, 383
Catanzaro, Marci, 384
cataracts, 331–34
  definition of, 331
  lens replacement methods for, 332–34
  photocoagulation and, 354
  surgical removal of, 331–32
catheterization:
  heart, 451
  incontinence and, 241
CCUs (coronary care units), 438, 439
chairs:
  in bedrooms, 124–26
  ejectors in, 190
  in kitchens, 130–31, 179–80
  Parkinson patients and, 400
chemotherapy, 281, 285–86, 324–25
  continuous infusion, 324–25
  insurance and, 325
child-safety caps, 207
circulatory / cardiovascular problems, 437
  heart attacks, 437–51
  hypertension, 452–67
  inactivity and, 438
cleaning supplies, 184–85
clearinghouses, national, 546–47
clipboards, 188
clothesline, travel, 183
clothing, 172–74
  aging and, 313–14
  incontinence and, 240–41
CNS (central nervous system), 381
codeine, 270
colchicine, 214
cold, exposure to, 314–15
cold therapy, 271–72
  arthritis and, 475
colitis, ulcerative, 426–29
colostomies, 250–51, 430–36
  care techniques for, 431
  ileostomies vs., 430–31
  see also ostomies
comas, diabetic, 352
combs, 168
commodes, 122, 170
community services:
  information resources on, 528–31
  in oral care, 247
  specific focuses of, 35, 55, 57

Complete Guide to Prescription and Non-prescription Drugs (Griffith), 208
compliance, patient's, 466–67
concerts, 186
condom catheters, 241
consumer movement, 31
containers, storage, 177
Continent (Kock) ileostomies, 429
continuous influsion chemotherapy, 324–25
contraceptives, oral, risks of, 415
Cooper, I. S., 159
COPD (chronic obstructive pulmonary disease), 495–501
  causes of, 495
  correct breathing in, 499
  dust and, 501
  early detection of, 497–98
  effect of, 496–97
  high-tech home care and, 281, 285
  incidence of, 495
  liquid intake in, 500
  normal breathing vs., 496
  oral care and, 500
  postural drainage in, 500
  progression of, 497
  treatment of, 497–98
  see also respiratory diseases
coronary bypass surgery, 450–51
counseling, *see* mental health services; social workers; therapy
counter-irritant analgesics, 217
Cousins, Norman, 145–50, 272
Crohn's disease, 284, 426–29
crutches, 162–63
  accessibility of, 190–91
  doors and, 118–19
cryoextraction, 332
cups, drinking from, 181
cushions:
  nonslip, 190
  swivel, 189
CVAs (cerebrovascular accidents), *see* stroke
cystic fibrosis, 537

daily routines, 139–91
  bathing / showering in, 170–71
  brushing teeth in, 166
  carrying items in, 157–58, 177
  chopping or blending in, 178
  chronic illness and, 158–60
  cooking in, 179
  cutting foods in, 178
  dentures cleaned in, 167
  dishwashing in, 183–84
  dressing in, 172–74
  eating and drinking in, 180–82
  energy conserved in, 157–58, 179–80
  energy cycles in, 151
  establishment of, 154
  flexibility in, 151–52
  flossing teeth in, 167
  fluids recorded in, 147
  food preparation in, 174–80
  grooming and personal care in, 166–71
  hair care in, 168
  health care charts in, 144–47
  household chores in, 152, 182–85
  ironing in, 182–83
  laundry in, 182–83
  makeup used in, 167
  making beds in, 184
  mobility in, 164–65
  mopping in, 183
  obstacles overcome in, 160–65
  opening containers in, 176–77
  out-of-doors times in, 152
  peeling or paring vegetables in, 178
  positive feelings promoted in, 145–51
  pouring liquids in, 178
  reading in, 188–89
  recreation activities in, 155–56, 186–87
  shaving in, 167
  sitting down in, 190
  sports in, 186–87
  standing up in, 190
  storage methods and, 134, 177
  sweeping in, 183
  symptoms noted in, 148–49
  table-setting in, 157–58, 179
  telephone calls in, 156
  television in, 155
  toileting in, 169–70
  travel in, 189–90
  treatment plans in, 142–44
  vacuuming in, 183
  vital signs recorded in, 146
  washing hands in, 166
  writing in, 188
day care centers, 82
  Alzheimer's patients in, 372
  information resources on, 517–19

decubitus ulcers, see pressure sores
dementia, 315
  aging associated with, 361–62
  diagnosis of, 362–63
  skin care and, 234
  see also Alzheimer's disease
dental floss, 167, 242, 247–48
  "flat," 248
dental tape, 247–48
dentistry, 244–45, 247
  information resources on, 536
  see also oral care, personal
Dentist's Desk Reference, The, 247
dentures, 243
  adherents for, 248–49
  cleaning of, 167, 246, 249
  names inscribed on, 245
depression, patient's, 67
  caretakers and, 37–38, 67–68
  dialysis and, 492–93
  enteral feeding and, 202–3
  exercise and, 230
  home health care success and, 105
  itching and, 234
  laughter and, 145–50
  medication for, 213
  narcotics and, 266
  parenteral feeding and, 202–3
  television and, 155
  terminal illnesses and, 289–90
dermatologists, 237
devices, home health care, 160–91
  cost of, 161
  home made, 161–62
  information resources on, 538–39
  insurance and, 161
  see also specific devices
diabetes, 207, 344–59
  comas in, 352
  complications in, 352–56
  definition of, 344
  dietary control in, 345–46
  diuretics and, 460
  in elderly, 358–59
  exercises and, 223, 346–47
  foot problems in, 355–56
  high-tech home care and, 281, 284
  incidence of, 344
  information resources on, 536–37
  insulin pumps used in, 284, 350–51
  insulin shock in, 351
  insulin used in, 207, 284, 347–49

kidney problems in, 354–55
  neuropathy in, 355–56
  oral health in, 245
  oral hypoglycemics in, 349–50
  retinopathy in, 352–54
  SBGM in, 357–58
  skin care and, 234, 235
  stroke and, 415
  symptoms of, 345
  tips for management of, 359
  treatments of, 345–51
  types of, 344–45, 349
  urine testing in, 357
Diabinese, 349–50
dialysis, 355, 488–93
  CAPD, 490
  coping with, 491–93
  early programs in, 489
  emotional upsets in, 492–93
  government support for, 489
  hemodialysis, 487, 488–89
  peritoneal, 489–90
  see also renal disease
diapers, disposable, 240–41
diastolic readings, 452–53, 455–56
disabilities, physical:
  abilities vs., 75–76
  ambulating capabilities and, 71
  amended baseline of wellness and,
    152–55
  functional profiles of, 106, 107–8
  information resources on, 558–60
  long-term, elderly and, 30–31
  nutritional therapy and, 78
  occupational therapy and, 72–75
  physical therapy and, 70–72
  respiratory therapy and, 76–78
  slow progression of, 80–81
  speech therapy and, 75–76
  strength and flexibility in, 71–72
discharge planning, 34–35, 52–54
  high-tech home care and, 280
  information available in, 53–54
  insurance coverage and, 35, 53
  social workers and, 66
  support services and, 141–42
dishes:
  bumper guard, 182
  washing of, 183–84
diuretics, 214, 459–60, 462–63
doors, width of, 118–19
dopamine, 390

dressing hooks, 173
DRGs (diagnosis-related groups), 34–35
drugs, *see* medications and drugs
drying racks, 183
dust, household, 501
Dycem, 182
dying patients, 288–305
  acceptance in, 290
  anger in, 289
  bad news related to, 290–91
  bargaining by, 289
  caregivers' stress and, 292–95
  death of, 298, 304
  denial in, 289
  depression in, 289–90
  guidelines in caring for, 295–96
  hospice care for, 298–305
  information resources and, 531–35
  pain control for, 290, 301, 302
  preparations of, 296–98
  stages of, 289–90
  stress experienced by, 291–92
Dymelor, 349–50
dynamic (isotonic) exercises, 229

elastic laces, 174
elastic thread, 172
elbow movement, exercises for, 225
elder abuse, 315–18
elderly:
  couples, 309–10
  diabetic, 358–59
  in family structure, 26–27
  group meal programs for, 83
  increasing number of, 27, 32
  life expectancy of, 27, 30
  long-term disabilities in, 30–31
  Medicare eligibility of, 57, 92, 100
  medications and, 205, 206–8, 217
  sexuality of, 249, 256
  sleep apnea in, 260
  social involvement of, 315
  see also aging process
electric blenders, 178
electric can openers, 176
electric outlets, 130
electric typewriters, 188
embroidery, 187
emphysema, *see* COPD; respiratory diseases
Emphysema Anonymous, Inc., 508
encephalitis, 391

Encyclopedia and Dictionary of Medicine, Nursing, and Allied Health (Miller et al.), 239
endocarditis, 246
end-of-dose akinesia, 396
enteral nutrition, 196–200, 284
  continuous drip feeding in, 199
  cost of, 203
  definition of, 196
  emotional support in, 202–3
  formula used in, 197–99
  health conditions associated with, 197
  infusion pumps in, 199
  special techniques for, 199–200
enterostomal therapists, 431
entertaining, patient's, 157–58
equipment, supplies, 538–39
  see also specific equipment and supplies
esophagostomy, cervical, 375
Essential Guide to Prescription Drugs, The (Long), 208
exercise, 222–32
  aerobic, 229–32
  Alzheimer's disease and, 223
  ankle, 226
  anxiety and, 230
  arthritis and, 223, 230, 474–76
  cool-downs after, 476
  depression and, 230
  diabetes and, 223, 346–47
  elbow, 225
  endurance, 476
  fatigue and, 222
  foot, 226
  heart attacks and, 438, 442–44, 446
  heart disease and, 230–31
  hip, 227
  hypertension and, 229, 231
  incontinence and, 241–42
  isometric, 228–29
  isotonic (dynamic), 229
  knee, 227
  MS and, 386
  neck, 224
  osteoporosis and, 231
  postsurgical recovery and, 231
  range-of-motion, 223–28, 418, 476
  regularity of, 229–30
  respiratory diseases and, 504
  shoulder, 224
  strain in, 229

exercise (*continued*)
  strengthening, 476
  stress and, 114
  stroke and, 231–32
  thumb and finger, 226
  toe, 226
  warm-ups, 228
  in water, 230
  wrist, 225
eye care, personal, 220–22
eye problems, 331–35
  cataracts, 331–34
  detached retinas, 335
  diabetic retinopathy, 352–54
  glaucoma, 334–35
  strokes and, 423–24

Fabrian Reading/Writing Aid, 188, 189
families:
  chronically ill patients and, 158–60
  critical role of, 49–50
  recovery periods and, 139–41
  stress experienced by, 37–38
  structural changes in, 26–27
  unforeseen events in, 37–39
  see also caregivers
fatigue, 258, 260
  energy conservation and, 157–58, 476–78
  exercise and, 222
  MS and, 387–88
faucets, 119, 121, 131
  gripping devices for, 132, 174–75
fecal incontinence, 238, 241
finger movement, exercises for, 226
flexibility, patient's, 71–72, 162
  exercise and, 223–29
  see also daily routines; *specific devices and tasks*
floor surfaces, 119
flossing teeth, 167, 242, 247–48
FLO-Trol invalid feeding cups, 181
fluroescein angiography, 352
Food and Drug Administration, U.S. (FDA), 218
food groups, basic, 192, 194
food preparation, *see* daily routines
food processors, 178
foot care, diabetes and, 356
foot movement, exercises for, 226
"fourth world," 109–10
Friendly Visiting Services, 66

friends, 33–34, 37–38
  critical role of, 49–50
  see also caregivers
Fries, James J., 470, 471
fungal infections, 215, 237

"gait training," 396
gardening, 156, 186
gas ranges, 131–33
gastrointestinal problems, 426–36
  IBDs, 426–29
  information resources on, 537–38
  ostomies, 429–33
gastrostomies, 375
gate control theory of pain, 267
genetics, Alzheimer's disease and, 369
GI (gastrointestinal) tract, 426–29
glasses, drinking from, 181
glass straws, bent, 181
glaucoma, 334–35
goals, patient's, 151, 155–58
  good feelings promoted by, 151
  planning in, 157–58
  recreational activities and, 155
Goldberg, Ann, 161
Goodrich, Jacqueline, 288–89
gooseneck mounts, 167, 187
gout, 214, 460, 473–74
grab bars, 120, 122, 123, 170, 171
Griffith, H. Winter, 208
gripping devices, 132, 174–75, 180–81
Griseofulvin, 215
group health insurance, 99
group meal programs, 83
group recreational activities, 156
group therapy, 56, 67
"Guide to Health Insurance for People with Medicare," 96–97
guilt feelings, 55, 114–15
  chronic illness and, 159–60
  of dying patients, 292
  expression of, 114–15
  human factor and, 207
  masturbation and, 254

hair, shampooing of, 168, 233
hair dryers, 168
handle loops, 134
hands, washing of, 166
Harold, Richard S., 247
Health and Human Services Department, U.S., 96–97

health care charts, 144–47
  sample of, 145
Health Insurance Association of America,
  86
health insurance plans (HIPs), 36
health maintenance organizations
  (HMOs), 36, 99–100
  routine medical checkups and, 89
hearing aids, 340–43
  types of, 341–42
Hearing Instruments, 339
hearing loss, 336–43
  in aging process, 310–11, 338–39
  caregivers' communication skills and,
    340
  causes of, 337–38
  checking for, 337
  hearing vs. understanding in, 340–41
  impact of, 336
  incidence of, 336
  information resources on, 539–41
  progressive, 336–37
  rehabilitative measures for, 339–40
heart attacks, 437–51
  emotional upsets after, 440–41, 445
  exercise after, 438, 442–44, 446
  fatalities due to, 438
  healing immediately after, 439–40
  inactivity and, 438
  life styles after, 445–46
  nutrition after, 441–42
  sexuality after, 252–53, 444–45
  silent coronaries, 439
  smoking and, 444
  warning signs of, 438–39
heart disease:
  exercise and, 230–31
  hypertension and, 453
  information resources on, 541–42
  isometric exercises and, 229
  oral care in, 246
  pain in, 267
  respiratory therapy for, 77–78
  sexual activity and, 252–53
  sleep apnea and, 260
  stroke and, 415
heat stress, 313–14
heat therapy, 271
  arthritis and, 475
Heavenrich, Ada Z., 339
hemodialysis, 487, 488–89
hemorrhages, cerebral, 414

Herndon, Robert M., 387–88
heroin, 266–67
high blood pressure, *see* hypertension
high-tech home health care, 280–87
  beneficial aspects of, 281–83
  chemotherapy in, 281, 285–86
  costs involved in, 283
  diabetes and, 281, 284
  emergencies and, 283
  emotional stability in, 282
  guidelines for, 286–87
  instruction in, 280–81, 282
  renal disease in, 281, 285
  respiratory disease in, 281, 285
  risks in, 282
  therapies used in, 281
hip movement, exercises for, 227
hip replacement surgery, 472–73
hobbies, 155–56, 186
  energy conserved in, 158
home health aides, 64–66
  elder abuse and, 317
  function of, 51
  home care team and, 50–52
  patients' relationships with, 65–66
  physical therapy and, 65, 71–72
  supervision of, 64–65
home health care, 25–48
  agencies, *see* agencies, home health
    care
  alternatives to, 37–47
  definitions of, 28–29
  early, 29–30
  family and friends in, 33–34, 37–38,
    49–50
  ideal candidates for, 104–5
  increasing consumer awareness and,
    31
  independence in, 26
  information resources on, 33–34, 511–
    66
  intensive, 33
  intermediate, 33
  minimal, 32
  models for, 30–32
  paying for, 36
  personal resources in, 29
  predictions for, 31–32, 48
  prevention orientation of, 31–32
  public and private funds for, 31, 36
  search for, 34–35
  team approach in, 50–52

home health care (*continued*)
  temporary vs. long-term, 69
  three pillars of, 63–79
  types of, 32–33
home health care professionals, 63–83
  caregivers and, 49–50
  continuity of care and, 141–42
  coordination of, 50–54, 68
  elder abuse and, 317
  health care charts and, 144–47
  in home setting, 140–41
  human element in, 68
  increasing availability of, 33–34
  primary, 63–68
  supplementary assistance and, 79–84
  support network of, 68–78
  team approach and, 50–52
  treatment plans and, 142–44
  see also specific professionals
Home Health Services and Staffing Association, 60
home life:
  disruption of, 113–14
  evaluation of, 105–10
  as "fourth world," 109–10
homemakers / housekeepers, 79–82
  agencies and, 81
  function of, 51
  home care team and, 50–52
  insurance coverage of, 81
  search for, 81–82
  supervision of, 81
hospice programs, 298–305
  admission requirements of, 300
  atmosphere in, 300
  compassion and affection in, 302–3
  cost of, 303–4
  death in, 304
  goals of, 299–300
  home care and, 298–99, 303
  information resources on, 532–35
  pain control in, 200, 301, 302
  routines in, 300–301
  visitation in, 300
hospital-based home care services:
  day care, 82
  discharge planning and, 53–54
  early, 30
  rehabilitation therapists in, 69
hospital charts, 144
hospitalization insurance coverage, 88–89

hospitals:
  discharge planning in, *see* discharge planning
  meals served in, 46
  morale problems in, 44
  paperwork in, 43–45
  professional hierarchies in, 45
  records kept in, 144
  regimented schedules in, 42–45
  rehabilitation departments in, 161
  staffs in, 44–45, 47
  see also housing facilities; nursing homes
housekeeping chores, 152, 182–85
housing facilities, 37–47
  behavioral changes in, 39–43
  information resources on, 37, 547–48
  meals in, 46
  Medicare coverage and, 96–97
  morale problems in, 44–45
  paperwork in, 43–45
  privacy in, 46–47
  professional hierarchies in, 45
  questions for evaluation of, 40–42
  regimented schedules in, 42–45
  staffs in, 44–45, 47
  types of, 38–39
  visits to, 37
Huntington's disease, 552–53
hyperglycemia, 352
hypertension (high blood pressure), 214, 452–67
  borderline, 415
  causes of, 454
  compliance problems in, 466–67
  effects of, 453–54
  exercises and, 229, 231
  home monitoring of, 460–66
  measurement of, 452–53, 455–56
  medications for, 458, 459–63
  misdiagnoses of, 456–57
  obesity and, 458
  during physical exam, 456–57
  racial predisposition toward, 454–55
  salt intake and, 459
  sleep apnea and, 260
  stress and, 454, 465–66
  stroke and, 414–15, 453
  symptoms of, 454
  treatment of, 457–65
  types of, 454
hypoglycemia, 351

hypoglycemics, oral, 349–50
hypothermia, 314–15

IBDs (inflammatory bowel diseases),
    426–29
  incidence of, 426
  medications for, 427
  support groups for, 429
  treatment of, 427–29
Ibuprofen, 266, 269
ice massage, 271–72
ileostomies, 429, 430–36
  care techniques for, 431
  colostomies vs., 430–31
  see also ostomies
impotence, 254–55
Impotents Anonymous, 255
incontinence, 237–42
  in Alzheimer's disease, 366–68
  causes of, 239
  cleanliness and dryness in, 239, 241,
      242
  disposable underclothes for, 240–41
  elderly and, 238, 240, 316–17
  exercise and, 241–42
  fecal vs. urinary, 238, 241
  incidence of, 238
  locomotor, 239
  nighttime, 240
  open discussion about, 239–40
  overflow, 239
  pressure sores and, 275
  regular episodes of, 240
  stress and, 238
  urge, 238–39
  in women vs. men, 238, 241–42
independence, patient's, 26, 152–91
  amended baseline of wellness and,
      152–55
  chronic illness and, 160
  and conservation of energy, 157–58,
      179–80
  in daily routines, 145–51, 160–65
  self-esteem tied to, 154–55
  see also personal health care
independent nurse practitioners, 63
infections:
  fungal, 215, 237
  heart, oral care and, 246
  incontinence and, 239, 241, 242
information resources, 35, 55, 57, 511–66

discharge planning and, 53–54
  see also specific topics
infusion pumps, 199
inhalation therapy, 76–78
inhalers, 77, 505
insomnia, 258–59
institutional facilities, see housing facili-
    ties; nursing homes
insulin infusion pumps, 284, 350–51
insulin injections, 207, 284, 347–49
  dietary controls and, 346
  insulin shock and, 351
  procedure for, 347–49
  types of, 347
insurance policies, 85–102
  ALS and, 380
  Alzheimer's disease and, 367
  appealing refusal of claim in, 102
  changes in, 86
  chemotherapy and, 325
  discharge planning and, 35, 53
  employer-provided, 56–57
  evaluation of, 87–92, 101–2
  group, 99
  home care devices and, 161
  home health care coverage and, 90–91
  homemakers and, 81
  home respiratory therapy and, 77–78
  hospice care and, 304
  hospitalization coverage in, 88–89
  limitations in, 56, 86
  major medical, 90, 99
  maximum amounts paid by, 89
  preexisting health conditions and, 89–
      90
  prevailing charges in, 89
  reimbursements in, 87–88, 101–2
  researching of, 86, 90–92, 102
  review of, 55, 56–57
  routine medical checkups and, 89
  supplemental, 98–100
  surgical-medical coverage in, 88, 89
  termination of coverage in, 101
  varying coverages under, 36
  visits covered by, 91–92
  see also Medicare
intensive home care, 33
interactions, drug, 208–12
  bioavailability in, 212–13
  definition of, 209
  food and nutrients in, 212–15
  potentiation in, 210–11

intermediate home care, 33
intravenous therapy, 280, 281, 283
IPPB (intermittent positive-pressure
    breathing) apparatus, 505
ironing, 182–83
iron supplements, 215
isometric exercises, 228–29
isosorbide dinitrate, 448–49
isotonic (dynamic) exercises, 229
itchiness, 234–35

Jane Brody's Nutrition Book (Brody), 196
jars, opening of, 176–77
Javits, Jacob, 159, 374, 379, 381
joint replacement surgery, 468, 472–73

Kaiser Permanente Aid, 36
karaya gum, 435
Kegel exercises, 241–42
kidney disease, *see* renal disease
kidneys, normal functions of, 494–95
kitchens, 129–34
    dangers in, 129
    devices in, 174–80
    faucets in, 131
    handle loops in, 134
    lazy Susans in, 133, 175
    lighting in, 130
    pegboard panels in, 133
    range of mobility in, 129–30
    reaching devices used in, 134, 175
    refrigerators in, 133
    seating in, 130–31, 179–80
    shelves in, 133
    sinks in, 131, 132
    storage aids in, 134, 177
    stoves in, 131–33
knee movement, exercise for, 227
knitting, 187

laudanum, 226
laughter, 145–50, 273
laundry, 182–83
    carts used for, 182
laxatives, 214
lazy Susans, 133, 175
L-dopa (levodopa), 213–14, 391–96
    drug holiday from, 393–96
    on-off phenomena in, 393
    side effects of, 392–93, 395
lesions, nonsymptomatic, 236
licensed practical nurses (LPNs), 64

licensure requirements:
    home care agencies and, 60–62
    physical therapists and, 72
life expectancy, 27
    elderly population and, 27, 32
Lifeline Foundation, 203
light switches, 130
living rooms, as bedrooms, 134–35, 153–
    54
living wills, 296–98
Living with Chronic Neurologic Disease
    (Cooper), 159
locomotor incontinence, 239
loners, 156
Long, James W., 208
Lorig, Kate, 470, 471

macronutrients, 192, 193
macular degeneration, 222
Madden, Peter, 493
major medical insurance, 90, 99
makeup, application of, 167
malnutrition, institutionally induced, 46
MAO (mono amine oxidase) inhibitors,
    213
massages, 271–73
    cancer treatment and, 329
    ice, 271–72
    trigger points in, 272–73
masturbation, 253–54
meals:
    group, 83
    institutional, 46
    medication and, 212–15
    nutritional therapy and, 78
    oral health and, 243
    see also daily routines
meals-on-wheels programs, 35, 66, 82–83
meats, preparation of, 178–79
Medicaid, 36, 100–101
    agencies certified by, 61
    waivers in, 101
Medic Alert program, 550
Medicare, 92–98
    agencies certified by, 61
    approved amounts in, 94–96
    chemotherapy and, 325
    deductibles in, 94
    eligibility for, 57, 92, 100
    essential details of, 93
    homebound patients and, 97–98
    home health care and, 31, 36, 96–98

home respiratory therapy and, 77
hospice programs and, 303–4
incontinence products and, 242
lifetime reserve in, 92
nursing home care and, 96–97
Parts A and B of, 92–94
renal disease and, 489, 491
subscriber's right to appeal in, 102
volume of hospital costs paid by, 92
Medicare supplement insurance, 99
medications and drugs, 204–19
angina and, 447–50
antiparkinsonism, 213–14, 391–96
arthritis and, 267, 468, 470–71, 478–85
asthma and, 503
bioavailability of, 212–13
chemotherapy, 281, 285–86, 324–25
child-safety caps on, 207
diabetes and, 207, 284, 347–51
elderly and, 205, 206–8, 217
essential facts on, 204–5
food interactions with, 212–15
generic vs. brand name, 204
glaucoma and, 334
hospice care and, 290, 301, 302
hypertension and, 458, 459–63
IBDs and, 427
information resources on, 204–5, 208
instructions for, 206
interactions among, 208–12
medical histories and, 205–6
memory loss and, 311–12
MS and, 385–86
new, 208–9
nutrient interactions with, 212–15
over-the-counter, 206, 210, 215–19
patients' reactions to, 205–6, 212
patients' resistance to, 207
potentiation and, 210–11
radiation treatment and, 323
respiratory diseases and, 503, 505
side effects of, 205
sleep difficulties and, 260
stress relieved by, 115
written records of, 210
memory loss:
aging process and, 311–12, 360–62
after stroke, 424
see also Alzheimer's disease
mental health services, 67–68, 549–50
see also social workers; therapy

micronutrients, 214
microwave ovens, 133
midbrain, pain as perceived in, 265
mineral oil, 214
minerals, 195–96
minimal home care, 32
mirrors, 167
MIUSA (Mobility International USA), 412
mobility, patients' range of:
in bathrooms, 118–19
bedbound patients and, 164–65
in bedrooms, 126–27
daily routines and, 164–65
doorways and, 118–19
exercises for, 223–28
in kitchens, 129–30
pressure sores and, 275
mopping, 183
morphine, 266–67, 270, 328
mouthwashes, 244
MRI (magnetic resonance imaging, 383
MS (multiple sclerosis), 381–89
autoimmune reaction theory of, 382
bladder problems in, 386
causes of, 382
combination reaction theory of, 382–83
constipation in, 386–87
cycles in, 385
description of, 381–82
diagnosis of, 383–84
emotional changes and, 388–89
fatigue in, 387–88
general health and, 385
information resources on, 553
life span and, 381
medications for, 385–86
nutrition in, 386
physical therapy in, 386
progression of, 384–85
quality of life as affected by, 384
rehabilitation therapy for, 386, 388
skin problems in, 387
slow virus theory of, 382
stress in, 387
support groups and, 388–89
symptoms of, 383–84
muscular dystrophy, information
resources on, 553–54
Muscular Dystrophy Association, 379, 380

myasthenia gravis, information resources on, 554
myocardial infarctions, *see* heart attacks
myotherapy, 272

NAPHT News, 487
naps, 152
insomnia and, 258
narcotic drugs, 266–67, 328
addiction to, 266
National Association for Patients on Hemodialysis and Transplantation, 487, 493
National Cancer Institute, 320
National Center for Health Statistics, 27
National Foundation for Ileitis and Colitis, 429
National Home Caring Council, Inc., 35, 61
National Institute on Aging, 32
National Institutes of Health, 421
National Kidney Foundation, 491
National Multiple Sclerosis Society, 385, 389
National Parkinson Fouhdation, 406
National Society to Prevent Blindness, 221, 222
National Spinal Cord Injury Association, 411
nausea, cancer treatment and, 326
nebulizers, 505
neck movement, exercises for, 226
neurological problems, 360–425
ALS, 373–81
Alzheimer's disease, 360–73
Huntington's disease, 552–53
information resources on, 551–55
MS, 381–89
muscular dystrophy, 553–54
myasthenia gravis, 554
Parkinson's disease, 389–406
spinal cord injuries, 406–12
stroke, 412–25
neuropathy, diabetic, 355–56
nitroglycerin, 267, 447–50
Niven, David, 374
nociceptors, 264–65
nonprofit home care agencies, 34
fees charged by, 59–60
funding for, 34
information resources on, 37
see also agencies, home health care

nurses, 63–64
differing experience among, 64
education as function of, 63, 64
home care team and, 50–52
home health aides and, 64–65
licensed practical, 64
in professional hierarchies, 45
role of, 51
supervision of, 63
nursing homes, 37–47
abuses in, 27–28
Alzheimer's patients in, 372
Medicare coverage and, 96–97
patients as viewed in, 44
services provided by, 38
see also housing facilities
nutrition, 192–203
arthritis and, 479
basic food groups in, 192, 194
cancer therapy and, 323–24, 326–27
diabetes and, 345–46
diuretics and, 460
drug interactions in, 212–15
empty calories in, 193
enteral, 196–200, 284
for heart attack patients, 441–42
IBDs and, 427
individuality in, 194
information resources on, 556–57
macronutrients in, 192, 193
micronutrients in, 214
minerals in, 195–96
moderation in, 193
MS and, 386
oral health and, 243
ostomies and, 435
parenteral, 196–97, 200–203, 281, 284
Parkinson's disease and, 402
pressure sores and, 275
radiation treatment and, 323–24
salt intake and, 459
variety in, 194–95
vitamins in, 194–95
nutritional therapy, 78

obesity:
arthritis and, 472
hypertension and, 458
Parkinson's disease and, 402
sleep apnea and, 260
occupational therapy, 72–75
ALS and, 378

amended baseline of wellness and,
   152–55
   function of, 51
   home care team and, 50–52
   home health aides and, 65
   home settings evaluated in, 72–73
   Parkinson's disease and, 397–98
   physical therapy and, 73
   in recovery periods, 152–55, 161
   stroke patients and, 419–20
ointments, topical, 216–17
oncologists, 330–32
one-handedness, 162
on-off phenomenon, 393
ophthalmologists, 220–21
ophthalmoscopes, 455
opium, 266, 270
oral care, personal, 242–49
   for bedridden patients, 246–47
   cancer treatment and, 246, 326
   community services for, 247
   COPD and, 500
   dental checkups and, 244–45
   denture adherents in, 248–49
   dentures in, 167, 243, 245–46, 249
   diabetes and, 245
   diet and, 243
   flossing in, 167, 242, 247–48
   for heart patients, 246
   information resources on, 536
   irrigating devices in, 248
   neglect of, 242
   postsurgical recovery and, 245–46
   speech abilities and, 243
   TMJ alignment in, 243–44
   toothbrushes in, 166, 244, 247
Orinase, 349–50
osteoarthritis, 471–72
osteoporosis, exercise and, 231
ostomies, 429–36
   care techniques for, 432–34
   diet and, 435
   embarrassment and, 430, 435–36
   information resources on, 537–38
   sexuality and, 435–36
   skin care and, 435
   support groups for, 436
overflow incontinence, 239
over-the-counter (OTC) drugs, 206, 210,
   215–19
   advertisements for, 219
   drug interactions with, 208–12

food / nutrient interactions with, 212–
   15
   increasing use of, 219
   labels on, 218–19
   physicians advised of, 206, 218
   risks of, 216–17
   sleep aids, 260
   standards set for, 218
oxygen systems, 505–7
   dangers of, 506

pacer boards, 76
pain, 263–66
   acute, 264
   as alarm network, 263, 264, 265
   autonomic nervous system and, 266
   chronic, 264
   definitions of, 263–64
   incidence of, 263
   neurological signals vs. sensations of,
      265–66
   nociceptors and, 264–65
   perception of, 264–66
   reflex actions and, 265
   stroke and, 415–16
pain control, 266–74
   in arthritis, see arthritis
   biofeedback in, 273
   in cancer treatment, 327–28
   cold therapy in, 271–72
   distraction as element in, 272
   drugs used in, 266–67, 268–70
   in dying patients, 290, 301
   gate control theory of, 267
   information resources on, 557
   laughter and, 147–50, 273
   TENS in, 271
Parafon Forte, 268
parenteral nutrition, 200–203, 281, 284
   cleanliness in, 201
   cost of, 203
   definition of, 196–97
   delivery systems in, 202
   emotional support needed in, 202–3
   formula used in, 201
   infusion vests in, 202
   total, 200–201, 324, 327
parking spaces, reserved, 190
Parkinson's disease, 159, 389–406
   activity levels in, 404–5
   bathrooms used in, 401
   causes of, 391–92

Parkinson's disease (*continued*)
  chairs as obstacles in, 400
  clothing in, 401–2
  constipation in, 402–3
  dependency in, 404
  description of, 389–90
  drug holiday in, 393–96
  early signs of, 390
  end-of-dose akinesia in, 396
  exercise in, 223, 396–97
  falling as risk in, 399–400
  festinating gait in, 390–91
  getting out of bed, 400–401
  incidence of, 391
  information resources on, 406, 554–55
  medication used for, 213–14, 391–96
  nutrition in, 402
  occupational therapy in, 397–98
  on-off phenomena in, 393
  psychological problems in, 403–4, 405–6
  routines essential in, 405
  speech therapy in, 76, 398
  tremors in, 389, 390
  walking difficulties in, 398–99
Parkinson's Educational Program
    (PEPUSA), 406
Parkinson's Patient, The, 405–6
passive patients, creation of, 112–13
patients:
  ambulating capabilities of, 71
  anger in, 67–68
  changing needs of, 112
  depression in, *see* depression
  ideal for home health care, 104–5, 107
  independence of, 26, 112, 165–91
  self-esteem of, 26, 46–47, 164–65
pegboard panels, 133, 177
penile implants, 255
pens, aids for writing with, 188
peritoneal dialysis, 489–90
personal health care, 220–62
  exercise and, 222–32
  incontinence and, 237–42
  oral health and, 242–49
  sexuality and, 249–56
  skin and, 232–37
  sleep difficulties and, 256–60
  vision and, 220–22
photocoagulation, 353–54
photography, 156

physical therapy, 70–72
  ALS and, 377–78
  goals of, 51, 70–71
  group, 397
  home care team and, 50–52
  home health aides and, 65, 71–72
  licensure requirements and, 72
  MS and, 386
  occupational therapy and, 73
  Parkinson's disease and, 223, 396–97
  range-of-motion exercises in, 223–28
  stroke patients and, 417–18
  therapists' assistants in, 71–72
physicians:
  caretakers and, 54, 78–79
  home care team and, 50–52, 78–79
  in institutional hierarchies, 45
  Medicare assignments and, 95–96
  medication prescribed by, 204–7
  patients' answers prepared for, 148–49
  patients as focus of, 54
  questions as "imposition" on, 204
  sexual advice given by, 249–50
*Physicians' and Pharmacists' Guide to
    Your Medicines, The,* 208
Pill Book, The (Silverman and Simon),
    208
pillows, 124
placemats, nonslip, 182
playing cards, 186
postural drainage, 77, 500
potentiation, 210–11
preparation for home health care, 103–35
  bathrooms, 117–23
  bedrooms, 123–29
  caregivers' role in, 110–16
  functional profiles in, 106, 107–8
  fundamental goals in, 116–17
  health problems evaluated in, 104,
    106, 107
  home life evaluated in, 105–10, 142
  kitchens, 129–34
  lighting, 130
  living rooms, 134–35
  patients' needs assessed in, 104–5,
    107, 112
  stress and, 113–16
  wastebaskets, 126
pressure sores, 274–79
  in ALS, 378

assessing risk of, 276–77
causes of, 274
development of, 274–76
incidence of, 275
prevention of, 278–79
size of, 275–76
treatment of, 277–78
preventive medicine, 31
privacy:
  institutional life and, 46–47
  patients' bedrooms and, 126
progressive diseases, 139, 158–60
  exercise and, 223
  primary requirement in, 160
  see also dying patients
propanolol, 460, 461
Proprietary Association, 218
proprietary home health care agencies,
  34, 59–63
  information resources on, 37
  see also agencies, home health care
pseudodementias, 362–63
purines, 473–74

quality of life, patient's:
  amended baseline of wellness and,
    152–55
  energy conservation and, 157–58, 476–
    78
  independence and, 26, 152–91
  MS and, 384
  occupational therapy and, 72–75
  see also recovery / readjustment periods
Questran, 214

radiation, solar, skin and, 232
radiation treatment:
  for cancer, 322–24
  oral care and, 246
rain gutter hooks, 189
rain ponchos, 174
range-of-motion exercises, 223–28, 418
  arthritis and, 476
  examples of, 224–27
  purpose of, 228
razors, handle extensions on, 167
reaching devices, 134, 175
reading, aids for, 188–89
recliners, 124–26
Recommended Daily Allowances, U.S.
  (USRDAs), 194

recovery / readjustment periods, 139–91
  amended baseline of wellness in, 152–
    55
  boredom avoided in, 151–52
  chronic illness and, 158–60
  continuity of care in, 141–42
  exercise in, 222–23, 231
  fluids recorded in, 147
  "good time" activities in, 151
  health care charts in, 144–47
  home health care professionals' visits
    before, 105–10, 142
  human spirit in, 145–50
  home health care professionals' visits
    before, 105–10, 142
  occupational therapists in, 152–55, 161
  out-of-doors time in, 152
  perspective maintained in, 158–60
  physicians' questions in, 148–49
  planning learned in, 157–58
  recreation and hobbies in, 155–56,
    186–87
  telephone calls in, 156
  television in, 155
  treatment plans in, 142–44
  vital signs recorded in, 146
recreation activities, 155–56, 186–87
  goals in, 155
  information resources on, 560–64
reflex actions, 265
refrigerators, 133
  handle loops on, 134
rehabilitation centers, 69
rehabilitation therapy, 68–78
  ALS and, 377–78
  heart attacks and, 438, 442–44, 446
  MS and, 386, 388
  overlap among, 69
  spinal cord injuries and, 409–10
  stroke patients and, 76–77, 416–20
  see also specific therapies
Reisberg, Barry, 364, 368
renal disease, 487–94
  CAPD in, 490
  hemodialysis in, 487, 488–89
  high-tech home care for, 281, 285
  hypertension and, 453–54
  information resources on, 548–49
  kidney malfunctioning in, 487–88
  Medicare and, 489, 491
  peritoneal dialysis in, 489–90

skin care and, 488
support groups for, 491, 492–93
technological advancements in, 487
transplants in, 490–91
see also dialysis
resource records, home health care, 57–58, 512
respiratory diseases, 495–508
activity levels in, 504
asthma, 77–78, 501–3
breathing aids in, 505
COPD, 495–501
exercise and, 504
high-tech home care and, 281, 285
information resources on, 564
medications for, 503, 505
oxygen systems in, 505–7
smoking and, 495, 497, 498, 504
stress and, 508
support groups for, 507–8
respiratory therapy, 76–78
insurance coverage of, 77–78
restaurants, dimly lit, 312
retinal examinations, 455
retinas, detached, 335
retinopathy, diabetic, 352–54
treatment of, 353–54
rheumatoid arthritis, 469–71
see also arthritis
"right to die," 379
RN Magazine, 384
rocker knives, 178, 180
Rogers, Sidney I., 233
Rupp, Ralph, 339, 342

salt intake, 459
sandwich holders, 182
SBGM (self blood glucose monitoring), 357–58
scalp care, 233
scissors, food, 178
scratching, 234
screw cap openers, 176
Scribner, Belding, 488
self-esteem, patient's:
independence and, 26
in institutional life, 46–47
mobility and, 164–65
oral health and, 243
self-help groups, 546–47
see also specific disorders

self-medication, *see* over-the-counter drugs
senility, *see* Alzheimer's disease; dementia
sexuality, 249–56
aging process and, 249, 256
arthritis and, 253
cancer treatment and, 330
definition of, 252
expression of, 251, 252
health care professionals' view of, 249–50
heart attacks and, 252–53, 444–45
information resources on, 564
impotence and, 254–55
masturbation and, 253–54
open communication about, 251–52
ostomies and, 435–36
shampoos, 168, 233
sheath catheters, 241
sheepskin bed pads, 279
shelves, 133
shingles, 234
shoe horns, 174
shoulder movement, exercises for, 224
shower heads, 121, 171
showers, 170–71
Silverman, Harold L., 208
Simon, Gilbert I., 208
sinks:
bathroom, 119
kitchen, 131, 132
knee room under, 131, 132
"sip and puff" units, 409–10
skin:
of elderly, 233–34, 242
functions of, 232–33
pigmentation of, 232
skin care, personal, 232–37
allergies and, 233, 236
arthritis and, 235
diabetes and, 234, 235
for dryness, 233, 234
functions of skin and, 232–33
incontinence and, 239, 241, 242
infections prevented by, 237
information resources on, 564–65
internal cancers and, 236
for itchiness, 234–35
lotions used in, 233
MS and, 387

for normal skin, 233
ostomies and, 435
physicians consulted in, 235
renal disease and, 488
shampooing in, 233
stroke and, 235
sun exposure and, 233–34
sleep apnea, 259–60
sleep difficulties, 256–60
   beds and, 257–58
   decreasing sleep requirements and, 259
   insomnia, 258–59
   involuntary dozing, 256–57
   medications and, 260
   overstimulation and, 258
   sleep apnea, 259–60
   sleep-wake cycles and, 258–59
smoking:
   heart attacks and, 444
   respiratory diseases and, 495, 497, 498, 504
   stroke and, 415
snacks, 182
soap on a rope, 166, 171
social workers, 66–68
   counseling offered by, 67–68
   function of, 51
   group therapy organized by, 67
   home care team and, 50–52
   private practices of, 67
   training of, 66
sodium, hypertension and, 459
speech:
   hearing loss and, 340–41
   oral health and, 243
   Parkinson's disease and, 398
speech discrimination tests, 341
speech therapy, 75–76
   aphasia and, 421–22
   function of, 51
   home care team and, 50–52
   information resources on, 566
   Parkinson's disease and, 76, 398
sphygmomanometers, 464
spinal cord, 407–8
spinal cord injuries, 406–12
   causes of, 406–8
   effects of, 409
   extent of, 408–9
   incidence of, 407

rehabilitation therapy and, 409–10
return home after, 410–12
support groups for, 411
sponges, long-handled, 166, 170
sports, 186–87
   information resources on, 560–64
states, licensure requirements and, 62
stocking helpers, 173–74
storage aids, 134, 177
stoves, 131–33
stress:
   in caregivers, 37–38
   disruptions of routines and, 113–14
   in dying patients, 291–92
   in dying patients' caregivers, 292–95
   energy consumed by, 158
   exercise and, 114
   guilt and, 114–15
   heat, 313–14
   hypertension and, 454, 465–66
   incontinence and, 238
   in institutionalized care, 42–45
   MS and, 387
   respiratory diseases and, 508
stroke, 412–25
   aphasia after, 420–22
   causes of, 413–14
   communication after, 420–23
   emotional instability after, 425
   exercise and, 231–32
   hypertension and, 414–15, 453
   incidence of, 412
   information resources on, 541–42
   little, 414, 416
   memory loss after, 424
   one-sided neglect after, 423–24
   physiological description of, 412–13
   predispositions to, 414–15
   racial factors in, 415
   rehabilitation after, 76–77, 416–20
   skin care and, 235
   speech therapy and, 421–22
   symptoms after, 417
   visual field deficits after, 423–24
   warning signs of, 415–16
Stroke Clubs, 422
"Stroke: Why Do They Behave That Way?", 422–23
sun, skin exposed to, 233–34
support groups:
   Alzheimer's disease and, 370–71

arthritis and, 486
cancer and, 330
IBDs and, 429
MS and, 388–89
ostomies and, 436
respiratory disease and, 507–8
spinal cord injuries and, 411
surgery:
cancer, 322–23
cataract removal, 331–32
coronary bypass, 450–51
Crohn's disease, 427–29
joint replacement, 468, 472–73
kidney transplants, 490–91
ostomies, 429–36
ulcerative colitis, 429
surgical-medical insurance coverage, 88, 89
sweeping, 183
Sygall, Susan, 412
systolic readings, 452–53, 456

taxes, health costs deductibility and, 102
teeth:
brushing of, 166, 242
see also oral care, personal
telephones, 156
cordless, 185, 187
devices for, 187
television, 155
aids for watching of, 189
TENS (transcutaneous electrical nerve stimulation), 271, 328
terminal illness, see dying patients; specific diseases
terry cloth mitts, 166
tetracycline, 213
thalamus, pain as perceived in, 265–66
theater-going, 186
therapy:
group, 56, 67
nutritional, 78
occupational, 72–75
physical, 70–72
psychological, 67–68, 549–50
sexuality and, 252
speech, 75–76
stress and, 115, 116
thiazides, 460, 462–63
thrombosis, 413–14
thumb movement, exercises for, 226

TIAs (transient ischemic attacks), 414, 416
TMJ (temporomandibular joint), 243–44
toaster ovens, 133
toe movement, exercises for, 226
toilets, 121–23
assistance devices for, 169–70
raised seats for, 122, 170
Tolinase, 349–50
toothbrushes:
battery-powered, 166, 247
suction-mounted, 244
toothpicks, 248
TPN (total parenteral nutrition), 200–201, 324, 327
tranquilizers, stress alleviated by, 113
transfer benches, 120–21
transplants, kidney, 490–91
transportation, patient's, 82, 83–84
devices for, 189
trapeze bars, 128, 185, 401
travel aids, 189–90
treatment plans, 142–44
tumors, brain, 414
Tylenol, 266, 268
typewriters, electric, 188

United Ostomy Association, 431, 434
"Un-Skru" jar openers, 176
urge incontinence, 238–39
uric acid, excessive, 473–74
urine testing, 357
utensils, kitchen, 180–81

vacuuming, 183
Valium, 210
vans, modified, 189
vegetables, 178–79
Velcro fasteners, 172, 173
Verapamil, 448–49
virectomy, 354
Visiting Nurse Association, 30
meals-on-wheels programs of, 83
visits, from home health care professional:
insurance coverage and, 91–92
before patient's arrival, 105–10, 142
questions expected in, 148–49
vitamins, 194–95
absorption of, 214
vitamin supplements, 195, 215

voice-controlled devices, 409–10
voluntary home health care agencies:
  early, 29–30
  meals-on-wheels, 35, 66, 82–83
  in search for home care, 35
  transportation services, 83–84

Waldrep, Kent, 411
Walker, Judy, 412
walkers, 162–63
  accessibility of, 190–91
  doors and 118–19
Warfarin, 215
washing, excessive, 234
wastebaskets, 126
Water Piks, 248
weight loss:
  in cancer treatment, 326–27
  sleep apnea and, 260

wheelchairs, 163–64
  accessibility of, 164
  in bathrooms, 118–19, 164
  in bedrooms, 126
  doors and, 118–19
  in kitchens, 129, 130–31
  lap boards for, 175, 179
  selection of, 163–64
  transportation and, 189–90
whirlpools, 72, 271
wills, living, 296–98
word processors, 188
wrist movement, exercise for, 225
writing, aids for, 188

"Your Medicare Handbook," 97

Zim jar openers, 176
Zyliss jar openers, 176

Here is a health book that should be in the home library of every American family.

There is a revolution taking place in medical care in the United States, as hospitals—under pressure from Medicare and private insurers to save money—discharge their patients more quickly than before. There are, as well, many handicapped and chronically ill patients for whom institutional care is not an option.

The new alternative for these patients is health care at home; and this book, the most comprehensive guide on home care yet available, will be a welcome resource for every family facing this situation. Written with expertise and compassion, its twenty-two fact-packed chapters cover all home-care situations—from postsurgical recuperation to recovery from stroke to daily living with a chronic illness or disability.

Jo-Ann Friedman tells you • how to determine what Medicare, Medicaid, and private insurers will and will not pay for • how to find the home care products you need • how to organize the home to care for a sick person • how to set up a support network and deal with doctors, home health aides, and therapists • how the caregiver can ease feelings of stress and guilt.

There is, as well, a unique Resource Directory, which provides the names, addresses, and phone numbers of organizations in every state which can provide help for a variety of home care needs.